Natural Feed Additives Used in the Poultry Industry

Edited by

Mahmoud Alagawany

&

Mohamed E. Abd El-Hack

Department of Poultry, Faculty of Agriculture
Zagazig University
Zagazig
Egypt

Natural Feed Additives Used in the Poultry Industry

Editors: Mahmoud Alagawany & Mohamed E. Abd El-Hack

ISBN (Online): 978-981-14-8845-0

ISBN (Print): 978-981-14-8843-6

ISBN (Paperback): 978-981-14-8844-3

Published by Bentham Science Publishers Pte. Ltd. Singapore. All Rights Reserved.

need for a court order if at any point you breach any terms of this License Agreement. In no event will any delay or failure by Bentham Science Publishers in enforcing your compliance with this License Agreement constitute a waiver of any of its rights.

3. You acknowledge that you have read this License Agreement, and agree to be bound by its terms and conditions. To the extent that any other terms and conditions presented on any website of Bentham Science Publishers conflict with, or are inconsistent with, the terms and conditions set out in this License Agreement, you acknowledge that the terms and conditions set out in this License Agreement shall prevail.

Bentham Science Publishers Pte. Ltd.
80 Robinson Road #02-00
Singapore 068898
Singapore
Email: subscriptions@benthamscience.net

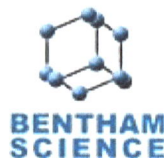

CONTENTS

FOREWORD

I was delighted when I received a request from Mahmoud Alagawany and Mohamed E. Abd El-Hack to write a brief foreword to the reprint of this book because, for several years, I have admired their incredible work. Moreover, as a consumer of poultry products, I always search the markets for organic products to keep my body away from the antibiotic residues. So, I believe that the topic of this book is much needed for all people who produce or consume poultry products in their food.

Looking through this magnificent book, I am amazed at the authors' talent and what they achieved with a pencil. It is more than a book of lovely illustrations. It is a mine of information, demonstrating their technique in the minutest detail and it is a source of inspiration and information for those who work in the poultry production field.

In shorts, Alagawany and Abd El-Hack's book is unique and indeed work to treasure for anyone interested in poultry production. So, read it, enjoy it and learn from it. Thank you, Alagawany and Abd El-Hack, for producing such a masterwork.

Vincenzo Tufarelli
DETO - Section of Veterinary
Science and Animal Production
University of Bari 'Aldo Moro' s.p.
Casamassima km 3, 70010 Valenzano
BA, Italy

PREFACE

Feed additives are non-nutritive preparations and formulations as well as useful microorganisms that are added to animal diets to enhance the growth, production, feed utilization, nutrient digestibility and absorption, immunity, public health, *etc*. This book on Natural Feed Additives Used in the Poultry Industry addresses recent information on the use of different natural feed additives in poultry nutrition with regard to growth, production and reproduction and health of poultry. This book contains 16 chapters contributed by 38 experts and scientists of animal and poultry nutrition, animal and poultry physiology, toxicology, pharmacology, and pathology, which highlights the significance of herbal plants and their extracts and derivatives, cold pressed and essential oils, fruits by-products, immunomodulators, organic acids, probiotics, nanoparticles and their role in poultry industry instead of the growth promoter antibiotics. This book provides details about the use of antibiotics as growth promoters in the poultry industry and the development of bacteria resistance to antibiotics. All chapters provide a holistic approach to how natural feed additives can provide an efficient solution to animal health, also covering the main categories of poultry, including broiler chickens, laying hens, quails, geese, ducks, and turkey. This book represents an up-to-date review of the existing knowledge on natural feed additives, both *in vitro* and *in vivo* and the basis for future research. This book is useful to the students of poultry sciences, nutritionists, scientists, veterinarians, pharmacologists, poultry breeders, and animal husbandry extension workers.

Mahmoud Alagawany

&

Mohamed E. Abd El-Hack
Department of Poultry, Faculty of Agriculture
Zagazig University
Zagazig
Egypt

List of Contributors

Ahmed Noreldin — Department of Histology and Cytology, Faculty of Veterinary Medicine, Damanhour University, Damanhour 22516, Egypt

Asmaa F. Khafaga — Department of Pathology, Faculty of Veterinary Medicine, Alexandria University, Edfina, 22758, Egypt

Ayman A. Swelum — Department of Theriogenology, Faculty of Veterinary Medicine, Zagazig University, Zagazig, 44511, Egypt

Ayman E. Taha — Department of Animal Husbandry and Animal Wealth Development, Faculty of Veterinary Medicine, Alexandria University, Edfina, 22578, Egypt

Elwy A. Ashour — Departmentof Poultry, Faculty of Agriculture, Zagazig University, Zagazig, 44511, Egypt

Feroza Soomro — Department of Animal Nutrition, Cholistan University of Veterinary and Animal Sciences Bahawalpu, Bahawalpu, Pakistan

Gaber E. Batiha — National Research Center for Protozoan Diseases, Obihiro University of Agriculture and Veterinary Medicine, Nishi 2-13, Inada-cho, 080-8555, Obihiro, Hokkaido, Japan
Department of Pharmacology and Therapeutics, Faculty of Veterinary Medicine, Damanhour University, Damanhour 22511, AlBeheira, Egypt

Gihan G. Moustafa — Forensic Medicine and Toxicology Department, Veterinary Medicine Faculty, Zagazig University, Zagazig, 44519, Egypt

Hamada A. M. Elwan — Animal and Poultry Production Department, Faculty of Agriculture, Minia University, El-Minya, 61519, Egypt

Husein Ohran — Department of Physiology, Veterinary Faculty, University of Sarajevo, Zmaja od Bosne 90, 71 000 Sarajevo, Bosnia and Herzegovina

Ilahi Bakhash Marghazani — Faculty of Veterinary and Animal Sciences, Lasbela University of Agriculture, Water and Marine Sciences, 3800 Uthal, Balochistan, Pakistan

Kuldeep Dhama — Division of Pathology, ICAR-Indian Veterinary Research Institute, Uttar Pradesh, 243 122, India

Mahmoud Alagawany — Poultry Department, Faculty of Agriculture, Zagazig University, Zagazig, 44519, Egypt

Maria Tabassum Chaudhry — Institute of Animal Nutrition, Northeast Agricultural University, Harbin, 150030, China

Mayada R. Farag — Forensic Medicine and Toxicology Department, Veterinary Medicine Faculty, Zagazig University, Zagazig, 44519, Egypt

Mohamed E. Abd El-Hack — Department of Poultry, Faculty of Agriculture, Zagazig University, Zagazig, 44511, Egypt

Mohamed Emam — Department of Nutrition and Clinical Nutrition, Faculty of Veterinary Medicine, Damanhour University, Damanhour, 22516, Egypt

Mohamed S. El-Kholy — Department of Poultry, Faculty of Agriculture, Zagazig University, Zagazig, 44511, Egypt

Mohamed T. El-saadony	Department of Agricultural Microbiology, Faculty of Agriculture, Zagazig University, Zagazig, 44511, Egypt
Mohammad Mehedi Hasan Khan	Department of Biochemistry and Chemistry, Sylhet Agricultural University, Sylhet, Bangladesh
Mohammed A. E. Naiel	Department of Animal Production, Faculty of Agriculture, Zagazig University, Zagazig, 44511, Egypt
Muhammad Arif	Department of Animal Sciences, College of Agriculture, University of Sargodha, Sargodha, 40100, Pakistan
Muhammad Asif Arain	Faculty of Veterinary and Animal Sciences, Lasbela University of Agriculture, Uthal-3800, Balochistan, Pakistan
Muhammad Saeed	Department of Veterinary Parasitology, Faculty of Animal Husbandry and Veterinary Sciences, Sindh Agriculture University, Tandojam, Pakistan
Muhammad Sajjad Khan	Cholistan University of Veterinary and Animal Sciences, Bahawalpur - 63100, Pakistan
Muhammad Umar	Faculty of Veterinary and Animal Sciences, Lasbela University of Agriculture, Uthal-3800, Balochistan, Pakistan
Nabela I. El-Sharkawy	Forensic Medicine and Toxicology Department, Veterinary Medicine Faculty, Zagazig University, Zagazig 44519, Egypt
Nahed Yehia	Reference Laboratory for Veterinary Quality Control on Poultry Production, Animal Health Research Institute, Agricultural Research Center, Egypt
Nasrullah	Faculty of Veterinary and Animal Sciences, Lasbela University of Agriculture, Uthal-3800, Balochistan, Pakistan
Rana M. Bilal	University College of Veterinary and Animal Sciences, The Islamia University of Bahawalpur, Pakistan
Rashed Chowdhury	Department of Biochemistry and Chemistry, Sylhet Agricultural University, Sylhet, Bangladesh
Sabry A.A. El-Sayed	Department of Nutrition and Clinical Nutrition, Faculty of Veterinary Medicine, Zagazig University, Zagazig, Egypt
Samar S. Negm	Fish Biology and Ecology Department, Central Lab for Aquaculture Research Abassa, Agriculture Research Centre, Giza, Egypt
Sameh A. Abdelnour	Department of Animal Production, Faculty of Agriculture, Zagazig University, Zagazig, 44511, Egypt
Sarah Y.A. Ahmed	Department of Microbiology, Faculty of Veterinary Medicine, Zagazig University, Zagazig, Egypt
Shaaban S. Elnesr	Poultry Production Department, Faculty of Agriculture, Fayoum University, Fayoum, 63514, Egypt
Zohaib A. Bhutto	Faculty of Veterinary and Animal Sciences, Lasbela University of Agriculture, Water and Marine Sciences, 3800 Uthal, Balochistan, Pakistan

CHAPTER 1

An Overview of Natural Feed Additive Alternatives to AGPs

Mahmoud Alagawany[*] and **Mohamed E. Abd El-Hack**[*]

Department of Poultry, Faculty of Agriculture, Zagazig University, Zagazig 44511, Egypt

Improving the growth rate and preventing infectious diseases of food-producing animals, including poultry, are critically required to satisfy the dietary needs of the growing population around the world. Antibiotics are drugs of low or medium molecular weights with variable biological and chemical characteristics. They could be produced naturally from microorganisms or synthesized in the laboratories. Antibiotics have been used extensively in the poultry sector for therapeutic purposes such as treatment and prevention of infectious diseases and reduction of their incidence by inhibiting the growth of microorganisms or destroying them to improve the bird's health. They also have been applied in sub-therapeutic levels as feed additives to promote the rates of growth, improve weight gain, enhance feed efficiency and increase egg production to provide adequate amounts of eggs and meat of good quality needed by consumers at reasonable costs. Anyway, the extensive use of such antibiotics in poultry diets raised concerns about increasing the incidence of resistant pathogens, which has an adverse effect not only on poultry performance but also on the health of humans.

In the last years, several substances have been used as good alternatives to antibiotic growth enhancers. Herbal plants and its derivatives (extracts, cold-pressed oils and essential oils), probiotics, fruits by-products, organic acids, nanomaterials, blends of such phytogenic feed additives have been accepted as suitable alternatives with distinct mechanisms. The beneficial uses of natural herbal plants in medical sciences have achieved great attention due to promising health benefits in comparison with synthetic pharmaceutics.

Due to its nutritional and immunological effects, such as improved feed efficiency, regulation of endogenous digestive enzymes, efficiency, regulation of endogenous digestive enzymes, immune response stimulation, antiviral, antibacterial, efficiency, regulation of endogenous digestive enzymes, efficiency,

---

[*] **Corresponding authors Magmoud Alagawany and Mohamed E. Abd El-Hack:** Poultry Department, Faculty of Agriculture, Zagazig University, Zagazig, Egypt; E-mails: mmalagwany@zu.edu.eg and m.ezzat@zu.edu.eg

regulation of endogenous digestive enzymes, immune response stimulation, antiviral, antibacterial, and antioxidant properties, medicinal plants seem to be of great importance.

Improving poultry production using probiotics as feed additives is one of the decent alternative options to antibiotics. Probiotics are described as "living microorganisms that confer a benefit on the host health when applied in adequate quantities". Probiotics as feed additives help in feed digestion by creating the nutrients in an available form for growing faster. Also, supplemented poultry diets with probiotics improved immunity status. Besides, fortified poultry diets with probiotics enhancing meat characterization and egg quality traits; while selected natural feed additives such as whole herbal plants, cold-pressed oil, essential oils proved to be able to reduce oxidative stress and inflammation in poultry, enhancing the digestibility of nutrient.

Also, organic acids are used as natural preservatives for food products and as hygiene promoters that affected microbial growth, which improved the freshness and shelf-life of food items. This book describes the benefits and the hazards of using antibiotics as growth promoters in poultry feeding and also discusses the valuable effects of natural feed additives on poultry production and health and their critical role in the poultry industry.

CHAPTER 2

Antibiotics as Growth Promoters in Poultry Feeding

Mayada R. Farag[1,*], Mahmoud Alagawany[2,*], Mohamed E. Abd El-Hack[2], Shaaban S. Elnesr[3], Gihan G. Moustafa[1], Kuldeep Dhama[4] and Nabela I. El-Sharkawy[1]

[1] *Forensic Medicine and Toxicology Department, Veterinary Medicine Faculty, Zagazig University, Zagazig 44519, Egypt*

[2] *Poultry Department, Faculty of Agriculture, Zagazig University, Zagazig 44519, Egypt*

[3] *Poultry Production Department, Faculty of Agriculture, Fayoum University, Fayoum 63514, Egypt*

[4] *Division of Pathology, ICAR-Indian Veterinary Research Institute, Izatnagar, Bareilly, 243 122, Uttar Pradesh, India*

Abstract: The improvement in the growth of birds through the use of antibiotics could be obtained by reducing the count of harmful microorganisms, providing beneficial ones by suitable growth media, decreasing the thickness of gut mucosa and regulating the motility of gut, leading to better absorption of nutrients. However, achieving these desirable goals is not devoid of risks. Where, the frequent and improper use of antibiotics can reverse their therapeutic advantages through giving the opportunity to any existent microorganism to develop antibiotic resistance, which can hinder the effectiveness of antibiotics as chemotherapeutic or prophylactic agents in poultry. Additionally, antibiotic resistance genes can be transmitted to the natural environment and contaminate soil, water and plants. Moreover, the indiscriminate application of antibiotics could result in the accumulation of noticeable amounts of drug residues (the parent compounds or their injurious metabolites) in the edible tissues of poultry, including eggs and meat, which are very important sources in human feeding. The residues of antibiotics in poultry products can result in various pathological conditions and hazardous impacts on human health, such as being sensitive to antimicrobials in addition to allergy, cell mutations, imbalanced microbiota in the intestine and the development of bacteria resistance to antibiotics. This chapter describes the benefits and the hazards of using antibiotics as growth promoters in poultry feeding.

Keywords: Antibiotics, Feed additives, Growth promoters, Poultry.

* Corresponding authors Mayada R. Farag: Forensic Medicine and Toxicology Department, Veterinary Medicine Faculty, Zagazig University, Zagazig - 44519, Egypt; E-mail: dr.mayadarf@gmail.com;
Mahmoud Alagawany: Poultry Department, Faculty of Agriculture, Zagazig University, Zagazig, Egypt; E-mail: mmalagwany@zu.edu.eg

INTRODUCTION

Antibiotics are among the most essential veterinary drugs associated with animal and poultry production as they could inhibit the growth of microorganisms or destroy them when used at low levels without damaging the host [1]. The antibiotics are used in the poultry industry for treatment (therapeutic) and prevention (prophylaxis) of diseases, modifying the body physiology, and for growth-promoting purposes [2]. The growth-promoting properties of antibiotics were first observed by Moore *et al.* [3]. They reported that birds exposed to streptomycin in their diet showed improved growth response. Some other experiments followed this study in chickens and different animal species with similar results [4 - 7]. Since then, the use of antibiotics as growth promoters became one of the most common well-established practices in the livestock industry and increased with animal production intensification. Antibiotics are utilized in poultry diet as feed additives to improve the growth, feed efficiency and productivity and to ensure food safety [8 - 10]. However, reaching these desirable objectives is related to some risks, where the inappropriate handling and use of these antibiotics have led to the accumulation of noticeable concentrations of harmful residues in edible poultry tissues and eggs [11]. Consumption of these residues can lead to various health problems and the development of antibiotic resistance in pathogens and/or commensal microorganisms, which may result in severe pathological conditions and consequently threaten the public health [12]. However, the transfer of antimicrobial resistance genes from animals to human pathogens is still unconfirmed. Several works showed a relationship between the improper use of antibiotics at sub-therapeutic levels and the development of antibiotic resistance in microflora [13 - 17].

Therefore, the antibiotic-treated birds should be held for specific withdrawal periods for the depletion of the antibiotic residues to safe levels in eggs and tissues. Moreover, applicable and straightforward screening methods should be developed for the detection of antimicrobial residues in edible tissues before reaching consumers [18]. Additionally, it is important to search for antibiotic alternatives such as probiotics, prebiotics, synbiotics, phytogenics and others to increase birds' productivity and help them perform their genetic potentials under commercial conditions [19]. The main objectives of the following sections are to provide an overview on the use of antibiotics as growth promoters in poultry production and to review the public health risks related to the residues of antibiotics (human health effects, antimicrobial resistance) and the techniques of their screening and detection in food from animal origins. Lastly, this chapter highlights the measures and recommendations to control or prevent antimicrobial residues in poultry tissues.

TYPES AND PROPERTIES OF ANTIBIOTICS

Antibiotics are all bacteriostatic, which could prevent the growth and division of the bacterial cell. Some of them can be bacteriocidal or even caused bacteriolysis. Antibiotics can exert their mode of actions through direct or indirect prevention of nucleic acid replication, interfering with protein development required for the growth of bacteria or interfering with the synthesis of the cell wall [20, 21]. The mechanism of the antimicrobial action of antibiotics is illustrated in Fig. (**1**). The most common types of antibiotics (aminoglycosides, beta-lactam antibiotics, tetracycline, polypeptide antibiotics, sulphonamides, quinolones, chloramphenicol, and macrolide antibiotics), their action mechanisms, the spectrum of activity and some specific characteristics are represented in Table **1** as extracted from Diaz-Sanchez *et al*. [22].

Table 1. Classes of antibiotics and their mechanisms of antimicrobial action, activity spectrum and some specific characters.

Class	Structure	Source	Action	Activity Spectrum	Characters
Aminoglycosides		Streptomyces spp.	Inhibit the synthesis of protein	Gram-negative	Form strong and irreversible bond with the ribosome by which they could inhibit bacterial re-growth.
Beta-Lactams		Fungal product	Inhibit the synthesis of cell wall	Gram-negative and some Gram-positive	Unstable in acidic media. Various bacterial strains secrete lactamases, which could break the cyclic bond in Beta-lactams chemical structure.
Glycopeptides		Chemically synthesized	Inhibit synthesis of peptidoglycan (act on cell wall or membrane)	Gram-positive enterococci	Restricted for use in food animals.
Polyether ionophores		Chemically synthesized	Increase the cell membrane leakage	Parasitic coccidia	Some of them are converted to inorganic arsenic by bacteria present in the liter.

(Table 1) cont.....

Class	Structure	Source	Action	Activity Spectrum	Characters
Lincosamides		*Streptomyces lincolnensis*	Reversibly bind to the 50S ribosomal subunit thereby inhibits protein synthesis	Gram-positive cocci	Can diffuse to tissues making them useful in treating bone and joint infections and necrotic enteritis.
Macrolides		Produced by a variety of bacteria	Reversibly bind to the 50S ribosomal subunit thereby inhibits protein synthesis	Gram-positive	Effective in treating Mycoplasma.
Polypeptides Amino-acid and peptide derivates		Fungi, bacteria, plants and eukaroytic cells	Interfere with cytoplasmic membrane and inhibit synthesis of cell wall	Bacilli such as *E. coli* and *Pasturella*	Include bacitracin, which is restricted for use at sub-therapeutic doses.
Quinolones and Fluoroquinolones		Chemically synthesized	Inhibit replication of DNA	Gram-positive Gram-negative	Used for prophylactic purposes and have been banned in poultry by the FDA in 2005.
Sulfonamides		Chemically synthesized	Inhibit synthesis of DNA, RNA and folic acid	Gram-positive Gram-negative	Used to treat the fowl typhoid and pullorum disease.
Tetracyclines		Streptomyces spp.	Inhibit the synthesis of protein	Gram-positive Gram-negative	Lead to plasmid-mediated resistance, can treat disease caused by vancomycin-resistant bacteria.

(Table 1) cont.....

Class	Structure	Source	Action	Activity Spectrum	Characters
Phenicols and amphenicols		Chemically synthesized	Inhibit the synthesis of protein	Gram-positive Gram-negative	Very stable, residual amounts of the drug can be left in different tissues and egg. It should not be used simultaneously with penicillin, cephalosporin's streptomycin.

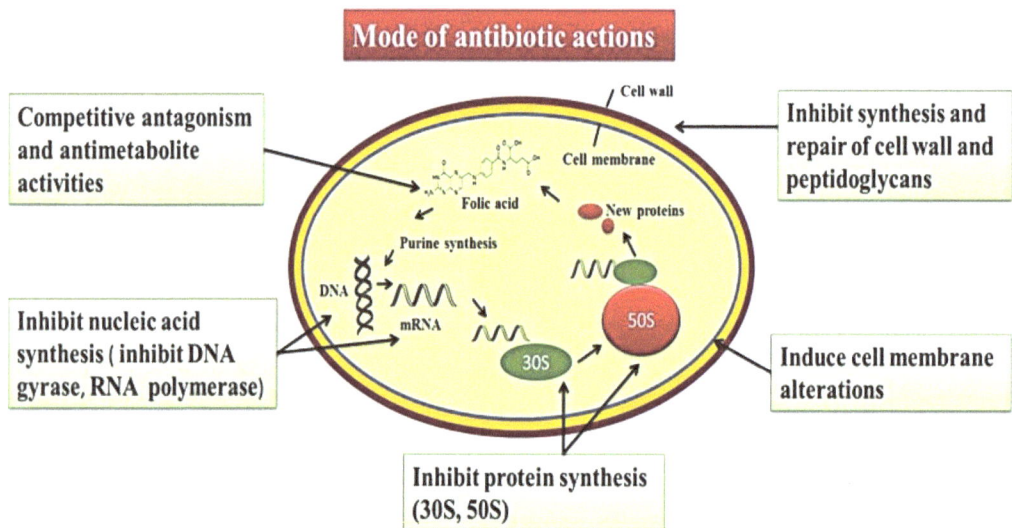

Fig. (1). Mechanism of antimicrobial action of antibiotics.

USES OF ANTIBIOTICS IN ANIMALS AND POULTRY

The antibiotics were used in food-producing animals for therapeutic purposes to control a bacterial infection, which leads to disease conditions without causing health effects to the host; or as prophylactic agents in sub-therapeutic concentration to prevent the possible infections in more susceptible animals. Moreover, antibiotics could be mixed with animal feed in subtherapeutic levels to inhibit the activity of natural microbiota in the digestive tract of animals and poultry for growth promotion [2, 10].

ANTIBIOTICS AS GROWTH PROMOTERS

The use of antimicrobials for growth promotion in farm animals was discovered in the late 1940s when tetracycline production wastes were fed to chickens as a vitamin B12 source. These wastes led to the rapid growth of birds compared to controls. Stokstad and Jukes [23] found that tetracycline residues were responsible for this rapid growth, not the vitamin contents. Since this discovery, antibiotics have been widely used in most food-producing animals to increase the rates of growth, feed conversion and egg production without veterinarian prescription [24, 25].

MECHANISM OF ACTION OF ANTIBIOTIC GROWTH PROMOTERS

There are various ideas that could be proposed to explain the growth-promoting properties of antibiotics; however, to date, the exact mechanism is not perfectly elucidated. A preliminary theory has related the efficacy of antibiotics as a growth promoter to its antimicrobial effect, which involved in reducing the overall diversity or number of microbiota in the gut [26, 27]. This leads to decreasing the competition between the host and microbiota for nutrients and also reduced the unwanted bacterial metabolites such as bile catabolism and amino acids [28, 29]. The addition of antibiotics to animal or birds diet at low doses could improve the physiological performances by enhancing the nutrient absorption *via* intestinal epithelia, promoting the synthesis of vitamins and growth factors and destroying the pathogens, thereby reducing the toxin release [30]. Moreover, the antibiotic growth promoters could increase productivity by enhancing the rate of growth and the efficiency of feed conversion and controlling some of the chronic conditions [31].

While, Niewold [32] proposed a contradicting theory, in which the growth-promoting impacts of antibiotic is related to its interaction with the immune system of the host rather than its microbial-inhibitory action. He suggested that antibiotic has an anti-inflammatory effect which could save the energy required for production. Where, antibiotic can decrease the host inflammatory responses and, consequently, the pro-inflammatory cytokines which are responsible for reduced appetite and enhanced catabolism of muscles.

With the development of molecular biology and bioinformatics, the shift in composition diversity and structure of microbiota became possible to be included in the livestock diet [33 - 35]. This shift may result in balanced microorganisms with less capability of inducing inflammatory responses in the host, maximize the harvesting of energy from different nutrients and improve the animal performance to its genetic potential [36, 37].

However, relating a specific type of bacteria to the enhancement of growth or the way of modifying microbiota to more beneficial onesis still a challenge for the researchers [38]. Some researchers showed that antimicrobial growth promoters could reduce the numbers of gut bacteria which produce bile salt hydrolase (BSH) enzyme (an enzyme catalyzes bile acids deconjugation and modifies the metabolism of lipid by the host) [29, 38, 39].

In another study on mice, antibiotics at sub-therapeutic levels altered the composition and metabolic activity of gut microorganisms through selecting the species of bacteria which can extract a higher calories proportion from complex carbohydrate (higher copy number of genes participated in carbohydrate metabolism into short-chain fatty acids (SCFA) [40]. They found that the phenotype with growth-promoting activity could be transferred to hosts free of germs by low doses of antibiotic-selected bacteria, indicating that the growth enhancement was related to the action of altered bacteria, not the antibiotic. Cox *et al.* [41] stated that early exposure to antibiotics at low doses in young mice affected the metabolism of the host by the development of age-related microorganisms and modifying the expressions of immune-related genes. Some properties of antibiotics as growth promoters in poultry are described in Fig. (**2**).

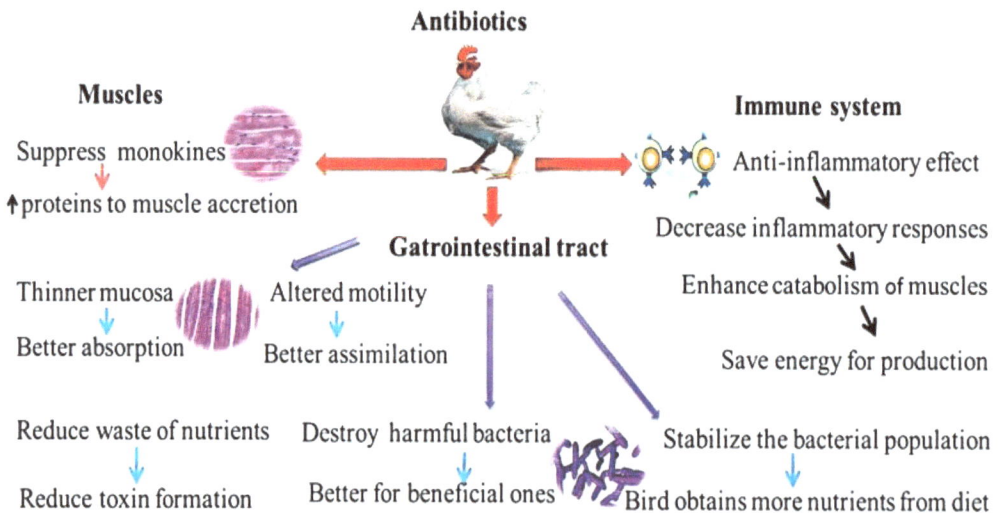

Fig. (2). Mechanism of action of antibiotic growth promoters in poultry.

PHARMACOLOGY AND TOXICOLOGY OF ANTIBIOTICS USED IN POULTRY PRODUCTION

Antibiotics are usually introduced to birds in their drinking water or feed. After administration, they are absorbed in the bird's GIT (gastrointestinal tract) and the rate of absorption depends on some factors including the physical and chemical characters of the drug, dietary sources and bivalent ions in the GIT [42]. The distribution of antibiotics in animal tissues is influenced by some other variables such as sex, age and species [43].

For example, the concentrations of Ampicillin, sulphadimidine and oxytetracycline have been reported to increase in the plasma immediately from the first day of administration and were detected in the kidney, liver and breast muscles on the second day [44]. Penicillin is metabolized in the liver and kidney and excreted in the urine. On the other hand, sulphonamides have various metabolic pathways and their main metabolite is an acetyl derivative and this class can affect the thyroids and the hypothalamic-pituitary axis as a primary mode of toxic action. Oxytetracycline showed a wide distribution in different body tissues and organs such as kidney, liver, bones and teeth with little or no metabolism [45]. Burrows *et al.* [46] stated that neomycin and gentamycin are not metabolized in the animal body but are depleted from fat and muscles and become persistent in the liver and kidney, affecting their functions. While streptomycin is not readily absorbed in GIT due to its high molecular mass and pass unchanged in feces.

CAUSES OF ANTIMICROBIAL RESIDUES IN TISSUES OF POULTRY

The purposes of using antibiotics in food producing animals are therapeutic, prophylactic or diagnostic ones. Therefore, it is of importance to ensure that the used drug would not be present in tissues above the safe Maximum Residue Limit (MRL) and the tissues should be free from residues of banned drugs [47, 48]. The authorized drugs should have a fixed MRL for the consumer's safety and it should not increase if the used veterinary practices were controlled. However, the presence of antimicrobial residues in edible poultry tissues and eggs and the unwanted impacts of such residues on the consumers are still an issue of public health concern.

One of the primary causes of antimicrobial residues in poultry products is the failure in determining the withdrawal period of the drug as this period varied greatly depending on the type of the drug, dose and administration route [49, 50]. Using of antibiotics contrary to the label directions or the use of off-label drugs, improper applications and management of antibiotics, continuous use of banned antibiotics, lack of treatment records, difficulties in identification of treated animals, absence of consumer awareness about the undesirable health effects associated with the consumption of antibiotics residues are other important causes for incidences of antibiotic residues [43, 51, 52].

The improper route of administration, overdose, longer duration, using of drugs that are not recommended for poultry (*e.g.*, the use of sulfonamides for laying birds and/or the use of hormones and beta-agonist compounds in poultry as general) can lead to toxic residues in edible poultry tissues or eggs [47].

POSSIBLE HEALTH RISKS RELATED TO ANTIBIOTIC RESIDUES

Residues of antibiotics in food from animal origins (meat, egg, or milk) represent one of the most critical public health concerns since man is the main consumer of such products with their toxic residues [53]. Public health hazards and pathological impacts of antibiotic residues (immunological, microbiological, or toxicological) have been stated in various researches worldwide [44, 50, 54 - 56].

ALLERGY OR HYPERSENSITIVITY REACTIONS

Various kinds of antibiotics could act as potent antigens or haptens, which can lead to an allergic reaction. For example, residues of ß-lactam antibiotic residues in meat or milk which induce hypersensitivity reactions in the form of IgE-mediated response which occurred directly after exposure to the antibiotic (as anaphylaxis, serum sickness, cutaneous reactions as urticaria, angioedema and bronchospasm) or non-IgE-mediated response such as hemolytic anemia, acute interstitial nephritis, thrombocytopenia, vasculitis, Stevens-Johnson syndrome, erythema multiforme and toxic epidermal necrolysis [57, 58]. Another example is the anaphylactic reactions (a delayed hypersensitivity response) caused by penicillin [59]. Additionally, the exposure to sulfonamide may induce some skin reactions such as mild rash or toxidermia [60]. On a similar ground, some kinds of macrolides (*e.g.*, clarithromycin and erythromycin) showed a tendency to induce allergic responses, which can modify the hepatic cells leading to hepatic injury [61]. Settepani [62] stated that residues of chloramphenicol in food could seldom induce fatal blood dyscrasia.

DISRUPTION OF NORMAL INTESTINAL MICROBIOTA

Intestinal microflora has important functions inside the body, such as controlling and preventing the colonization of pathogenic microorganisms in the GIT [63]. However, some researchers have concluded that the administration of antimicrobial agents at subtherapeutic levels produced some alterations and changes in the ecological compositions, reduced the number, or killed some important species of the gut microflora leading to gastrointestinal disturbance [64, 65]. The degree of changes varied depending on the antibiotic dose, administration route, bioavailability, length of exposure and the biotransformation of the antibiotic in the body, including metabolism, distribution and excretion [66]. Streptomycin, flunixin and tylosin are reported to induce such effects [67]. Some antibiotics (particularly of broad-spectrum activity) or their residues can lead to the elimination of intestinal microflora, providing a free field for fungi and yeast multiplication resulting in pathogenic conditions or altered the drug resistance of intestinal microflora [68, 69].

DEVELOPMENT OF ANTIMICROBIAL RESISTANCE

The drug resistance has been observed after exposure to a new antibiotic class or repeated exposure to sublethal doses [70]. Bacteria can resist the antimicrobial action by different mechanisms such as inactivating the enzyme, altering the binding sites on the drug targets, efflux activities and decreasing the cell wall permeability. The bacterial resistance against antibiotics could be intrinsic or acquired. The intrinsic resistance is associated with the bacterial chromosome inherent characters such as gene mutations and induction of enzymes production [71]. The acquired one could result from resistance gene transmission from the environment and/or horizontal transfer from other bacterial species [72, 73]. The mechanism of antimicrobial resistance is represented in Fig. (3).

The transfer of antibiotic-resistant strains of bacteria represents a health hazard in peoples consumed food of animal origins (meat, egg, milk) contaminated with the toxic residues of antibiotics. As the microorganisms from animal origins, can replace the human microflora or supplement and superimpose loads to the reservoir of resistance genes already exist in human [67].

The overuse of antimicrobial drugs around the world can also lead to the emergence of antibiotic-resistant genes (ARGs) [74]. The utilizing of the antimicrobials in food animals can select for antibiotic-resistant bacteria, which may spread to humans through the food (food borne-pathogens), leading to inadequate responses to treatment [75]. For example, using fluoroquinolones in the poultry sector resulted in the development of resistant strains of *Salmonella spp.* and *Campylobacter spp.* which have been isolated from the poultry tissues [76 - 78]. Moreover, the use of broad-spectrum antibiotics in both humans and animals resulted in the development of the multi-resistant *Escherichia coli*, which created a problem of transmitting their ARGs to the next generations [79]. Table **2** summarizes the antibiotic resistance of some selected microorganisms in poultry.

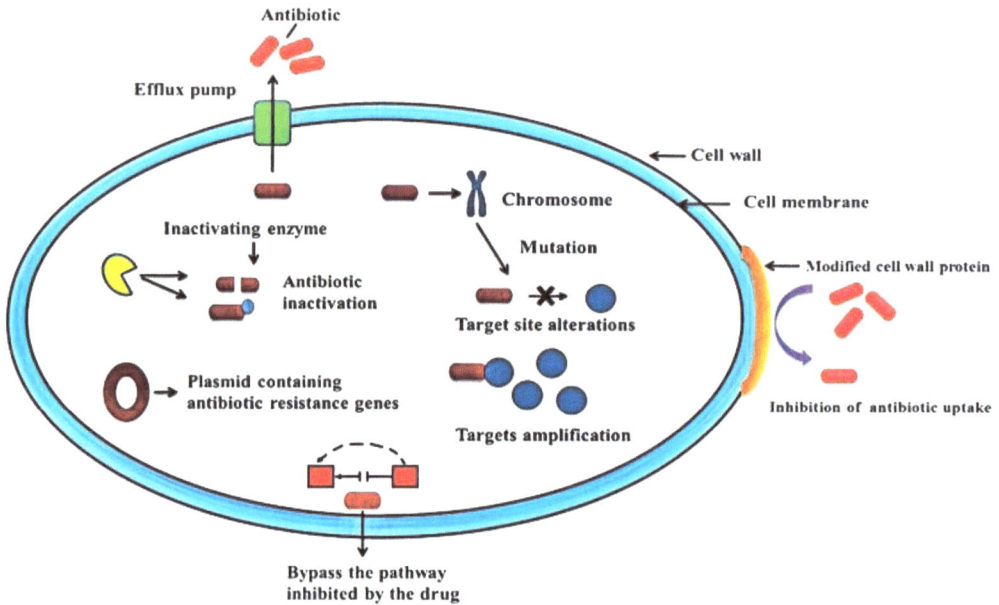

Fig. (3). Antimicrobial resistance.

OTHER HEALTH EFFECTS

Moreover, the administration of antibiotic residues can result in hearing loss, hepatotoxicity, nephrotoxicity, bone marrow toxicity, reproductive toxicity, immunotoxicity, carcinogenicity, mutagenicity and teratogenicity [67, 130, 131].

IMPACT OF ANTIMICROBIAL RESIDUES ON ENVIRONMENT AND SOIL MICROBES

Antibiotics can contaminate the environment in different ways *viz.*, during the process of manufacturing, throwing the drug containers and unused drugs or through the animal wastes and manure. Large amounts of antibiotics are excreted by animals in feces and urine as parent compounds or toxic metabolites as a considerable amount of antibiotics are not completely absorbed from GIT [132, 133]. The antibiotic concentration is varied greatly depending on the dilution, duration of exposure and the sampling time after exposure. The highest and most frequently detected residues in animal wastes are those belonging to the tetracycline group, followed by fluoroquinolone [133, 134] while penicillin is unstable in wastes and could be degraded by the soil microorganisms [135].

Table 2. Antibiotic resistance of some selected microorganisms in poultry.

Bacterial Species	Characters	Responsible For	Resistant To	References
Staphylococcus	Gram-positive facultative anaerobe.	*Staphylococcus*, pododermatitis (bumblefoot) and septicemia in chicken and turkeys Coagulase-negative species have also been implicated in human and animal infections.	Methicillin resistant *Staphylococcus aureus* (MRSA) is resistant to almost all antibiotic used against *Staphylococcus* with high resistance to oxacillin and tetracycline.	[80 - 85]
Pseudomonas	Gram-negative aerobic bacteria.	Pseudomoniasis in poultry where infections in eggs destroy embryos *P. aeruginosa* causes respiratory infection, sinusitis, keratitis/keratoconjuctivitis and septicemia, pyogenic infections, septicemia, endocarditis and lameness.	Cephalosporins,carbapenems, penicillins, quinolones, onobactam and aminoglycoside, β-lactam antibiotics (meropenem, imipenem, aztreonam, and ceftazidime), tetracycline, tobramycin, nitrofurantoin, ceftriaxone, sulfamethoxazole-trimethoprim, meropenem, ciproloxacin, erythromycin and colistin, ampicillin sulbactam, ceftazidime, cefoperazone and rifampicin.	[86 - 92]
Escherichia	Gram-negative.	Gastrointestinal illnesses.	Tetracycline, amoxicillin, amoxicillin oxytetracycline, streptomycin, sulfamethoxazole and trimethoprim. Ceftriaxone, cefotaxime, gentamycin cotrimoxazole tetracycline and ampicillin. Resistant genes have been found in *E. coli* include bla-TEM, sul2, sul3, aadA, strA, strB, catA1, tetB which conveyed resistance to tetracycline, sulfamethoxazole, nalidixic acid, streptomycin, trimethoprim, ampicillin, ciproloxacin, spectinomycin, neomycin, chloramphenicol, and gentamicin.	[93 - 96]
Salmonella	Gram-negative, facultative anaerobic.	Salmonellosis, pullorum disease in poultry.	Streptomycin, sulfonamides lorfenicol and ampicillin.	[16, 80, 97]

(Table 2) cont.....

Bacterial Species	Characters	Responsible For	Resistant To	References
Streptococcus.	Gram-positive.	Mastitis in cattle, septicemia in pigeons, and meningitis, septicemia, and endocarditis in humans.	The isolates were resistant to tetracycline and had tet(M) and/or tet(L) and/or tet(O) genes.	[98, 99]
Campylobacter	Gram-negative.	foodborne gastroenteritis.	tetracycline, erythromycin, gentamycin, ampicillin, ciproloxacin, nalidixic acid, chloramphenicol, β-lactams, quinolones, aminoglycosides, trimethoprim- ulfamethoxazole and imipenem - tet(O) gene, tet(A) gene and mutations in the gyrA genes were found to be associated with the observed antibiotic resistance.	[100 - 107]
Yersinia	Gram-negative.	Enteritis.	cephalotin and ampicillin.	[108, 109]
Clostridium	Gram-positive obligate anaerobic.	botulism caused by *C. botulinum*, pseudomembranous colitis caused by *C. diicile*, cellulitis and gas gangrene caused by *C. perfringens*, tetanus caused by *C. tetani* and fatal post-abortion infections caused by *C. sordellii.*	Gentamycin, streptomycin, oxolinic acid, lincomycin, erythromycin and spiramycin., sulfamethoxazole-trimethoprim, doxycycline, perloxacin, colistin and neomycin, chlortetracycline.	[110 - 113]
Bacillus	Gram-positive, obligate aerobic or facultative anaerobic.	*B. anthracis* causes anthrax and *B. cereus* causes food poisoning. pneumonia, endocarditis, ocular and musculoskeletal infections.	penicillin, amoxicillin, amoxicillin-clavulanate, colistin, cefoperazone, sulfamethizole, metronidazole, and ampicillin and carbenicillin.	[114 - 116]
Mycobacterium	Mycobacteria are acid-fast, aerobic, nonmotile.	*M. tuberculosis, M. bovis, M. africanum, M. macroti cause tuberculosis* and *M. leprae* cause leprosy.	penicillin and rifampicin.	[117, 118]
Klebsiella	Gram-negative, non-motile.	septicaemia, meningitis, urinary tract infections, pneumonia, diarrhea.	ampicillin, nalidixic acid, tetracycline, and trimethoprim amoxicillin, cotrimoxazole and augmentin.	[119 - 121]

(Table 2) cont.....

Bacterial Species	Characters	Responsible For	Resistant To	References
Enterococcus	Gram-positive.	urinary tract infections, bacteremia, meningitis, endocarditis.	β-lactam antibiotics, minoglycosides, vancomycin, tetracycline, erythromycin, oloxacin, ampicillin, ampicillin/sulbactam, lincomycin, and penicillin.	[122 - 125]
Proteus	Gram-negative.	nosocomial urinary and septic infections.	nalidixic acid, doxycycline and tetracycline, norloxacin, ampicillin, amikacin, ceftriaxone, and ciproloxacin.	[126 - 129]

Antibiotics can also contaminate the terrestrial and aquatic ecosystems *via* the discharges of effluents from the farms with the bioactive drug residues [136].

The persistence of antimicrobial residues in the different environments depends on some factors such as physiochemical characters of the residue, characteristics of the environment (soil, water, or air) and climatic conditions including humidity, rainfall and temperature [137]. For example, tetracyclines and fluoroquinolones persist in soil for long periods while sulphonamides [138] while, sulphonamides showed relative stability and found in the bioavailable form in the environment.

The presence of antimicrobial residues in the soil can affect the microbial communities in such soil, depending on the type and amount of residues and the bacterial species present [139, 140]. These residues can change the structures and abundance of the microbial communities and their activity in degrading the environmental contaminants and inhibit their ecological roles such as the transformation of nitrogen, methanogenesis, and reduction of sulfate in aquatic and soil environments [141].

TECHNIQUES FOR SCREENING OF ANTIBIOTIC RESIDUES IN EDIBLE POULTRY TISSUES

There are various analytical techniques available for screening and confirmation of antimicrobial residues in animal products, which are varied according to the types of residues and analyzed food. The analytical techniques include biological, immunological and chromatographic techniques. Microbiological methods are used to monitor the veterinary drug residues in foods derived from animals [50, 56] and are commonly used for detecting the residues of antibiotics in slaughtered animals in Europe [142]. Immunological techniques are sensitive and specific screening techniques based on antigen-antibody reaction. One example is the enzyme-linked immunosorbent assay (ELISA), which showed high efficacy in the screening of antibiotic residues in meat, particularly tetracycline and tylosin [143, 144]. The other example is the radioimmunoassay technique, which can measure the radioactivities of immunological complexes by a counter [145].

Chromatographic methods which are confirmatory techniques used for screening of sample that requires further investigations such as liquid chromatography which enables the quantitative and qualitative multi-residues screening in animal tissues however its use showed a rapid decrease in the last two decades [146]. Another technique is the high-performance liquid chromatography (HPLC), which can analyze multiple antimicrobial residues in a short time with fully automated equipment. It has been used for the screening of antibiotics in fish, meat and internal organs [147, 148]. Moreover, the coupling of HPLC with mass spectrometry (MS/LC) could effectively reduce the time of analysis for better confirmation of the samples, which were positive in initial screening suggesting its simultaneous use for screening and confirmation purposes [149, 150]. Liquid chromatography-tandem mass spectrometry (LC-MS/MS) and Ultra-performance liquid chromatography-Mass spectrometry (UPLC-MS) have also been used widely for quantitative and confirmatory analysis of antibiotic residues in meat, egg as well as milk [151 - 154].

In recent years, for food safety purposes, modern screening technologies have been developed, such as biosensors. These instruments are made up of two elements, which are bioreceptor (biological recognition element) and transducer (can convert the recognized events into measurable signals) [155]. Biosensors have been reported to be rapid, inexpensive, highly selective and easily handled instruments (not need skilled persons) [156]. Biosensors can be classified based on the types of bioreceptors, which can be organic molecules (antibody, protein, enzyme, or nucleic acid) or living biological systems (tissues, cells, or a whole organism) [157].

The enzyme-based biosensor, which is commonly applied for herbicides analysis, has been used for the detection of penicillin [158]; however, the studies on its application for other antibiotics are still few. On the other hand, the cellular biosensor has been reported to be applied for fast and effective detection of multiple antibiotic residues either separately, such as beta-lactam antibiotics [159, 160], tetracyclines [161, 162], quinolones [159] or simultaneously as chloramphenicol and quinolones [163]. The transducer biosensors have various common types such as mass-based, electrochemical or optical biosensors.

Surface Plasmon Resonance (SPR) based biosensors, Microdialysis and Solid

Phase Micro-Extraction (SPME) methods are also from the modern screening techniques which are capable of analyzing the drug residues in animal tissues [48, 164]. The antibiotic residues in animal products (milk, meat, muscle, liver and kidney) have been detected in several studies by the use of different screening methods, as summarized in Table **3**.

Table 3. Detection of antibiotic residues in animal products by different techniques.

Detection Method	Antibiotic Found	Sample	Residue (PBB)	Reference
ELISA	Quinolone	Chicken	30.81	[153]
		Beef	6.64	
	Enrofloxacin	Liver-Poultry	10-10690	[165]
		Liver-Cattle	30-3610	
		Liver-Sheep	20-1320	
		Milk	16-134.5	[166]
	Gentamicin	Milk	90	[167]
	Streptomycin		80	
	Chloramphenicol	Chicken	12.64- 226.62	[168]
HPLC	Oxytetracycline	Cured meat	42-360	[169]
	Penicillin	Milk	0-28	[170]
HPLC-DAD	Quinolone	Milk	0.6-22.0	[171]
	Tetracycline		17.4-149.1	
	Sulphonamides		13.5-147.9	
HPLC-FL	Tetracycline	Cattle tissue	176.3	[152]
		Triceps muscle	176.3	
		Gluteal muscle	405.3	
		Diaphragm	96.8	
		Kidney	672.40	
		Liver	651.30	
LC-MS	Enrofloxacin and Tetracycline	Chicken	-	[153]
		Pork	-	

(Table 3) cont.....

Detection Method	Antibiotic Found	Sample	Residue (PBB)	Reference
LC-MS/MS	Doxycycline	Poultry muscle	847.7	[154]
	Minocycline	Porcine muscle	-	[172]
	Tilmicosin Cloxacillin and Ceftiofur	Bovine milk	-	[154]
	β-lactams	Milk	-	[173]
	Sulphonamides			
	Tetracycline			
	Macrolides			
	Cephalosporin			
UPLC-MS/MS	Flumequine	Milk	2.58	[174]
	Sulfapyridine		1.77	
	Sulfamethoxazole		4.2	
	Lincomycin		11.25	
Biosensors	β-lactams (β-Ls)	Milk - serum	nanogram per milliliter (ng/ml)	[175, 176]
	tetracycline			
	streptogramin			
	macrolide			

RECOMMENDATIONS AND MEASURES FOR CONTROL AND PREVENTION OF ANTIBIOTIC RESIDUES IN POULTRY TISSUES

Prevention of antimicrobial residues in food from animal origins is an important issue, particularly for veterinarians in the regulatory and pharmaceutical sectors responsible for the assessment of the fates of chemicals and drugs which enter the food chain of the human through consumption of edible tissues [164]. There are some valuable steps that should be followed to achieve this purpose, as reported in previous literature. These steps include: improving the awareness of organizations and individuals about the problems and health risks associated with antibiotic residues in animal products including meat and eggs [21, 164] following the appropriate periods of withdrawal strictly to reach the safe concentrations of antibiotics for consumers and this should be enforced by the government or other regulatory bodies [44, 177], reducing the unnecessary use of antibiotics and management of the farms with the best available hygiene practices [178]. Additionally, inactivation of antibiotic residues could be reached by proper cooking, processing and preservation (refrigeration and pasteurization) of the animal products [56, 179]. The concentration of antibiotic residues in edible animal products could be lowered by using resin, activated charcoal and UV irradiation [179]. Moreover, simple, rapid and inexpensive screening techniques and field testes should be developed for the detection of antimicrobial residues in edible tissues before reaching consumers [18, 179, 180]. Proper monitoring procedures are essential to control the irrational use of antibiotics in animal feed and environment and to avoid the emergence of antimicrobial resistance Cheng *et al.* [181].

The heat treatment of animal foodstuffs may inactivate antibiotics [61]. Many of the studies have reported that degradation of β-lactams, quinolones, sulfonamides, macrolides, tetracyclines, and aminoglycosides are temperature-dependent and prolonged heating time helps to induce more degradation [182]. Introducing of novel alternatives with the same beneficial impacts of antibiotics growth promoters such as synbiotics, prebiotics, probiotics and organic acids should be considered [19].

Promotion and development of ethnoveterinary practices obtained from herbal plants as alternatives to antibiotics are also highly recommended due to their availability, accessibility, safety, efficacy, affordability and ease of production and preparation [183]. Ethno-pharmacology can also combat the problems of antibiotic resistance and residues accumulation in animal products [184].

CONCLUSIONS

Antibiotics have been used extensively in the poultry industry for the treatment or prevention of infectious diseases. Subtherapeutic levels of antibiotics have been applied as feed additives to promote the growth rate, increase weight gain, and improve feed utilization and egg production. But, the indiscriminate application of antibiotics could result in the accumulation of residues in edible tissues and eggs, which represent an essential source in human feeding. Such residues can pose health hazards to consumers, such as hypersensitivity and development of antibiotic resistance. The antibiotic-resistant bacterial strains (pathogenic and nonpathogenic) can be disseminated into the environment and transmitted to humans *via* the food chain leading to severe problems for public health. The occurrence of antibiotic residues is mainly related to the improper use (using f extra-label or illegal drugs) and the failure in determining the specific withdrawal period. Therefore, for therapeutic purposes, antibiotics should be used in proper doses for proper periods. Additionally, the indiscriminate use of antibiotics at subtherapeutic levels for growth-promoting purposes should be prohibited by regulatory bodies. The withdrawal period should be followed and the rules associated with the permissible limits of antimicrobial residues should be strictly enforced. More so, developing sensitive and reliable techniques to monitor the antibiotic residues is important to save the consumer health and to decrease the contamination of the environment. Promotion of ethnoveterinary practices and keeping the best available hygienic conditions are necessary to obtain safe animal products and to reduce the emergence of antibiotic resistance in pathogenic microorganisms.

CONSENT FOR PUBLICATION

Not Applicable.

CONFLICT OF INTEREST

The author confirms that this chapter contents have no conflict of interest.

ACKNOWLEDGEMENTS

Declared none.

REFERENCES

[1]   Bacanlı M, Başaran N. Importance of antibiotic residues in animal food. Food Chem Toxicol 2019; 125: 462-6.
        [http://dx.doi.org/10.1016/j.fct.2019.01.033] [PMID: 30710599]

[2]   Prajwal S, Vasudevan VN, Sathu T, Irshad A, Nayankumar SR. Kuleswan Pame antibiotic residues in food animals: Causes and health effects Pharma. Innov J 2017; 6: 1-4.

[3]   Moore PR, Evenson A, Luckey TD, McCoy E, Elvehjem CA, Hart EB. Use of sulfasuxidine, streptothricin, and streptomycin in nutritional studies with the chick. J Biol Chem 1946; 165(2): 437-41.
        [PMID: 20276107]

[4]   Groschke AC, Evans RJ. Effects of antibiotics, synthetic vitamins, vitamin B12 and an APF supplement on chick growth. Poult Sci 1950; 29: 616-8.
        [http://dx.doi.org/10.3382/ps.0290616]

[5]   Jukes TH, Stokstad ELR, Taylor RR, Cunha TJ, Edwards HM, Meadows GB. Growth-promoting effects of aureomycin on pigs. Arch Biochem Biophys 1950; 26: 324-5.

[6]   Luecke RW, Newland HW, McMillen WN, Thorp F Jr. The effects of antibiotics fed at low levels on the growth of weaning pigs. J Anim Sci 1950; 9: 662.

[7]   Rusoff LL, Davis AV, Alford JA. Growth-promoting effect of aureomycin on young calves weaned from milk at an early age. J Nutr 1951; 45(2): 289-300.
        [http://dx.doi.org/10.1093/jn/45.2.289] [PMID: 14889330]

[8]   Choct M. Alternatives to in-feed antibiotics in monogastric ani-mal industry. ASA Tech Bull 2001; 30: 1-6.

[9]   Dahiya JP, Wilkie DC, Van Kessel AG, Drew MD. Potential strategies for controlling necrotic enteritis in broiler chickens in post-antibiotic era. Anim Feed Sci Technol 2006; 129: 60-88.
        [http://dx.doi.org/10.1016/j.anifeedsci.2005.12.003]

[10]   Swatantra S, Shukla S, Tandia N, Kumar N, Paliwal R. Antibiotic Residues: A global challenge. Pharma Sci Monitor 2014; 5(3): 184-97.

[11]   Sanz D, Razquin P, Condón S, Juan T, Herraiz B, Mata L. Incidence of antimicrobial residues in meat using a broad spectrum screening strategy. Eur J Nutr Food Saf 2015; 5(3): 156-65.

[http://dx.doi.org/10.9734/EJNFS/2015/13795]

[12]   Vragović N, Bazulić D, Njari B. Risk assessment of streptomycin and tetracycline residues in meat and milk on Croatian market. Food Chem Toxicol 2011; 49(2): 352-5.
        [http://dx.doi.org/10.1016/j.fct.2010.11.006] [PMID: 21074594]

[13]   Witte W. Medical consequences of antibiotic use in agriculture. Science 1998; 279(5353): 996-7.
        [http://dx.doi.org/10.1126/science.279.5353.996] [PMID: 9490487]

[14]   Wegener HC, Aarestrup FM, Jensen LB, Hammerum AM, Bager F. Use of antimicrobial growth promoters in food animals and *Enterococcus faecium* resistance to therapeutic antimicrobial drugs in Europe. Emerg Infect Dis 1999; 5(3): 329-35.
        [http://dx.doi.org/10.3201/eid0503.990303] [PMID: 10341169]

[15]   M'ikanatha NM, Sandt CH, Localio AR, *et al.* Multidrug-resistant *Salmonella* isolates from retail chicken meat compared with human clinical isolates. Foodborne Pathog Dis 2010; 7(8): 929-34.
        [http://dx.doi.org/10.1089/fpd.2009.0499] [PMID: 20443729]

[16]   Medeiros MA, Oliveira DC, Rodrigues Ddos P, Freitas DR. Prevalence and antimicrobial resistance of *Salmonella* in chickencarcasses at retail in 15 Brazilian cities. Pan Am J Public Health 2011; 30: 555-60.
        [http://dx.doi.org/10.1590/S1020-49892011001200010]

[17]   Cosby DE, Cox NA, Harrison MA, Wilson JL, Buhr RJ, Fedorka-Cray PJ. *Salmonella* and antimicrobial resistance in broilers: a review. J Appl Poult Res 2015; 24: 408-26.
        [http://dx.doi.org/10.3382/japr/pfv038]

[18]   Abasi MM, Rashidi MR, Javadi A, Amirkhiz MB, Mirmahdavi S, Zabihi M. Levels of tetracycline residues in cattle meat, liver, and kidney from a slaughterhouse in Tabriz, Iran. Turk J Vet Anim Sci 2009; 33: 345-9.

[19]   Gadde U, Kim WH, Oh ST, Lillehoj HS. Alternatives to antibiotics for maximizing growth performance and feed efficiency in poultry: a review. Anim Health Res Rev 2017; 18(1): 26-45.
        [http://dx.doi.org/10.1017/S1466252316000207] [PMID: 28485263]

[20]   Landoni MF, Albarellos G. The use of antimicrobial agents in broiler chickens. Vet J 2015; 205(1): 21-7.
        [http://dx.doi.org/10.1016/j.tvjl.2015.04.016] [PMID: 25981931]

[21]   Alhaji NB, Haruna AE, Muhammad B, Lawan MK, Isola TO. Antimicrobials usage assessments in commercial poultry and local birds in North-central Nigeria: Associated pathways and factors for resistance emergence and spread. Prev Vet Med 2018; 154: 139-47.
        [http://dx.doi.org/10.1016/j.prevetmed.2018.04.001] [PMID: 29685438]

[22]   Diaz-Sanchez S, Moscoso S, Solís de los Santos F, Andino A, Hanning I. Antibiotic use in poultry; A driving force for organic poultry production. Food Prot Trends 2015; 35(6): 440-7.

[23]   Stokstad ELR, Jukes TH, Pierce J, Page AC Jr, Franklin AL. The multiple nature of the animal protein factor. J Biol Chem 1949; 180(2): 647-54.
        [PMID: 18135798]

[24]   Chapman HD, Johnson ZB. Use of antibiotics and roxarsone in broiler chickens in the USA: analysis for the years 1995 to 2000. Poult Sci 2002; 81(3): 356-64.
        [http://dx.doi.org/10.1093/ps/81.3.356] [PMID: 11902412]

[25]   Castanon JIR. History of the use of antibiotic as growth promoters in European poultry feeds. Poult Sci 2007; 86(11): 2466-71.
        [http://dx.doi.org/10.3382/ps.2007-00249] [PMID: 17954599]

[26]   Dennis SM, Nagaraja TG, Bartley EE. Effects of lasalocid or monensin on lactate-producing or -using rumen bacteria. J Anim Sci 1981; 52(2): 418-26.
        [http://dx.doi.org/10.2527/jas1981.522418x] [PMID: 7275867]

[27]　Nagaraja TG, Taylor MB, Harmon DL, Boyer JE. *In vitro* lactic acid inhibition and alterations in volatile fatty acid production by antimicrobial feed additives. J Anim Sci 1987; 65(4): 1064-76.
[http://dx.doi.org/10.2527/jas1987.6541064x] [PMID: 3667452]

[28]　Gaskins HR, Collier CT, Anderson DB. Antibiotics as growth promotants: mode of action. Anim Biotechnol 2002; 13(1): 29-42.
[http://dx.doi.org/10.1081/ABIO-120005768] [PMID: 12212942] .

[29]　Knarreborg A, Lauridsen C, Engberg RM, Jensen SK. Dietary antibiotic growth promoters enhance the bioavailability of alpha-tocopheryl acetate in broilers by altering lipid absorption. J Nutr 2004; 134(6): 1487-92.
[http://dx.doi.org/10.1093/jn/134.6.1487] [PMID: 15173416]

[30]　Prescott JF, Baggot JD. Antimicrobial Therapy in Veterinary Medicine. Ames, IA: Iowa State University Press 1993; pp. 250-525.

[31]　Taylor DJ. The pros and cons of antimicrobial use in animal husbandry. Baillie Are's. Clin Infect Dis 1999; 5: 269-87.

[32]　Niewold TA. The nonantibiotic anti-inflammatory effect of antimicrobial growth promoters, the real mode of action? A hypothesis. Poult Sci 2007; 86(4): 605-9.
[http://dx.doi.org/10.1093/ps/86.4.605] [PMID: 17369528]

[33]　Dumonceaux TJ, Hill JE, Hemmingsen SM, Van Kessel AG. Characterization of intestinal microbiota and response to dietary virginiamycin supplementation in the broiler chicken. Appl Environ Microbiol 2006; 72(4): 2815-23.
[http://dx.doi.org/10.1128/AEM.72.4.2815-2823.2006] [PMID: 16597987]

[34]　Pedroso AA, Menten JFM, Lambais MR, Racanicci AMC, Longo FA, Sorbara JOB. Intestinal bacterial community and growth performance of chickens fed diets containing antibiotics. Poult Sci 2006; 85(4): 747-52.
[http://dx.doi.org/10.1093/ps/85.4.747] [PMID: 16615359]

[35]　Lin J, Hunkapiller AA, Layton AC, Chang YJ, Robbins KR. Response of intestinal microbiota to antibiotic growth promoters in chickens. Foodborne Pathog Dis 2013; 10(4): 331-7.
[http://dx.doi.org/10.1089/fpd.2012.1348] [PMID: 23461609]

[36]　Huyghebaert G, Ducatelle R, Van Immerseel F. An update on alternatives to antimicrobial growth promoters for broilers. Vet J 2011; 187(2): 182-8.
[http://dx.doi.org/10.1016/j.tvjl.2010.03.003] [PMID: 20382054]

[37]　Lin J. Effect of antibiotic growth promoters on intestinal micro-biota in food animals: a novel model for studying the relationship between gut microbiota and human obesity? Front Microbiol 2011; 2: 53.
[http://dx.doi.org/10.3389/fmicb.2011.00053] [PMID: 21833309]

[38]　Lin J. Antibiotic growth promoters enhance animal production by targeting intestinal bile salt hydrolase and its producers. Front Microbiol 2014; 5: 33.
[http://dx.doi.org/10.3389/fmicb.2014.00033] [PMID: 24575079]

[39]　Guban J, Korver DR, Allison GE, Tannock GW. Relationship of dietary antimicrobial drug administration with broiler performance, decreased population levels of Lactobacillus salivarius, and reduced bile salt deconjugation in the ileum of broiler chickens. Poult Sci 2006; 85(12): 2186-94.
[http://dx.doi.org/10.1093/ps/85.12.2186] [PMID: 17135676]

[40]　Cho I, Yamanishi S, Cox L, *et al.* Antibiotics in early life alter the murine colonic microbiome and adiposity. Nature 2012; 488(7413): 621-6.
[http://dx.doi.org/10.1038/nature11400] [PMID: 22914093]

[41]　Cox LM, Yamanishi S, Sohn J, *et al.* Altering the intestinal microbiota during a critical developmental window has lasting metabolic consequences. Cell 2014; 158(4): 705-21.
[http://dx.doi.org/10.1016/j.cell.2014.05.052] [PMID: 25126780]

[42]   Ramadan A, Hanafy MSM, Afifi NA. Effect of pantothenic acid on disposition kinetics and tissue residues of sulphadimidine in chickens. Res Vet Sci 1992; 52(3): 337-41.
[http://dx.doi.org/10.1016/0034-5288(92)90034-Y] [PMID: 1620967]

[43]   Geidam YA, Usman H, Musa HI, Anosike F, Adeyemi Y. Ox tetracycline and Procain Penicillin residues in tissues of slaughtered cattle in Maiduguri, Borno state, Nigeria. Terrestrial Agua. Environ Toxicol 2009; 3(2): 68-70.

[44]   Alhendi AB, Homeida AAM, Galli ES. Drug residues in broiler chicken fed with antibiotics in ration. Vet Arh 2000; 70: 199-205.

[45]   El Atabani AI, El-Ghareeb WR, Elabbasy MT, Ghazaly EI. Oxytetracycline residues in marketed Frozen beef livers at Sharkia, Egypt ElAtabani, A. Benha Vet Med J 2014; 26(1): 104-12.

[46]   Burrows GE, Barto PB, Martin B. Comparative pharmacokinetics of gentamicin, neomycin and oxytetracycline in newborn calves. J Vet Pharmacol Ther 1987; 10(1): 54-63.
[http://dx.doi.org/10.1111/j.1365-2885.1987.tb00077.x] [PMID: 3586124]

[47]   Kabir J, Umoh VJ, Audu E, Okoh J, Umoh U, Kwaga JKP. Veterinary drug use inpoultry farms and determination of antimicrobial drug residues in commercial eggs and slaughtered chicken in Kaduna State. Nigeria Food Control 2004; 15: 99-105.
[http://dx.doi.org/10.1016/S0956-7135(03)00020-3]

[48]   Haughey SA, Baxter GA. Biosensor screening for veterinary drug residues in foodstuffs. J AOAC Int 2006; 89(3): 862-7.
[http://dx.doi.org/10.1093/jaoac/89.3.862] [PMID: 16792087]

[49]   Dipeolu MA. Problems and prospects of antibiotics residues in meat products in Nigeria. Vom J Vet Sci 2004; 1(1): 63-7.

[50]   Olatoye IO, Ehinwomo AA. Oxytetracycline Residues in Edible tissues of cattle slaughtered in Akure, Nigeria. Intern J Food Safety 2009; 11: 62-6.

[51]   Muriuki FK, Ogara WO, Njeruh FM, Mitema ES. Tetracycline residue levels in cattle meat from Nairobi salughter house in Kenya. J Vet Sci 2001; 2(2): 97-101.
[http://dx.doi.org/10.4142/jvs.2001.2.2.97] [PMID: 14614278]

[52]   Sasanya JJ, Okeng JW, Ejobi F, Muganwa M. Use of sulfonamides in layers in Kampala district, Uganda and sulfonamide residues in commercial eggs. Afr Health Sci 2005; 5(1): 33-9.
[PMID: 15843129]

[53]   Shareef AM, Jamel ZT, Yonis KM. Detection of antibiotic residues in stored poultry products. Iraqi J Vet Sci 2009; 23(1): 45-8.

[54]   FAO Food Nutrition Paper. Residues of some veterinary drugs in animals and foods. 1999; 41: pp. 97-199.

[55]   Cunha BA. Antibiotic side effects. Med Clin North Am 2001; 85(1): 149-85.
[http://dx.doi.org/10.1016/S0025-7125(05)70309-6] [PMID: 11190350]

[56]   Javadi A, Mirzaei H, Khatibi SA. Effect of roasting process on antibiotic residues inedible tissues of poultry by FRT method. J Anim Vet Adv 2009; 8(12): 2468-72.

[57]   Granowitz EV, Brown RB. Antibiotic adverse reactions and drug interactions. Crit Care Clin 2008; 24(2): 421-442, xi.
[http://dx.doi.org/10.1016/j.ccc.2007.12.011] [PMID: 18361954]

[58]   Padol AR, Malapure CD, Domple VD, Kamdi BP. Occurrence, public health implications and detection of antibacterial drug residues in cow milk. Environ We Int J Sci Tech 2015; 10: 7-28.

[59]   Thong BY, Tan TC. Epidemiology and risk factors for drug allergy. Br J Clin Pharmacol 2011; 71(5): 684-700.
[http://dx.doi.org/10.1111/j.1365-2125.2010.03774.x] [PMID: 21480948]

[60]   Choquet-Kastylevsky G, Vial T, Descotes J. Allergic adverse reactions to sulfonamides. Curr Allergy Asthma Rep 2002; 2(1): 16-25.
[http://dx.doi.org/10.1007/s11882-002-0033-y] [PMID: 11895621]

[61]   Darwish WS, Eldaly EA, El-Abbasy MT, Ikenaka Y, Nakayama S, Ishizuka M. Antibiotic residues in food: the African scenario. Jpn J Vet Res 2013; 61 (Suppl.): S13-22.
[PMID: 23631148]

[62]   Settepani JA. The hazard of using chloramphenicol in food animals. J Am Vet Med Assoc 1984; 184(8): 930-1.
[PMID: 6715222]

[63]   Vollaard EJ, Clasener HAL. Colonization resistance. Antimicrob Agents Chemother 1994; 38(3): 409-14.
[http://dx.doi.org/10.1128/AAC.38.3.409] [PMID: 8203832]

[64]   Carman RJ, Van Tassell RL, Wilkins TD. The normal intestinal microflora: ecology, variability and stability. Vet Hum Toxicol 1993; 35(1) (Suppl. 1): 11-4.
[PMID: 8236752]

[65]   Edlund C, Nord CE. Effect of quinolones on intestinal ecology. Drugs 1999; 58(2) (Suppl. 2): 65-70.
[http://dx.doi.org/10.2165/00003495-199958002-00013] [PMID: 10553709]

[66]   Cerniglia CE, Kotarski S. Approaches in the safety evaluations of veterinary antimicrobial agents in food to determine the effects on the human intestinal microflora. J Vet Pharmacol Ther 2005; 28(1): 3-20.
[http://dx.doi.org/10.1111/j.1365-2885.2004.00595.x] [PMID: 15720510]

[67]   Beyene T. Veterinary drug residues in food-animal products: its risk factors and potential effects on public health. J Vet Sci Technol 2016; 7(1): 285.

[68]   Ram C, Bhavadasan MK, Vijaya GV. Antibiotic residues in milk. Indian J Dairy Biosci 2000; 11: 151-4.

[69]   Larkin C, Poppe C, McNab B, McEwen B, Mahdi A, Odumeru J. Antibiotic resistance of *Salmonella* isolated from hog, beef, and chicken carcass samples from provincially inspected abattoirs in Ontario. J Food Prot 2004; 67(3): 448-55.
[http://dx.doi.org/10.4315/0362-028X-67.3.448] [PMID: 15035356]

[70]   Landers TF, Cohen B, Wittum TE, Larson EL. A review of antibiotic use in food animals: perspective, policy, and potential. Public Health Rep 2012; 127(1): 4-22.
[http://dx.doi.org/10.1177/003335491212700103] [PMID: 22298919]

[71]   Davies J. Microbes have the last word. A drastic re-evaluation of antimicrobial treatment is needed to overcome the threat of antibiotic-resistant bacteria. EMBO Rep 2007; 8(7): 616-21.
[http://dx.doi.org/10.1038/sj.embor.7401022] [PMID: 17603533]

[72]   McDermott PF, Walker RD, White DG. Antimicrobials: modes of action and mechanisms of resistance. Int J Toxicol 2003; 22(2): 135-43.
[http://dx.doi.org/10.1080/10915810305089] [PMID: 12745995]

[73]   Randall LP, Cooles SW, Osborn MK, Piddock LJV, Woodward MJ. Antibiotic resistance genes, integrons and multiple antibiotic resistance in thirty-five serotypes of *Salmonella enterica* isolated from humans and animals in the UK. J Antimicrob Chemother 2004; 53(2): 208-16.
[http://dx.doi.org/10.1093/jac/dkh070] [PMID: 14729766]

[74]   Yasser M, Kwon A, Kim R. Monitoring antibiotic residues and corresponding antibiotic resistance genes in an agroecosystem. J Chem 2015; 2015: 1-7.
[http://dx.doi.org/10.1155/2015/974843.] [PMID: 974843]

[75]   Phillips I, Casewell M, Cox T, *et al.* Does the use of antibiotics in food animals pose a risk to human health? A critical review of published data. J Antimicrob Chemother 2004; 53(1): 28-52.

[http://dx.doi.org/10.1093/jac/dkg483] [PMID: 14657094]

[76]   Boothe DH, Arnold JW. Resistance of bacterial isolates from poultry products to therapeutic veterinary antibiotics. J Food Prot 2003; 66(1): 94-102.
        [http://dx.doi.org/10.4315/0362-028X-66.1.94] [PMID: 12540187]

[77]   Hayes JR, English LL, Carr LE, Wagner DD, Joseph SW. Multiple-antibiotic resistance of *Enterococcus spp.* isolated from commercial poultry production environments. Appl Environ Microbiol 2004; 70(10): 6005-11.
        [http://dx.doi.org/10.1128/AEM.70.10.6005-6011.2004] [PMID: 15466544]

[78]   Aarestrup FM. Veterinary drug usage and antimicrobial resistance in bacteria of animal origin. Basic Clin Pharmacol Toxicol 2005; 96(4): 271-81.
        [http://dx.doi.org/10.1111/j.1742-7843.2005.pto960401.x] [PMID: 15755309]

[79]   McEwen SA, Black WD, Meek AH. Antibiotic residues (bacterial inhibitory substances) in the milk of cows treated under label and extra-label conditions. Can Vet J 1992; 33(8): 527-34.
        [PMID: 17424060]

[80]   Barrow GI, Feltham RKA. Cowan and Steel's Manual for the Identiication of Medical Bacteria. 3rd ed. Cambridge, UK: Cambridge University Press 2009; p. 331.

[81]   Koksal F, Yasar H, Samasti M. Antibiotic resistance patterns of coagulase-negative *Staphylococcus* strains isolated from blood cultures of septicemic patients in Turkey. Microbiol Res 2009; 164(4): 404-10.
        [http://dx.doi.org/10.1016/j.micres.2007.03.004] [PMID: 17475456]

[82]   Boamah VE, Agyare C, Odoi H, Adu F, Gbedema SY, Dalsgaard A. Prevalence and antibiotic resistance of coagulase-negative *Staphylococci* isolated from poultry farms in three regions of Ghana. Infect Drug Resist 2017; 10: 175-83.
        [http://dx.doi.org/10.2147/IDR.S136349] [PMID: 28652785]

[83]   Stapleton PD, Taylor PW. Methicillin resistance in *Staphylococcus aureus*: mechanisms and modulation. Sci Prog 2002; 85(Pt 1): 57-72.
        [http://dx.doi.org/10.3184/003685002783238870] [PMID: 11969119]

[84]   Suleiman A, Zaria LT, Grema HA, Ahmadu P. Antimicrobial resistant coagulase positive *Staphylococcus* aureus from chickens in Maiduguri, Nigeria. Sokoto J Vet Sci 2013; 11: 51-5.
        [http://dx.doi.org/10.4314/sokjvs.v11i1.8]

[85]   Waters AE, Contente-Cuomo T, Buchhagen J, *et al.* Multidrug-resistant *Staphylococcus aureus* in US meat and poultry. Clin Infect Dis 2011; 52(10): 1227-30.
        [http://dx.doi.org/10.1093/cid/cir181] [PMID: 21498385]

[86]   Skerman SV, McGowan V, Sneath P. Approved Lists of Bacterial Names (Amended) Approved List of Bacteria Names. Washington, DC: ASM Press 1989; p. 196.

[87]   de Vos P, Garrity GM, Jones D, *et al.* Bergey's Manual of Systematic Bacteriology. New York: Springer 2009; p. 1450.

[88]   Sams AR. Poultry Meat Processing. Boca Raton: CRC Press 2001; p. 345.

[89]   Basseti M, Merelli M, Temperoni C, Astilean A. New antibiotics for bad bugs: where are we?. Ann Clin Microbiol Antimicrob 2013; 12: 22.
        [http://dx.doi.org/10.1186/1476-0711-12-22.]

[90]   Zhang R, Liu Z, Li J, *et al.* Presence of VIM-positive Pseudomonas species in chickens and their surrounding environment. Antimicrob Agents Chemother 2017; 61(7): 1-5.
        [http://dx.doi.org/10.1128/AAC.00167-17] [PMID: 28438943]

[91]   Aniokete U, Iroha CS, Ajah MI, Nwakaeze AE. Occurrence of multi-drug resistant Gram-negative bacteria from poultry and poultry products sold in Abakaliki. J Agric Sci Food Technol 2016; 2: 119-24.

[92]   Sharma S, Galav V, Agrawal M, Faridi F, Kumar B. Multi-drug resistance patern of bacterial lora obtained from necropsy samples of poultry. J Anim Health Prod 2017; 5: 165-71.

[93]   Tenaillon O, Skurnik D, Picard B, Denamur E. The population genetics of commensal *Escherichia coli*. Nat Rev Microbiol 2010; 8(3): 207-17.
[http://dx.doi.org/10.1038/nrmicro2298] [PMID: 20157339]

[94]   van den Bogaard AE, Stobberingh EE. Epidemiology of resistance to antibiotics. Links between animals and humans. Int J Antimicrob Agents 2000; 14(4): 327-35.
[http://dx.doi.org/10.1016/S0924-8579(00)00145-X] [PMID: 10794955]

[95]   van den Bogaard AE, London N, Driessen C, Stobberingh EE. Antibiotic resistance of faecal *Escherichia coli* in poultry, poultry farmers and poultry slaughterers. J Antimicrob Chemother 2001; 47(6): 763-71.
[http://dx.doi.org/10.1093/jac/47.6.763] [PMID: 11389108]

[96]   Adelowo OO, Fagade OE, Agersø Y. Antibiotic resistance and resistance genes in *Escherichia coli* from poultry farms, southwest Nigeria. J Infect Dev Ctries 2014; 8(9): 1103-12.
[http://dx.doi.org/10.3855/jidc.4222] [PMID: 25212074]

[97]   Bell C, Kyriakides A. Salmonella A Practical Approach to the Organism and its Control in Foods. Oxford: Blackwell Science 2007; p. 338.

[98]   de Herdt P, Devriese LA, de Groote B, Ducatelle R, Haesebrouck F. Antibiotic treatment of *Streptococcus bovis* infections in pigeons. Avian Pathol 1993; 22(3): 605-15.
[http://dx.doi.org/10.1080/03079459308418947] [PMID: 18671044]

[99]   Nomoto R, Tien HT, Sekizaki T, Osawa R. Antimicrobial susceptibility of *Streptococcus gallolyticus* isolated from humans and animals. Jpn J Infect Dis 2013; 66(4): 334-6.
[http://dx.doi.org/10.7883/yoken.66.334] [PMID: 23883848]

[100] Sackey BA, Mensah P, Collison E, Sakyi-Dawson E. *Campylobacter, Salmonella, Shigella* and *Escherichia coli* in live and dressed poultry from metropolitan accra. Int J Food Microbiol 2001; 71(1): 21-8.
[http://dx.doi.org/10.1016/S0168-1605(01)00595-5] [PMID: 11764888]

[101] Allos BM, Allos BM. *Campylobacter jejuni* Infections: update on emerging issues and trends. Clin Infect Dis 2001; 32(8): 1201-6.
[http://dx.doi.org/10.1086/319760] [PMID: 11283810]

[102] Wilson IG. Antibiotic resistance of *Campylobacter* in raw retail chickens and imported chicken portions. Epidemiol Infect 2003; 131(3): 1181-6.
[http://dx.doi.org/10.1017/S0950268803001298] [PMID: 14959786]

[103] Randall LP, Ridley AM, Cooles SW, *et al.* Prevalence of multiple antibiotic resistance in 443 *Campylobacter spp.* isolated from humans and animals. J Antimicrob Chemother 2003; 52(3): 507-10.
[http://dx.doi.org/10.1093/jac/dkg379] [PMID: 12917241]

[104] Rożynek E, Dzierżanowska-Fangrat K, Korsak D, *et al.* Comparison of antimicrobial resistance of *Campylobacter jejuni* and *Campylobacter coli* isolated from humans and chicken carcasses in Poland. J Food Prot 2008; 71(3): 602-7.
[http://dx.doi.org/10.4315/0362-028X-71.3.602] [PMID: 18389707]

[105] Nguyen TNM, Hotzel H, Njeru J, *et al.* Antimicrobial resistance of *Campylobacter* isolates from small scale and backyard chicken in Kenya. Gut Pathog 2016; 8(1): 39.
[http://dx.doi.org/10.1186/s13099-016-0121-5] [PMID: 27570543]

[106] Kumar VA, Steffy K, Chatterjee M, *et al.* Detection of oxacillin-susceptible mecA-positive *Staphylococcus aureus* isolates by use of chromogenic medium MRSA ID. J Clin Microbiol 2013; 51(1): 318-9.
[http://dx.doi.org/10.1128/JCM.01040-12] [PMID: 23135944]

[107]   Karikari AB, Obiri-Danso K, Frimpong EH, Krogfelt KA. Antibiotic resistance of *Campylobacter* recovered from faeces and carcasses of healthy livestock. BioMed Res Int 2017; 2017: 4091856.
[http://dx.doi.org/10.1155/2017/4091856] [PMID: 28194411]

[108]   Annamalai T, Venkitanarayanan K. Expression of major cold shock proteins and genes by *Yersinia enterocolitica* in synthetic medium and foods. J Food Prot 2005; 68(11): 2454-8.
[http://dx.doi.org/10.4315/0362-028X-68.11.2454] [PMID: 16300089]

[109]   Dallal MMS, Doyle MP, Rezadehbashi M, *et al.* Prevalence and antimicrobial resis-tance proiles of *Salmonella serotypes*, *Campylobacter* and *Yersinia spp.* isolated from retail chicken and beef, Tehran, Iran. Food Control 2010; 21(4): 388-92.
[http://dx.doi.org/10.1016/j.foodcont.2009.06.001]

[110]   Péchiné S, Collignon A. Immune responses induced by Clostridium difficile. Anaerobe 2016; 41: 68-78.
[http://dx.doi.org/10.1016/j.anaerobe.2016.04.014] [PMID: 27108093]

[111]   Num SM, Useh NM. Clostridium: Pathogenic roles, industrial uses and medicinal prospects of natural products as ameliorative agents against pathogenic species. Jordan J Biol Sci 2014; 7(2): 81-94.
[http://dx.doi.org/10.12816/0008220]

[112]   Osman KM, Elhariri M. Antibiotic resistance of Clostridium perfringens isolates from broiler chickens in Egypt. Rev Sci Tech 2013; 32(3): 841-50.
[http://dx.doi.org/10.20506/rst.32.2.2212] [PMID: 24761735]

[113]   Fan YC, Wang CL, Wang C, Chen TC, Chou CH, Tsai HJ. Incidence and antimicrobial susceptibility to Clostridium perfringens in premarket broilers in Taiwan. Avian Dis 2016; 60(2): 444-9.
[http://dx.doi.org/10.1637/11315-110915-Reg] [PMID: 27309285]

[114]   Fagerlund A, Lindbäck T, Granum PE. *Bacillus cereus* cytotoxins Hbl, Nhe and CytK are secreted *via* the sec translocation pathway. BioMed Cen Microbiol 2010; 10
http://www.biomedcentral.com/1471-2180/10/304

[115]   Floriştean V, Cretu C, Carp-Cărare M. Bacteriological characteristics of *Bacillus cereus* isolates from poultry. Bulletin of University of Agricultural Sciences and Veterinary Medicine Cluj-Napoca 2007; 64: 1-2.

[116]   Bashir M, Malik MA, Javaid M, Badroo GA. Prevalence and characterization of *Bacillus cereus* in meat and meat products in and around Jammu region of Jammu and Kashmir, India. Int J Curr Microbiol Appl Sci 2017; 6(12): 1094-106.
[http://dx.doi.org/10.20546/ijcmas.2017.612.124]

[117]   Barrow WW. Treatment of mycobacterial infections. Rev Sci Tech 2001; 20(1): 55-70.
[http://dx.doi.org/10.20506/rst.20.1.1264] [PMID: 11288520]

[118]   Reza M, Lijon M, Khatun M, Islam M. Prevalence and antibiogram proile of *Mycobacterium spp.* in poultry and its environments. J Adv Vet Anim Res 2015; 2(4): 458.
[http://dx.doi.org/10.5455/javar.2015.b118]

[119]   Podschun R, Ullmann U. Klebsiella spp. as nosocomial pathogens: epidemiology, taxonomy, typing methods, and pathogenicity factors. Clin Microbiol Rev 1998; 11(4): 589-603.
[http://dx.doi.org/10.1128/CMR.11.4.589] [PMID: 9767057]

[120]   Ajayi AO, Egbebi AO. Antibiotic susceptibility of *Salmonella typhi* and *Klebsiella pneumoniae* from poultry and local birds in Ado-Ekiti, Ekiti-state. Nigeria. Ann Biol Res 2011; 2(3): 431-7.

[121]   Fielding BC, Mnabisa A, Gouws PA, Morris T. Antimicrobial-resistant Klebsiella species isolated from free-range chicken samples in an informal settlement. Arch Med Sci 2012; 8(1): 39-42.
[http://dx.doi.org/10.5114/aoms.2012.27278] [PMID: 22457672]

[122]   Teixeira LM, De Janeiro R, Merquior VLC. *Enterococcus*. In: Filippis I, McKee M, Eds. Molecular Typing in Bacterial Infections. New York: Springer Science 2013; pp. 17-27.

[http://dx.doi.org/10.1007/978-1-62703-185-1_2]

[123] Fisher K, Phillips C. The ecology, epidemiology and virulence of *Enterococcus*. Microbiology (Reading) 2009; 155(Pt 6): 1749-57.
[http://dx.doi.org/10.1099/mic.0.026385-0] [PMID: 19383684]

[124] Kolář M, Pantůček R, Bardoň J, *et al.* Occurrence of antibiotic-resistant bacterial strains isolated in poultry. Vet Med 2002; 47: 52-9.
[http://dx.doi.org/10.17221/5803-VETMED]

[125] Vignaroli C, Zandri G, Aquilanti L, Pasquaroli S, Biavasco F. Multidrug-resistant enterococci in animal meat and faeces and co-transfer of resistance from an *Enterococcus durans* to a human *Enterococcus faecium.* Curr Microbiol 2011; 62(5): 1438-47.
[http://dx.doi.org/10.1007/s00284-011-9880-x] [PMID: 21286720]

[126] Różalski A, Torzewska A, Moryl M, *et al. Proteus spp.* – An opportunistic bacterial pathogen–Classiication, swarming growth, clinical signiicance and virulence factors. Acta Univ Lodz Folia Biol Oecol 2012; 8(1): 1-17.
[http://dx.doi.org/10.2478/fobio-2013-0001]

[127] Ahmed DA. Prevalence of *Proteus spp.* in some hospitals in Baghdad City. Iraq J Sci 2015; 56(1): 665-72.

[128] Nemati M. Antimicrobial resistance of Proteus isolates from poultry. Eur J Exp Biol 2013; 3(6): 499-500.

[129] Nahar A, Siddiquee M, Nahar S, Anwar KS, Ali SI, Islam S. Multidrug resistant-Proteus mirabilis isolated from chicken droppings in commercial poultry farms: Bio-security concern and emerging public health threat in Bangladesh. Biosaf Health Educ 2014; 2(2): 120-5.
[http://dx.doi.org/10.4172/2332-0893.1000120]

[130] El-Makawy A, Radwan HA, Ghaly IS, El-Raouf AA. Genotoxical, teratological and biochemical effects of anthelmintic drug oxfendazole Maximum Residue Limit (MRL) in male and female mice. Reprod Nutr Dev 2006; 46(2): 139-56.
[http://dx.doi.org/10.1051/rnd:2006007] [PMID: 16597420]

[131] Jing T, Gao XD, Wang P, *et al.* Determination of trace tetracycline antibiotics in foodstuffs by liquid chromatography-tandem mass spectrometry coupled with selective molecular-imprinted solid-phase extraction. Anal Bioanal Chem 2009; 393(8): 2009-18.
[http://dx.doi.org/10.1007/s00216-009-2641-z] [PMID: 19214484]

[132] Boxall ABA, Fogg LA, Blackwell PA, Kay P, Pemberton EJ, Croxford A. Veterinary medicines in the environment. Rev Environ Contam Toxicol 2004; 180: 1-91.
[http://dx.doi.org/10.1007/0-387-21729-0_1] [PMID: 14561076]

[133] Massé DI, Saady NM, Gilbert Y. Potential of biological processes to eliminate antibiotics in livestock manure: an overview. Animals (Basel) 2014; 4(2): 146-63.
[http://dx.doi.org/10.3390/ani4020146] [PMID: 26480034]

[134] Pan X, Qiang Z, Ben W, Chen M. Residual veterinary antibiotics in swine manure from concentrated animal feeding operations in Shandong Province, China. Chemosphere 2011; 84(5): 695-700.

[135] Berendsen BJA, Wegh RS, Memelink J, Zuidema T, Stolker LA. The analysis of animal faeces as a tool to monitor antibiotic usage. Talanta 2015; 132: 258-68.
[http://dx.doi.org/10.1016/j.talanta.2014.09.022] [PMID: 25476307]

[136] Bates J, Jordens JZ, Griffiths DT. Farm animals as a putative reservoir for vancomycin-resistant enterococcal infection in man. J Antimicrob Chemother 1994; 34(4): 507-14.
[http://dx.doi.org/10.1093/jac/34.4.507] [PMID: 7868403]

[137] Kemper N. Veterinary antibiotics in the aquatic and terrestrial environment. Ecol Indic 2008; 8: 1-13.
[http://dx.doi.org/10.1016/j.ecolind.2007.06.002]

[138] Bansal OP. A laboratory study on degradation of tetracycline and chlortetracycline in soils of aligarh district as influenced by temperature, water content, concentration of farm yield manure, nitrogen and tetracyclines. Proc Natl Acad Sci, India, Sect B Biol Sci 2012; 82(4): 503-9.
[http://dx.doi.org/10.1007/s40011-012-0062-9]

[139] Zielezny Y, Groeneweg J, Vereecken H, Tappe W. Impact of sulfadiazine and chlorotetracycline on soil bacterial community structure and respiratory activity. Soil Biol Biochem 2006; 38(8): 2372-80.
[http://dx.doi.org/10.1016/j.soilbio.2006.01.031]

[140] Hammesfahr U, Heuer H, Manzke B, Smalla K. Thiele- Bruhn S. Impact of the antibiotic sulfadiazine and pig manure on the microbial community structure in agricultural soils. Soil Biol Biochem 2008; 40(7): 1583-91.
[http://dx.doi.org/10.1016/j.soilbio.2008.01.010]

[141] Keen PL, Patrick DM. Tracking change: A look at the ecological footprint of antibiotics and antimicrobial resistance. Antibiotics (Basel) 2013; 2(2): 191-205.
[http://dx.doi.org/10.3390/antibiotics2020191] [PMID: 27029298]

[142] Bogaerts R, Wolf F. Standardized method for the detection of residues of antibacterial substances in fresh meat. Fleischwirtschaft (Frankf) 1980; 60: 672-3.

[143] Mahgoub O, Kadim IT, Ann Mothershaw AI, Zadjali SA, Annamalai K. Use of enzyme-linked immune sorbent assay (ELISA) for detection of antibiotic and anabolic residues in goat and sheep meat. World J Agric Sci 2006; 2: 298-302.

[144] Kadim IT, Mahgoub O, Al-Marzooqi W, Al-Magbaly R, Annamal K, Khalaf S. Enzyme-linked immunosorbent assay for screening antibiotic and hormone residues in broiler chicken meat in Sultanate of Oman. J Muscle Foods 2009; 21(2): 243-54.
[http://dx.doi.org/10.1111/j.1745-4573.2009.00179.x]

[145] Samarajeewa U, Wei CI, Huang TS, Marshall MR. Application of immunoassay in the food industry. Crit Rev Food Sci Nutr 1991; 29(6): 403-34.
[http://dx.doi.org/10.1080/10408399109527535] [PMID: 2039597]

[146] Toldrá F, Milagro R. Methods for rapid detection of chemical and veterinary drug residues in animal foods. Trends Food Sci Technol 2006; 17: 482-9.
[http://dx.doi.org/10.1016/j.tifs.2006.02.002]

[147] Cinquina AL, Roberti P, Giannetti L, *et al.* Determination of enrofloxacin and its metabolite ciprofloxacin in goat milk by high-performance liquid chromatography with diode-array detection. Optimization and validation. J Chromatogr A 2003; 987(1-2): 221-6.
[http://dx.doi.org/10.1016/S0021-9673(02)01800-9] [PMID: 12613815]

[148] Kirbis A, Marinsek J, Flajs VC. Introduction of the HPLC method for the determination of quinolone residues in various muscle tissues. Biomed Chromatogr 2005; 19(4): 259-65.
[http://dx.doi.org/10.1002/bmc.435] [PMID: 15828062]

[149] Hewitt SA, Kearney M, Currie JW, Young PB, Kennedy DG. Screening and confirmatory strategies for the surveillance of anabolic steroid abuse within Northern Ireland. Anal Chim Acta 2002; 473: 99-109.
[http://dx.doi.org/10.1016/S0003-2670(02)00750-X]

[150] Thevis M, Opfermann G, Schänzer W. Liquid chromatography/electrospray ionization tandem mass spectrometric screening and confirmation methods for beta2-agonists in human or equine urine. J Mass Spectrom 2003; 38(11): 1197-206.
[http://dx.doi.org/10.1002/jms.542] [PMID: 14648827]

[151] Plozza T, Trenerry VC, Zeglinski P, Nguyen H, Johnstone P. The confirmation and quantification of selected aminoglycoside residues in animal tissue and bovine milk by liquid chromatography tandem mass spectrometry. Int Food Res J 2011; 18(3): 1077-84.

[152] Mesgari Abbasi M, Nemati M, Babaei H, Ansarin M, Nourdadgar AOS. Solid-Phase extraction and

simultaneous determination of tetracycline residues in edible cattle tissues using an HPLC-FL method. Iran J Pharm Res 2012; 11(3): 781-7.
[PMID: 24250505]

[153] Kim DP, Degand G, Douny C, *et al.* Preliminary evaluation of antimicrobial residue levels in marketed pork and chicken meat in the red river delta region of Vietnam. Food Public Health 2013; 3(6): 267-76.

[154] Jank L, Martins MT, Arsand JB, *et al.* Liquid chromatography-tandem mass spectrometry multiclass method for 46 antibiotics residues in milk and meat: Development and validation. Food Anal Methods 2017; 10(7): 2152-64.
[http://dx.doi.org/10.1007/s12161-016-0755-4]

[155] Velusamy V, Arshak K, Korostynska O, Oliwa K, Adley C. An overview of foodborne pathogen detection: in the perspective of biosensors. Biotechnol Adv 2010; 28(2): 232-54.
[http://dx.doi.org/10.1016/j.biotechadv.2009.12.004] [PMID: 20006978]

[156] Gaudin V. Advances in biosensor development for the screening of antibiotic residues in food products of animal origin - A comprehensive review. Biosens Bioelectron 2017; 90: 363-77.
[http://dx.doi.org/10.1016/j.bios.2016.12.005] [PMID: 27940240]

[157] Vo-Dinh T, Cullum B. Biosensors and biochips: advances in biological and medical diagnostics. Fresenius J Anal Chem 2000; 366(6-7): 540-51.
[http://dx.doi.org/10.1007/s002160051549] [PMID: 11225766]

[158] Kirian BR, Kale KU. Transformed E coli JM 109 as a biosensor for penicillin. Indian J Pharm Sci 2002; 83(3): 205-8.

[159] Ben-Yoav H, Elad T, Shlomovits O, Belkin S, Shacham-Diamand Y. Optical modeling of bioluminescence in whole cell biosensors. Biosens Bioelectron 2009; 24(7): 1969-73.
[http://dx.doi.org/10.1016/j.bios.2008.10.035] [PMID: 19131239]

[160] Ferrini AM, Mannoni V, Carpico G, Pellegrini GE. Detection and identification of beta-lactam residues in milk using a hybrid biosensor. J Agric Food Chem 2008; 56(3): 784-8.
[http://dx.doi.org/10.1021/jf071479i] [PMID: 18211013]

[161] Bahl MI, Hansen LH, Sørensen SJ. Construction of an extended range whole-cell tetracycline biosensor by use of the tet(M) resistance gene. FEMS Microbiol Lett 2005; 253(2): 201-5.
[http://dx.doi.org/10.1016/j.femsle.2005.09.034] [PMID: 16239081]

[162] Virolainen NE, Pikkemaat MG, Elferink JWA, Karp MT. Rapid detection of tetracyclines and their 4-epimer derivatives from poultry meat with bioluminescent biosensor bacteria. J Agric Food Chem 2008; 56(23): 11065-70.
[http://dx.doi.org/10.1021/jf801797z] [PMID: 18998699]

[163] Shapiro E, Baneyx F. Stress-activated bioluminescent *Escherichia coli* sensors for antimicrobial agents detection. J Biotechnol 2007; 132(4): 487-93.
[http://dx.doi.org/10.1016/j.jbiotec.2007.08.021] [PMID: 17897748]

[164] Muhammed F, Aktar M, Rahman ZU, Javed I, Anwar MI. Role of veterinarians in providing Residue-free veterinary food. Pak Vet J 2009; 29(1): 42-6.

[165] Sultan IA. Detection of Enrofloxacin in livers of livestock animals obtained from a slaughterhouse in Mosul City. J Vet Sci Technol 2014; 5(2): 1-3.
[http://dx.doi.org/10.4172/2157-7579.1000168]

[166] Gaurav A, Gill JPS, Aulakh RS, Bedi JS. ELISA based monitoring and analysis of tetracycline residues in cattle milk in various districts of Punjab. Vet World 2014; 7: 26-9.
[http://dx.doi.org/10.14202/vetworld.2014.26-29]

[167] Zeina K, Pamela AK, Fawwak S. Quantification of antibiotic residues and determination of antimicrobial resistance profiles of microorganisms isolated from bovine milk in Lebanon. Food Nutr Sci 2013; 4: 1-9.

[http://dx.doi.org/10.4236/fns.2013.47A001]

[168]   Yibar A, Cetinkaya F, Soyutemiz GE. ELISA screening and liquid chromatography-tandem mass spectrometry confirmation of chloramphenicol residues in chicken muscle, and the validation of a confirmatory method by liquid chromatography-tandem mass spectrometry. Poult Sci 2011; 90(11): 2619-26.
[http://dx.doi.org/10.3382/ps.2011-01564] [PMID: 22010249]

[169]   Senyuva H, Ozden T, Sarica DY. High-performance liquid chromatographic determination of Oxytetracycline residue in cured meat products. Turk J Chem 2000; 24: 395-400.

[170]   Abebew D, Belihu K, Zewde G. Detection and determination of Oxytetracycline and Penicillin G antibiotic residue levels in bovine bulk milk from Nazareth dairy farms, Ethiopia. Ethiop Vet J 2014; 18(1): 1-15.

[171]   Elizabeta DS, Zehra HM, Biljana SD, Pavle S, Risto U. Screening of veterinary drug residues in milk from individual farms in Macedonia. Maced Vet Rev 2011; 34(1): 5-13.

[172]   Park JA, Jeong D, Zhang D. Simple extraction method requiring no cleanup procedure for the detection of minocycline residues in porcine muscle and milk using triple quadrupole liquid chromatography-tandem mass spectrometry. Appl Biol Chem 2016; 59(2): 297-303.
[http://dx.doi.org/10.1007/s13765-016-0158-7]

[173]   Martins-Junior HA, Tereza A. Kussumi, Alexandre Y, Wang, Lebre DT. A Rapid method to determine antibiotic residues in milk using liquid chromatography coupled to electrospray tandem mass spectrometry. J Braz Chem Soc 2007; 18(2): 397-405.
[http://dx.doi.org/10.1590/S0103-50532007000200023]

[174]   Han RW, Zheng N, Yu ZN, *et al.* Simultaneous determination of 38 veterinary antibiotic residues in raw milk by UPLC-MS/MS. Food Chem 2015; 181: 119-26.
[http://dx.doi.org/10.1016/j.foodchem.2015.02.041] [PMID: 25794729]

[175]   Weber CC, Link N, Fux C, Zisch AH, Weber W, Fussenegger M. Broad-spectrum protein biosensors for class-specific detection of antibiotics. Biotechnol Bioeng 2005; 89(1): 9-17.
[http://dx.doi.org/10.1002/bit.20224] [PMID: 15580576]

[176]   Kivirand K, Kagan M, Rinken T. Biosensors for the detection of antibiotic residues in milk, Biosensors - Micro and Nanoscale Applications, Toonika Rinken, IntechOpen. September 24th 2015. Available from: https://www.intechopen.com/books/biosensors-micro-and- nanoscale-applications/ biosensors-for-the-detection-of-antibiotic-residues-in-milk
[http://dx.doi.org/10.5772/60464.]

[177]   Booth NH, McDonald LE. Toxicology of drug and chemical residues. Veterinary Pharmacology and Therapeutics. 6th ed. USA: Iowa State University Press 1988; pp. 1149-95.

[178]   Moreno L, Lanusse C. Veterinary drug residues in meat-related edible tissues. New Aspects of Meat Quality. United Kingdom: Woodhead Publishing Limited 2017; pp. 581-603.
[http://dx.doi.org/10.1016/B978-0-08-100593-4.00024-2]

[179]   Nisha AR. Antibiotic residues: A global health hazard. Vet World 2008; 1(12): 375-7.
[http://dx.doi.org/10.5455/vetworld.2008.375-377]

[180]   Ghidini S, Zanardi E, Varisco G, Chizzolini R. Prevalence of molecules of β-lactam antibiotics in bovine milk in Lombardia and Emilia Romagna (Italy). Ann Fac Medic Vet Di Parma 2002; 22: 245-52.

[181]   Cheng G, Hao H, Xie S, *et al.* Antibiotic alternatives: the substitution of antibiotics in animal husbandry? Front Microbiol 2014; 5: 217.
[http://dx.doi.org/10.3389/fmicb.2014.00217] [PMID: 24860564]

[182]   Tian L, Khalil S, Bayen S. Effect of thermal treatments on the degradation of antibiotic residues in food. Crit Rev Food Sci Nutr 2017; 57(17): 3760-70.
[http://dx.doi.org/10.1080/10408398.2016.1164119] [PMID: 27052471]

[183] Wanzala W, Zessin KH, Kyulec NM, Baumann MPO, Mathias E, Hassanali A. Ethnoveterinary medicine: A critical review of its evolution, perception, understanding and the way forward. Livest Res Rural Dev 2005; 17(11): 1-41.

[184] Ranganathan V. Ethno veterinary practices for combating antimicrobial resistance. Int J Sci Environ Technol 2017; 1(6): 840-4.

CHAPTER 3

The Role of Garlic and Rosemary Herbs in Poultry Nutrition

Hamada A. M. Elwan[1], Shaaban S. Elnesr[2], Mayada R. Farag[3], Rana M. Bilal[4], Mohamed E. Abd El-Hack[5] and Mahmoud Alagawany[5,*]

[1] *Animal and Poultry Production Department, Faculty of Agriculture, Minia University, El-Minya 61519, Egypt*

[2] *Poultry Production Department, Faculty of Agriculture, Fayoum University, Fayoum 63514, Egypt*

[3] *Forensic Medicine and Toxicology Department, Veterinary Medicine Faculty, Zagazig University, Zagazig 44519, Egypt*

[4] *University College of Veterinary and Animal Sciences, The Islamia University of Bahawalpur, Pakistan*

[5] *Poultry Department, Faculty of Agriculture, Zagazig University, Zagazig 44519, Egypt*

Abstract: The use of herbal plants as natural remedies is gaining immense global popularity in feeding systems of humans and animals including avian species due to their promising health benefits. Among the livestock sector, poultry production and regulations are in a continuous development, particularly in the field of nutrition, genetic, refinement, management and disease prevention, which could be probably achieved through regulation of the nutritional needs and the poultry production prerequisites. Therefore, this section is directed toward the use of herbs as a therapeutic and sustainable production tool, because of their health and economic benefits. This chapter will discuss and highlight the valuable impacts and the latest features of supplementing the livestock rations with garlic and rosemary herbs, including their promising natural growth promoting activities and useful applications in improving, performance, feed efficiency and nutrient digestibility in addition to enhancing antioxidant capacity and immunological responses and this would be helpful for veterinarians, scientists, pharmacists, physiologists, pharmaceutical industries, nutritionists and poultry breeders.

Keywords: Beneficial effects, Garlic and rosemary, Mechanism of action, Poultry, Sources.

* **Corresponding author Mahmoud Alagawany:** Poultry Department, Faculty of Agriculture, Zagazig University, Zagazig 44519, Egypt; E-mail: mmalagwany@zu.edu.eg

INTRODUCTION

Several medicinal plants can be considered as potential feed additives resources in poultry production due to the presence of phytochemicals with powerful antioxidant properties [1 - 4]. Garlic (*Allium sativum* L.) is a perennial herb with a pear which is divided into segments or cloves and is commonly used as medicinal plant in all regions of the world to prevent and treat a broad class of diseases extending from infection to heart diseases (Fig. **1**). Garlic is believed to be among the 20 main vegetables, with different uses globally. It is being used as a crude vegetable intended for cooking or eating or as a constituent of many modern herbal and other chemical-based drugs. Also, it is suggested as a very unique and one of the wealthiest resources of total phenolic contents in the diet of human beings [5]. Recently, multiple investigations have proved the notable biological roles of garlic, such as anticancer, antioxidant, cardioprotective, immuno modulatory, anti-inflammatory anti-bacterial, antifungal anti-diabetic and anti-obesity properties [6 - 11]. Garlic has also been acknowledged as broiler supplement due to its role in improving the digestion and immune response of birds [12]. These characteristics were ascribed to the bioactive elements in garlic, such as allicin, diallyldisulphide and alliine with antibacterial and antioxidant activities [13 - 15]. Moreover, the lipo-soluble garlic organosulfur components, for example, n-acetyl cysteine or S-ethyl cysteine and diallyldisulphide have been reported to reduce lipid oxidation levels [16].

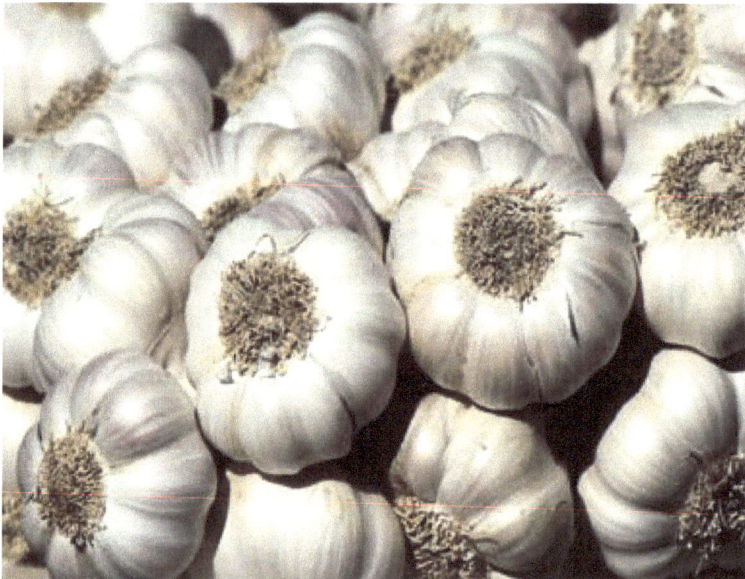

Fig. (1). Garlic plant.

Rosemary (*Rosmarinus officinalis* L.) is a member of the family *Lamiaceae* (Fig. 2) which is associated with the Mediterranean countries. The plant has pink, purple, white or blue flowers and is currently spreading globally due to its medical and industrial uses [17].

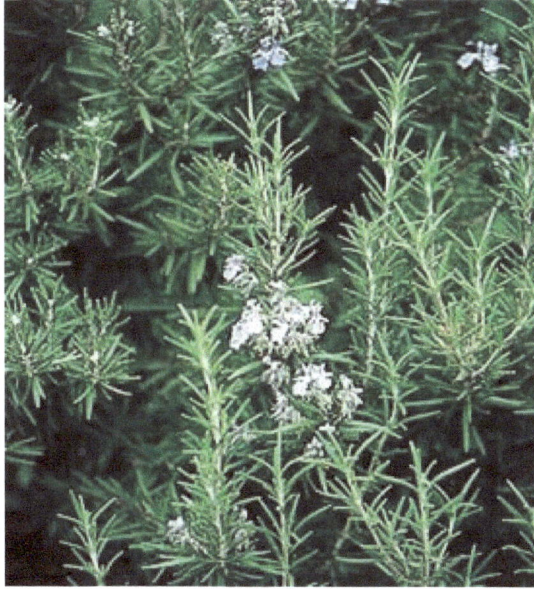

Fig. (2). Rosemary plant.

Since ancient times, rosemary has been used as a drug to treat the kidneys and dysmenorrhea. Moreover, it has also been used to relieve signs of breathing and lung-related sicknesses/problems. Moreover, the extracts of rosemary are used to treat anxiety and stress [18]. In today's scenario, several herbal extracts and essential oils have become a great point of interest because of their possible applications as an alternative to different drugs [19]. Rosemary oil has also been shown to improve meat production as well as egg quality traits [20 - 22]. Rosemary products may inhibit oxidative damage and bring blood cholesterol contents in a normal range. Carnosol, carnosic acid and esters are the principal biologically active constituents of rosemary oil [23]. Data from various studies indicated that carnosine acid, a valuable phenolic components in rosemary oil can serve as antioxidants as tocopherol [21], and showed a higher antioxidant activity than some synthetic antioxidants [24]. This chapter describes the beneficial applications and new aspects of garlic and rosemary herbs, including its useful applications, health benefits.

GARLIC AND ROSEMARY CHEMICAL COMPOSITION AND STRUCTURE

Garlic has a special interest because of its availability for poultry farmers. It is well established that this herb may positively alter the growth performance of broiler chickens and decrease mortality due to its antimicrobial and antioxidant effects [25 - 27]. These properties are the result of the actions of garlic bioactive compounds mainly organic sulfur compounds such as aliine, allicin, alyude, allylpropyldisulfide, diallyltrisulfide, sallilcistein and others [28 - 32]. The garlic and its co-products also contain enzymes (peroxidase, myrosinasis and allinase, *etc.*), amino acids, vitamins (A, B, C, D, and E) and minerals (potassium, calcium, iodine, sodium, selenium, magnesium, phosphorus) [33].

Rosemary is considered as a powerful anti-oxidant agent and its chemical analysis showed different types of flavonoids and volatile oils such as carnosol, carnosic acid [34, 35]. Interestingly, carnosic acid is much higher (3%) than carnosol in the antioxidant activity, and also higher (7%) than curved hydroxyanisole and curved hydroxytoluene [24].

MECHANISM OF ACTION

Garlic (*Allium sativum*) is frequently used to treat several ailments such as cardiac and blood vessel diseases and hypertension due to its ability to reduce the excessive cholesterol level [36, 37]. The active ingredients in garlic consist of allicin (dial thiosulfinate), which is the main organosulfur compound. Its extraction process can be performed by cutting or crushing garlic, thus allowing the garlic allinase enzyme to transform alliin to allicin which then rots to diallyl disulfide, and diallyltrisulfide that make up the organic polysulfides [38]. Garlic also has a positive influence on the body and reduces blood pressure that seems to be an impact of several mechanisms/factors. Kim-Park *et al.* [39] reported that the first suggested mechanism of garlic action is its capability to promote the vasodilation and the activity of nitric oxide (NO) either directly or indirectly, which led to lowering blood pressure. Garlic could also support the action of arginine, a known precursor in the NO production [40, 41]. *Allium sativum* has also been reported to prevent the synthesis of renin-angiotensin-aldosterone and prostaglandin. The variance in this balance favors vasodilatation. This, in part, is thought to be due to inhibition of angiotensin-converting enzyme (ACE) activity [42]. The primary result is the decrease of the vasoconstrictor angiotensin II (ATII). Second, a decline in ATII would reduce adrenal aldosterone production [43]. This reduction in the production of aldosterone can eventually reduce the reabsorption of sodium and water from the distal convoluted renal tubules and therefore reduced the amount of plasma [44, 45]. Third, although the decreases in

ATII may lessen the availability of vasodilatory prostaglandin (PGE2), improved levels of bradykinin (inhibited by ACE) may promote PGE2. Garlic is also believed to prevent cyclooxygenase action that would enable thromboxane B2, a known vasoconstrictor, to be generated [46]. The decrease in bradykinin metabolism *via* garlic ACE inhibition has also been acknowledged to promote NO output and support vasodilatation [47]. In addition, the final mechanism of associated garlic vasodilation is its ability to increase hydrogen sulfide (H_2S) production [48].

Rosmarinus officinalis L. showed various pharmacological effects such as the ability to reduce asthma, atherosclerosis, cataracts, chronic renal colic, hepatotoxicity, peptic ulcer, inflammatory ailments and ischaemic heart disease [49, 50]. In addition to the anti-oxidant and anti-inflammatory properties of rosmarinic acid [51, 52]. Rosemary can also control hypercholesterolemia and oxidative stress and relief the physical and mental exhaustion [53]. Rosmarinic acid can reduce the myocardial blood pressure and lipid peroxidation in the heart and brain and act as antiulcer agent [52, 54, 55]. Additionally, carnosic acid and carnosol showed anti-angiogenic and neuroprotective effects [56]. Moreover, rosemary showed antiatherosclerosis [57], anticancer, antiproliferative [58 - 60], antiviral [61], antimicrobial [62], hepatoprotective [63], nephroprotective [64] radioprotective, and antimutagenic [65] activities. In addition to its role in the reduction of blood sugar [66], muscle relaxation, treatment of skin allergies [67] and its ability to deal with depressive behaviour [68].

BENEFICIAL EFFECTS OF GARLIC AND ROSEMARY HERBS

Growth Enhancer

For many centuries ago, herbs were used in the management of many sicknesses, such as diabetes, cardiac problems, hypertension and obesity [69 - 71].

The scientific literature suggested that the inclusion of garlic and its co-products can beneficially alter the poultry performance. Garlic supplementation (0.5%) to the broiler diet increased the feed intake and enhanced bird's growth performance [72, 73].

Ademola *et al.* [74] showed no difference in the average live weight of broiler chickens, which fed on 5,000 mg garlic/kg diet. Ademola *et al.* [75] observed that during the finishing phase of growth of the chickens, 1.5% garlic and 2% ginger decreased the final live body weight. Ziton [76] stated that the supplementation of the control diet with 2, 3 or 4% garlic as a dry powder resulted in a better weight gain. Kumar *et al.* [77] stated that 250 ppm of garlic could improve the body weight of broiler chicks. Also, Lewis *et al.* [78] found that body weight gain was increased in broiler chickens fed low levels of commercial garlic products.

Aji *et al.* [79] found that garlic and onion supplementation (50 and 100 mg/kg diet) increased the body weight of birds. However, no variation in body weights was observed in birds treated with 25 mg of both herbs. Issa *et al.* [80] showed that garlic powder had no significant effects on the broiler's weight gain. Fayed *et al.* [81] found that 0.5 kg/ton dietary garlic promoted final body weights. Elagib *et al.* [82] speculated that broilers fed on a diet containing 3% garlic powder had the highest body weight gain. Similarly, dietary supplementation of a mixture of 1.0 g/kg (neem leaf powder) and 0.5 g/kg (garlic powder) showed a beneficial impact on body weight gains [83]. Ramiah *et al.* [72] also proposed that birds fed diets supplemented with garlic (0.5%) had greater body weight than control birds. Inclusion of a mixture from 1.50% garlic plus 0.25% ginger increased the final body weight of birds. The birds were fed a diet supplemented with 3% of garlic powder showed a greater body weight gain than other dietary groups [84].

Noman *et al.* [85] stated that broilers supplemented with garlic extract (1 and 2%) increased body weight gain during the period from 7 to 35 days compared to the control group. Similarly, Puvača *et al.* [86] reported that broiler chicks reared on a basal diet containing 0.5% garlic showed increased final body weight. El-katcha *et al.* [87] observed that allicin supplementation at 25, 50, 75 or 100 mg/kg diet for broilers for five continuous weeks significantly increased body gain. Low dietary garlic (0.125 and 0.25%) significantly improved the feed intake of birds compared to the group that was fed the high doses 0.5, 1, and 2% of garlic. The improvement in the feed efficiency of broilers was recorded by feeding on a diet containing 0.3% garlic [88]. Similarly, the addition of garlic-based growth promoter in broiler diet at level of 250 ppm improved feed efficiency [77]. Moreover, the dietary garlic (200 mg/kg) positively influenced feed efficiency of broilers [89]. On the other hand, Ashayerizadeh *et al.* [90] and Ghasemi *et al.* [91] reported that the supplementation of garlic preparation failed to produce a significant impact on the feed efficiency of broilers and layers chicks.

Pourali *et al.* [92] found that the addition of garlic powder 200 mg/kg diet improved average daily feed intake in broiler chickens. Also, Racesi *et al.* [93] indicated that the diet supplemented with garlic powder at levels from 1 to 3% resulted in significantly better feed intake compared to the control diet. However, Aji *et al.* [79] mentioned that the administration of 100 mg of garlic did not affect feed intake of broiler chickens. Javendel *et al.* [94] showed that diets with a 2% garlic meal supplement had a higher feed conversion ratio (FCR) in comparison to broilers fed diets containing 0.125,0.50 or1.0% garlic meal. Further, Onu [95] indicated that the broilers supplemented with 0.25% (garlic and ginger) showed an improved feed efficiency compared to the control birds.

Elagib *et al*. [82] documented that broiler chicks supplemented with a diet having 3% garlic powder exhibited maximum feed consumption with the best feed efficiency. Safa *et al*. [84] speculated that a broiler diet contains a 3% level of garlic powder showed the highest total feed intake and FCR compared to the other experimental diets. However, they found that broiler chicks fed diet incorporated with 1.75% mixture level (garlic 1.50% + ginger 0.25%) showed the best FCR in comparison with other experimental diets. Adjei *et al*. [96] stated that daily feed intake of broiler chicks fed allicin (0.10 g/kg) was better than other fed diets with 0, 0.15 and 0.20 g allicin/kg diet or control diets supplemented with antibiotics. Also, El-katcha *et al*. [87] added dietary allicin at a concentration of 25, 50 or 75mg/kg for 5 weeks and found a significant improvement in the feed efficiency.

Immunomodulator

Dietary inclusion of garlic at 200 gm/kg promoted the bursa of Fabricius weight in broilers [97]. But, Elagib *et al*. [82] found that both thymus and bursa of Fabricius exhibited non-significant change among the different treatments (0, 3 and 5%). Sameh and Ramadan [98] revealed that broilers fed garlic (200 g/kg) had the highest weight of bursa (0.13) compared to the control, ginger, thyme and antibiotic groups. Elagib *et al*. [82] stated that broiler spleen's weight was reduced when the diet having 3 and 5% garlic compared to 0% level. While El-katcha *et al*. [87] observed that dietary garlic extract at a concentration of 0.1, 0.2, 0.3 or 0.4 mg/kg for 5 consecutive weeks did not significantly increase spleen weight compared with the control.

The dietary garlic extract (0.2 mg/kg) significantly promoted both the thymus gland and bursa weight. Yang *et al*. [99] observed no significant change in broiler chicks white blood cells, including neutrophils, eosinophils, monocytes and lymphocytes when birds were raised on a diet containing varying concentrations of garlic such as 0, 3 and 5%. Fadlalla *et al*. [25] showed that total white blood cells were improved with the higher doses of garlic such as 0.3% compared to other groups. Mohebbifar and Torki [100] found that there was no effect of garlic supplementation (200 mg/kg diet) on heterophils in Ross broiler chicken. Seyed *et al*. [101] found that there was no significant difference in heterophils/lymphocytes ratio (H/L) and white blood cell concentration due to supplementation of broiler chicks with garlic (1%). Concerning the impact of garlic bioactive compounds (allicin) on broiler health and performance, it was recorded that dietary allicin supplementation at 50 mg/kg showed an insignificant increase in heterophil and the neutrophil percentage by about 1.1 and 4.7% and showed an increased H/L ratio relative to the control group birds. However, supplementation of 100 mg allicin/kg diet showed a numerical decrease in neutrophil and heterophil and reduced H/L ratio.

Rosemary is often used to control asthma, eczema, and arthritis. Moreover, it is also capable of controlling breast tumors. Amin and Hamza [102] revealed that mice immunity was increased by rosemary addition probably due to the various active ingredients in rosemary such as saponins, flavonoids and organic acids that can improve the binding of RBCs to B memory cells and the antibody production. Rosemary has acidic anti-inflammatory activities *in vivo*, therefore, it can improve secondary antibody reactions. Mice treated with 50 mg rosemary/kg body weight showed high antibody response against sheep red blood cells (SRBCs). While, 100 mg of rosemary extract/kg, showed no immunosuppression compared to the non-treated group. The humoral immune response can be determined as an increase in the level of total antibodies or antibodies specific to a non-pathogenic antigen such as SRBCs [103, 104]. Animals can produce immunoglobulins against foreign blood cells. These natural immunoglobulins are not derived from the previous contact with RBC abroad but are the result of exposure to similar or identical epitopes found in nature [105]. Hou *et al.* [106] reported that 100 mg rosemary/kg diet caused an increase in the spread of Con A-induced T cells, while the lower doses of rosemary had no significant effect.

On the contrary, Xiao-Ming *et al.* [107] reported that rosemary addition failed to show any significant impact on the spread of bacterial lipopolysaccharide (LPS)-induced B cells. It is evident that rosemary may promote immunoglobulins, *i.e* IgM and IgG excretion, without disturbing the propagation of B cells. Rosemary components, such as carnosol and carnosine acid showed similar effects [108].

Moreover, rosemary has been used in the food industry as a flavouring additive in the culinary and as a dietary supplement, which is attributed to its potent antioxidant action [109]. Rosemary may elevate the immune function of the body with low antioxidant or protein [103].

Blood Biochemistry

The dietary addition of 5% medicinal plants (ginger, cinnamon and garlic) did not affect the blood profile (globulin, total protein and albumin contents) of turkey [110]. Fadlalla *et al.* [25] observed that the contents of total protein were higher in chicks fed a basal diet containing 0.3, 0.45, and 0.6% garlic as a growth promoter.

Moreover, they found that albumin exhibited optimum values in the chicks supplemented with 0.3% garlic. While no significant change in contents of serum total protein, globulin and albumin were detected when broilers fed on garlic with

0.3, 0.45, and 0.6%. Onu [95] found that dietary supplementation with garlic and ginger at 0.25% increased the concentration of serum creatinine of the rabbits compared to the control. Oleforuh-Okoleh *et al.* [111] found that there was a statistically significant rise in the globulin, total protein and albumin of the chicks fed ginger or garlic treated diet compared to the control. Lee *et al.* [112] reported that broiler chickens fed the garlic supplemented diets exhibited higher blood levels of total protein compared with those fed the control diet. El-katcha *et al.* [87] stated that feeding of 50 mg/kg garlic extract (allicin) for five consecutive weeks significantly improved blood serum albumin and total protein concentrations.

Liver and Kidney Functions as Affected by Garlic and Rosemary

Mahdi *et al.* [113] showed that there was a reduction in serum glutamic oxaloacetic transaminase (GOT) and glutamic-pyruvic transaminase (GPT) of turkey birds fed dietary garlic, ginger and cinnamon at the level of 5% of each herb. El-katcha *et al.* [87] observed that allicin inclusion in broiler diet (25, 50 or 75 mg/kg) for 5 weeks significantly reduced the serum concentration of GPT by about 7.5%, 12.7%, and 8.6%, respectively, while higher inclusion rate of allicin (100 mg/kg) increased serum GPT concentration by about 3.1% when compared with the control. Onu [95] found that dietary supplementation of garlic and ginger at in broiler diet significantly improved the concentration of serum urea of the rabbits compared to the control. Mahdi *et al.* [113] observed that there is no effect on creatinine level by using a mixture of medicinal plants containing garlic, ginger and cinnamon at the level of 5% of each addition in turkey diets. El-katcha *et al.* [87] indicated that allicin supplementation at 25 mg/kg diet for five consecutive weeks significantly reduced blood serum uric acid concentration of broilers when compared with the control. They also observed that allicin supplementation at 25, 50 and 75 mg/kg significantly reduced blood serum creatinine concentration when compared with the control. Mohamed *et al.* [114] observed that dietary supplementation of allicin at 50 or 75 mg/kg diet significantly increased blood serum uric acid concentration when compared with the control.

Hypocholesterolemic Effect

Globally, herbal medicines and its products are demanded as an alternative medicine because they are actively participating in the cure and treatments of various diseases. It is said that herbal extracts may be beneficial in regulating the normal blood glucose and triglyceride levels. Moreover, they also protect the body from cancer by increasing host immune response [115]. El Deeb *et al.* [116]

and Herrero *et al.* [117] reported that the stem and leaves of rosemary have ample quantity of biologically active phytochemicals. Moreover, rosemary also contains various polyphenol compounds, such as isorosmanolcarnosol, carnosic acid, rosmanol, 7-methyl-epirosmanol, rosmadial and colic acid, with high *in vitro* significant antioxidant activity. Rosemary contains some antioxidant phenols, which have proven to be a defense against oxidative stress of oxidative substances and free radicals [118, 119]. In recent decades, there are growing evidence on the crucial role of traditional medicinal plants in preventing or controlling certain metabolic disorders such as diabetes, heart disease and cancer [120]. Additionally, rosemary and its constituents have antioxidant potential as reported in various *in vitro* and *in vivo* studies [121 - 123].

Konjufca *et al.* [9] stated that supplementation of 2% garlic powder to the diet of broilers was enough to reduce plasma total cholesterol. Also, Mansoub [32] reported that dietary supplementation with garlic (1 g/kg) reduced the total cholesterol of broilers. Issa *et al.* [80] showed that, in the 5th week of post-treatment with 0.4% garlic, there was a decrease in total cholesterol contents compared with the control. They also observed that garlic powder (GP) significantly reduced the levels of triacylglycerol (TG). Moreover, 0.2 and 0.4% of GP lowered TG contents and 0.2% garlic reduced triglycerides of broilers compared to the control group. Also, Jimoh *et al.* [124] noticed that supplementation levels of garlic at 2.0 and 2.5 g/kg decreased serum concentration of triacylglycerol in broilers. They also demonstrated the inclusion of garlic with 0.5, 1.0, 1.5, 2.0 and 2.5 g/kg decreased the total serum cholesterol. Similarly, Puvača *et al.* [86] reported that the inclusion of GP at a concentration of 0.5% decreased the concentration of total cholesterol. El-katcha *et al.* [87] indicated that dietary of 0.2, 0.3 or 0.4 mg/kg garlic extract for 5 consecutive weeks significantly reduced blood serum triglycerides concentration by about 25.7%, 7.5% and 19.0%, respectively when compared with the control. El-katcha *et al.* [87] observed that application of garlic extract at 0.4, 0.3, 0.2 or 0.1 mg/kg diet for five consecutive weeks significantly reduced cholesterol concentration of broiler chickens by about 12.9, 11.9, 7.9 and 14.2%, respectively compared with the control. However, Lee *et al.* [112] found that broiler chickens fed fermented garlic at the level of 0.5% exhibited higher blood cholesterol compared with those fed the control diet.

Several studies have shown the antioxidant, diuretics, anti-inflammatory and antimicrobial, anticarcinogenic, hypoglycemic, and hypolipidaemic activities of rosemary and related such activities to the presence of phenolic compounds, particularly the flavonoids and the phenolic acids. Polyphenols are also known for their capacity to prevent oxidative fatty acid degradation [125 - 127].

Labban *et al*. [128] suggest that phenolic compounds from *Rosmarinus officinalis* protect against hyperglycemia and oxidative stress induced by hypercholesterolemia and increase the function of the antioxidant enzymes. They also added that the powder of the rosemary leaves has antioxidant properties and a beneficial effect on the content of glutathione reductase, malondialdehyde, vitamin C, and B-carotene. Supplementation with these natural extracts was useful in limiting the pathophysiology of much oxidative damage and inflammation-related disorders. The rosemary leaves powder also enhanced the serum lipid profile and helped in minimizing cardiovascular disease and lipid peroxidation [129 - 133].

Antioxidant Enzyme Effect

Garlic has been reported to have anti-oxidant, anti-cancer, anti-inflammatory, anti-diabetic, anti-allergic, immunomodulatory and cardioprotective effects [134 - 139]. Rosemary, as a natural anti-oxidant, disturbs the sequence of lipid oxidation may be due to its potent anti-oxidant compounds [132, 133]. Furthermore, results from *in vivo* and *in vitro* studies indicate that rosemary could control free radicals production and inhibit lipid peroxidation. The extract of rosemary plant has important components such as icing acid, α-tocopherol and diterpene, which make it a potent antioxidant compound [101]. Moreover, it is said that its anti-inflammatory effects are attributed to the presence of organic isoprenoids such as sterol, isoprene, mono and diterween, carotenoids and tocopherols [140, 141]. Furthermore, its anti-oxidant properties are a result of their promotion of the biosynthesis of glutathione, a known compound that prevents loss of main cellular components caused by free radicals [38]. In addition, other important volatile compounds with powerful bioactive abilities are ajoenes, which possess sulfoxide and disulfide functional group [142].

Garlic contains an active component alliin (S-allyl cysteine sulfoxide), which has antioxidant properties, which prevent cardiac and neurodegenerative diseases [143]. Moreover, garlic essential oil also possesses orgnanosulpher compounds such asallicin, 1,2-vinyldithiin, allixin S-allyl-cysteine and sulphides such as dipropyl mono-, di-, tri, diallyl-, methyl allyl-, and tetra-sulfides which are formed after thiosulfinates degradation [144, 145]. In a report by Borlinghaus *et al.* [137] it was observed that garlic bioactive molecules are very effective against pathogenic microbes with a unique defensive mechanism. Garlic may inhibit the harmful effects of fungi and bacteria. Further, it has been found as an antiprotozoal agent as it displayed a strong trypanocidal activity.

Rosemary contains strong compounds such as 1,8-cineole, α-pinene, camphor and bornyl acetate, which have many unique functions. Rosemery oil has a distinctive and refreshing aroma and because of this it is also utilized in the perfume industry. Moreover, reports suggest that rosemary and garlic have good anti-microbial and anti-bacterial properties and can control a variety of diseases [146 - 152].

CONCLUSION

This chapter summarized many studies to point out the beneficial effects of garlic and rosemary on health and nutritional issues. It can be stated that garlic and rosemary and their multiple extracts exert significant antioxidant, antifungal, antibacterial and immunomodulatory effects. They can enhance the healing process of serious diseases. Regarding poultry performance, the addition of garlic and rosemary or their extracts into diets could increase feed efficiency and general performance traits. Another very significant conclusion is that garlic and rosemary could partially or fully substitute antibiotics in poultry diets.

CONSENT FOR PUBLICATION

Not Applicable.

CONFLICT OF INTEREST

The author confirms that this chapter contents have no conflict of interest.

ACKNOWLEDGEMENTS

Declared none.

REFERENCES

[1]   Alagawany M, Elnesr SS, Farag MR, *et al.* Use of licorice (Glycyrrhizaglabra) herb as a feed additive in poultry: Current knowledge and prospects. Animals (Basel) 2019; 9(8): 536.
[http://dx.doi.org/10.3390/ani9080536]

[2]   Khafaga AF, Abd El-Hack ME, Taha AE, Elnesr SS, Alagawany M. The potential modulatory role of herbal additives against Cd toxicity in human, animal, and poultry: a review. Environ Sci Pollut Res Int 2019; 26(5): 4588-604.
[http://dx.doi.org/10.1007/s11356-018-4037-0] [PMID: 30612355]

[3]   Abd El-Hack ME, Elnesr SS, Alagawany M, *et al.* Impact of green tea (*Camellia sinensis*) and epigallocatechin gallate on poultry. World PoultSci J 2020; 76(76): 49-63.
[http://dx.doi.org/https://doi.org/10.1080/00439339.2020.1729672]

[4]   Cuvelier ME, Richard H, Berset C. Comparison of the antioxidative activity of some acid-phenols: structure-activity relationship. Biosci Biotechnol Biochem 1992; 56: 324-5.
[http://dx.doi.org/10.1271/bbb.56.324]

[5]   Martins N, Petropoulos S, Ferreira IC. Chemical composition and bioactive compounds of garlic (*Allium sativum* L.) as affected by pre- and post-harvest conditions: A review. Food Chem 2016; 211: 41-50.
[http://dx.doi.org/10.1016/j.foodchem.2016.05.029] [PMID: 27283605]

[6]   Boonpeng S, Siripongvutikorn S, Sae-Wong C, Sutthirak P. The antioxidant and anti-cadmium toxicity properties of garlic extracts. Food Sci Nutr 2014; 2(6): 792-801.
        [http://dx.doi.org/10.1002/fsn3.164] [PMID: 25493198]

[7]   Hayat S, Cheng Z, Ahmad H, Ali M, Chen X, Wang M. Garlic, from remedy to stimulant: Evaluation of antifungal potential reveals diversity in phytoalexinallicin content among garlic cultivars; allicin containing aqueous garlic extracts trigger antioxidants. Front Plant Sci 2016; 7: 1235.
        [http://dx.doi.org/10.3389/fpls.2016.01235] [PMID: 27610111]

[8]   Singh MP, Panda H. Medicinal Herbs with Their Formulations, vol: 1: *Allium sativum*. Delhi: Daya Publishing House 2005.

[9]   Konjufca VH, Pesti GM, Bakalli RI. Modulation of cholesterol levels in broiler meat by dietary garlic and copper. Poult Sci 1997; 76(9): 1264-71.
        [http://dx.doi.org/10.1093/ps/76.9.1264] [PMID: 9276889]

[10]   Weber ND, Andersen DO, North JA, Murray BK, Lawson LD, Hughes BG. *In vitro* virucidal effects of *Allium sativum* (garlic) extract and compounds. Planta Med 1992; 58(5): 417-23.
        [http://dx.doi.org/10.1055/s-2006-961504] [PMID: 1470664]

[11]   Ankri S, Mirelman D. Antimicrobial properties of allicin from garlic. Microbes Infect 1999; 1(2): 125-9.
        [http://dx.doi.org/10.1016/S1286-4579(99)80003-3] [PMID: 10594976]

[12]   Demir E, Kiline K, Yildirim Y. Use of antibiotic growth promoter and two herbal natural feed additives with and without exogenous enzymes in wheat base broiler diets. South Afr Anim Sci 2005; 35: 61-72.

[13]   Amagase H, Milner JA. Impact of various sources of garlic and their constituents on 7,12-dimethylbenz[a]anthracene binding to mammary cell DNA. Carcinogenesis 1993; 14(8): 1627-31.
        [http://dx.doi.org/10.1093/carcin/14.8.1627] [PMID: 8353846]

[14]   Tsao S, Yin M. *In vitro* activity of garlic oil and four diallyl sulphides against antibiotic-resistant Pseudomonas aeruginosa and Klebsiella pneumoniae. J Antimicrob Chemother 2001; 47(5): 665-70.
        [http://dx.doi.org/10.1093/jac/47.5.665] [PMID: 11328781]

[15]   Yamasaki T, Li L, Lau B. Garlic compounds protect vascular endothelial cells from hydrogen peroxide-induced oxidant injury. Phytother Res 1994; 8: 408-12.
        [http://dx.doi.org/10.1002/ptr.2650080706]

[16]   Yin MC, Cheng WS. Antioxidant and antimicrobial effects of four garlic-derived organosulfur compounds in ground beef. Meat Sci 2003; 63(1): 23-8.
        [http://dx.doi.org/10.1016/S0309-1740(02)00047-5] [PMID: 22061980]

[17]   Solomon H. The Therapeutic Potential of Rosemary (*Rosmarinus officinalis*) Diterpenes for Alzheimer's Disease. Evid-Based Compl Alt 2016: 2680409.
        [http://dx.doi.org/10.1155/2016/2680409] [PMID: 2680409]

[18]   Oluwatuyi M, Kaatz GW, Gibbons S. Antibacterial and resistance modifying activity of *Rosmarinus officinalis*. Phytochemistry 2004; 65(24): 3249-54.
        [http://dx.doi.org/10.1016/j.phytochem.2004.10.009] [PMID: 15561190]

[19]   Agunu A, Yusuf S, Andrew GO, Zezi AU, Abdurahman EM. Evaluation of five medicinal plants used in diarrhoea treatment in Nigeria. J Ethnopharmacol 2005; 101(1-3): 27-30.
        [http://dx.doi.org/10.1016/j.jep.2005.03.025] [PMID: 15908152]

[20]   Galobart J, Barroeta AC, Baucells MD, Codony R, Ternes W. Effect of dietary supplementation with rosemary extract and alpha-tocopheryl acetate on lipid oxidation in eggs enriched with omega3-fatty acids. Poult Sci 2001; 80(4): 460-7.
        [http://dx.doi.org/10.1093/ps/80.4.460] [PMID: 11297285]

[21]   Mc Carthy TL, Kerry JP, Kerry JF, Lynch PB, Buckley DJ. Assessment of the antioxidant potential of

natural food and plant extracts in fresh and previously frozen pork patties. Meat Sci 2001; 57(2): 177-84.
[http://dx.doi.org/10.1016/S0309-1740(00)00090-5] [PMID: 22061361]

[22] Govaris A, Florou-Paneri P. The inhibitory potential of feed supplementation with rosemary and/or alpha-tocopheryl acetate on microbial growth and lipid oxidation of turkey breast during refrigerated storage. Lebensm Wiss Technol 2007; 40: 331-7.
[http://dx.doi.org/10.1016/j.lwt.2005.10.006]

[23] Boutekedjiret C, Bentahar F, Belabbes R, Bessiere JM. Extraction of rosemary essential oil by steam distillation and hydrodistillation. Flavour Fragrance J 2003; 18: 481-4.
[http://dx.doi.org/10.1002/ffj.1226]

[24] Richheimer SL, Bernart MW, King GA, Kent MC, Bailey DT. Antioxidant activity of lipid-soluble phenolic diterpenes from rosemary. J Am Oil Chem Soc 1996; 73(4): 507-14.
[http://dx.doi.org/10.1007/BF02523927]

[25] Fadlalla IMT, Mohammed BH, Bakhiet AO. Effect of feeding garlic on the performance and immunity of broilers. Asian J Polit Sci 2010; 4: 182-9.

[26] Stanaćev V, Milošević N, Kovčun S, *et al.* Effect of different garlic levels in broiler chicken food on production parameters. Contemporary Agric 2010; 59: 86-91.

[27] Sivam GP. Protection against *Helicobacter pylori* and other bacterial infections by garlic. J Nutr 2001; 131(3s): 1106S-8S.
[http://dx.doi.org/10.1093/jn/131.3.1106S] [PMID: 11238826]

[28] Suriya R, Zulkifli I, Alimon AR. The effect of dietary inclusion of herbs as growth promoter in broiler chickens. J Anim Vet Adv 2012; 11: 346-50.
[http://dx.doi.org/10.3923/javaa.2012.346.350]

[29] Choi IH, Park WY, Kim YJ. Effects of dietary garlic powder and α-tocopherol supplementation on performance, serum cholesterol levels, and meat quality of chicken. Poult Sci 2010; 89(8): 1724-31.
[http://dx.doi.org/10.3382/ps.2009-00052] [PMID: 20634529]

[30] Amagase H. Clarifying the real bioactive constituents of garlic. J Nutr 2006; 136(3) (Suppl.): 716S-25S.
[http://dx.doi.org/10.1093/jn/136.3.716S] [PMID: 16484550]

[31] Kemper KJ. Garlic (*Allium sativum*) Longwood Herbal Task Force 2000. http://www.mcp.edu/herbal/default.htm

[32] Mansoub NH. Comparative effects of using garlic as probiotic on performance and serum composition of broiler chickens. Ann Biol Res 2011; 2(3): 486-90.

[33] Grela RR, Klebaniuk R. Chemical composition of garlic preparation and its utilization u piglet diets. Med Welt 2007; 63: 792-5.

[34] Peng Y, Yuan J, Liu F, Ye J. Determination of active components in rosemary by capillary electrophoresis with electrochemical detection. J Pharmaceut Biomed 2005; 39(3–4): 431-7.
[http://dx.doi.org/10.1016/j.jpba.2005.03.033]

[35] Angelini LG, Carpanese G, Cioni PL, Morelli I, Macchia M, Flamini G. Essential oils from Mediterranean lamiaceae as weed germination inhibitors. J Agric Food Chem 2003; 51(21): 6158-64.
[http://dx.doi.org/10.1021/jf0210728] [PMID: 14518938]

[36] Ackermann RT, Mulrow CD, Ramirez G, Gardner CD, Morbidoni L, Lawrence VA. Garlic shows promise for improving some cardiovascular risk factors. Arch Intern Med 2001; 161(6): 813-24.
[http://dx.doi.org/10.1001/archinte.161.6.813] [PMID: 11268223]

[37] Yeh GY, Davis RB, Phillips RS. Use of complementary therapies in patients with cardiovascular disease. Am J Cardiol 2006; 98(5): 673-80.
[http://dx.doi.org/10.1016/j.amjcard.2006.03.051] [PMID: 16923460]

[38]   Banerjee SK, Mukherjee PK, Maulik SK. Garlic as an antioxidant: the good, the bad and the ugly. Phytother Res 2003; 17(2): 97-106.
[http://dx.doi.org/10.1002/ptr.1281] [PMID: 12601669]

[39]   Kim-Park S, Ku DD. Garlic elicits a nitric oxide-dependent relaxation and inhibits hypoxic pulmonary vasoconstriction in rats. Clin Exp Pharmacol Physiol 2000; 27(10): 780-6.
[http://dx.doi.org/10.1046/j.1440-1681.2000.03333.x] [PMID: 11022969]

[40]   Kim KM, Chun SB, Koo MS, *et al.* Differential regulation of NO availability from macrophages and endothelial cells by the garlic component S-allyl cysteine. Free Radic Biol Med 2001; 30(7): 747-56.
[http://dx.doi.org/10.1016/S0891-5849(01)00460-9] [PMID: 11275474]

[41]   Morihara N, Sumioka I, Moriguchi T, Uda N, Kyo E. Aged garlic extract enhances production of nitric oxide. Life Sci 2002; 71(5): 509-17.
[http://dx.doi.org/10.1016/S0024-3205(02)01706-X] [PMID: 12052435]

[42]   Sharifi AM, Darabi R, Akbarloo N. Investigation of antihypertensive mechanism of garlic in 2K1C hypertensive rat. J Ethnopharmacol 2003; 86(2-3): 219-24.
[http://dx.doi.org/10.1016/S0378-8741(03)00080-1] [PMID: 12738090]

[43]   Palmer BF. Managing hyperkalemia caused by inhibitors of the renin-angiotensin-aldosterone system. N Engl J Med 2004; 351(6): 585-92.
[http://dx.doi.org/10.1056/NEJMra035279] [PMID: 15295051]

[44]   Garty H. Mechanisms of aldosterone action in tight epithelia. J Membr Biol 1986; 90(3): 193-205.
[http://dx.doi.org/10.1007/BF01870126] [PMID: 3016278]

[45]   Verrey F, Schaerer E, Zoerkler P, *et al.* Regulation by aldosterone of Na^+,K^+-ATPase mRNAs, protein synthesis, and sodium transport in cultured kidney cells. J Cell Biol 1987; 104(5): 1231-7.
[http://dx.doi.org/10.1083/jcb.104.5.1231] [PMID: 3032984]

[46]   Al-Qattan KK, Khan I, Alnaqeeb MA, Ali M. Thromboxane-B2, prostaglandin-E2 and hypertension in the rat 2-kidney 1-clip model: a possible mechanism of the garlic induced hypotension. Prostaglandins Leukot Essent Fatty Acids 2001; 64(1): 5-10.
[http://dx.doi.org/10.1054/plef.2000.0232] [PMID: 11161580]

[47]   Liu YH, Yang XP, Sharov VG, *et al.* Effects of angiotensin-converting enzyme inhibitors and angiotensin II type 1 receptor antagonists in rats with heart failure. Role of kinins and angiotensin II type 2 receptors. J Clin Invest 1997; 99(8): 1926-35.
[http://dx.doi.org/10.1172/JCI119360] [PMID: 9109437]

[48]   Benavides GA, Squadrito GL, Mills RW, *et al.* Hydrogen sulfide mediates the vasoactivity of garlic. Proc Natl Acad Sci USA 2007; 104(46): 17977-82.
[http://dx.doi.org/10.1073/pnas.0705710104] [PMID: 17951430]

[49]   al-Sereiti MR, Abu-Amer KM, Sen P. Pharmacology of rosemary (*Rosmarinus officinalis* Linn.) and its therapeutic potentials. Indian J Exp Biol 1999; 37(2): 124-30.
[PMID: 10641130]

[50]   Hsieh CL, Peng CH, Chyau CC, Lin YC, Wang HE, Peng RY. Low-density lipoprotein, collagen, and thrombin models reveal that Rosemarinus officinalis L. exhibits potent antiglycative effects. J Agric Food Chem 2007; 55(8): 2884-91.
[http://dx.doi.org/10.1021/jf0631833] [PMID: 17385882]

[51]   Scheckel KA, Degner SC, Romagnolo DF. Rosmarinic acid antagonizes activator protein-1-dependent activation of cyclooxygenase-2 expression in human cancer and nonmalignant cell lines. J Nutr 2008; 138(11): 2098-105.
[http://dx.doi.org/10.3945/jn.108.090431] [PMID: 18936204]

[52]   Karthik D, Viswanathan P, Anuradha CV. Administration of rosmarinic acid reduces cardiopathology and blood pressure through inhibition of p22phox NADPH oxidase in fructose-fed hypertensive rats. J Cardiovasc Pharmacol 2011; 58(5): 514-21.

[http://dx.doi.org/10.1097/FJC.0b013e31822c265d] [PMID: 21795992]

[53]   Fernández LF, Palomino OM, Frutos G. Effectiveness of *Rosmarinus officinalis* essential oil as antihypotensive agent in primary hypotensive patients and its influence on health-related quality of life. J Ethnopharmacol 2014; 151(1): 509-16.
[http://dx.doi.org/10.1016/j.jep.2013.11.006] [PMID: 24269249]

[54]   Amaral GP, de Carvalho NR, Barcelos RP, *et al.* Protective action of ethanolic extract of *Rosmarinus officinalis* L. in gastric ulcer prevention induced by ethanol in rats. Food Chem Toxicol 2013; 55: 48-55.
[http://dx.doi.org/10.1016/j.fct.2012.12.038] [PMID: 23279841]

[55]   Posadas SJ, Caz V, Largo C, *et al.* Protective effect of supercritical fluid rosemary extract, *Rosmarinus officinalis*, on antioxidants of major organs of aged rats. Exp Gerontol 2009; 44(6-7): 383-9.
[http://dx.doi.org/10.1016/j.exger.2009.02.015] [PMID: 19289162]

[56]   Kayashima T, Matsubara K. Antiangiogenic effect of carnosic acid and carnosol, neuroprotective compounds in rosemary leaves. Biosci Biotechnol Biochem 2012; 76(1): 115-9.
[http://dx.doi.org/10.1271/bbb.110584] [PMID: 22232247]

[57]   Sinkovic A, Suran D, Lokar L, *et al.* Rosemary extracts improve flow-mediated dilatation of the brachial artery and plasma PAI-1 activity in healthy young volunteers. Phytother Res 2011; 25(3): 402-7.
[PMID: 20734322]

[58]   Yesil-Celiktas O, Sevimli C, Bedir E, Vardar-Sukan F. Inhibitory effects of rosemary extracts, carnosic acid and rosmarinic acid on the growth of various human cancer cell lines. Plant Foods Hum Nutr 2010; 65(2): 158-63.
[http://dx.doi.org/10.1007/s11130-010-0166-4] [PMID: 20449663]

[59]   Menghini L, Genovese S, Epifano F, Tirillini B, Ferrante C, Leporini L. Antiproliferative, protective and antioxidant effects of artichoke, dandelion, turmeric and rosemary extracts and their formulation. Int J Immunopathol Pharmacol 2010; 23(2): 601-10.
[http://dx.doi.org/10.1177/039463201002300222] [PMID: 20646355]

[60]   Kontogianni VG, Tomic G, Nikolic I, *et al.* Phytochemical profile of *Rosmarinus officinalis* and Salvia officinalis extracts and correlation to their antioxidant and anti-proliferative activity. Food Chem 2013; 136(1): 120-9.
[http://dx.doi.org/10.1016/j.foodchem.2012.07.091] [PMID: 23017402]

[61]   Nolkemper S, Reichling J, Stintzing FC, Carle R, Schnitzler P. Antiviral effect of aqueous extracts from species of the Lamiaceae family against Herpes simplex virus type 1 and type 2 *in vitro*. Planta Med 2006; 72(15): 1378-82.
[http://dx.doi.org/10.1055/s-2006-951719] [PMID: 17091431]

[62]   Bernardes WA, Lucarini R, Tozatti MG, *et al.* Antibacterial activity of the essential oil from *Rosmarinus officinalis* and its major components against oral pathogens. Z Naturforsch C J Biosci 2010; 65(9-10): 588-93.
[http://dx.doi.org/10.1515/znc-2010-9-1009] [PMID: 21138060]

[63]   Ramadan KS, Khalil OA, Danial EN, Alnahdi HS, Ayaz NO. Hypoglycemic and hepatoprotective activity of *Rosmarinus officinalis* extract in diabetic rats. J Physiol Biochem 2013; 69(4): 779-83.
[http://dx.doi.org/10.1007/s13105-013-0253-8] [PMID: 23625639]

[64]   El Saied Azab A. Nephro-protective effects of curcumin, rosemary, and propolis against gentamicin-induced toxicity in Guinea pigs: morphological and biochemical study. Am J ClinExp Med 2014; 2: 28.
[http://dx.doi.org/10.11648/j.ajcem.20140202.14]

[65]   Del Baño MJ, Castillo J, Benavente-García O, *et al.* Radioprotective-antimutagenic effects of rosemary phenolics against chromosomal damage induced in human lymphocytes by gamma-rays. J Agric Food Chem 2006; 54(6): 2064-8.

[http://dx.doi.org/10.1021/jf0581574] [PMID: 16536576]

[66]   Al-Hader AA, Hasan ZA, Aqel MB. Hyperglycemic and insulin release inhibitory effects of *Rosmarinus officinalis*. J Ethnopharmacol 1994; 43(3): 217-21.
[http://dx.doi.org/10.1016/0378-8741(94)90046-9] [PMID: 7990497]

[67]   Tabassum N, Hamdani M. Plants used to treat skin diseases. Pharmacogn Rev 2014; 8(15): 52-60.
[http://dx.doi.org/10.4103/0973-7847.125531] [PMID: 24600196]

[68]   Machado DG, Cunha MP, Neis VB, *et al. Rosmarinus officinalis* L. hydroalcoholic extract, similar to fluoxetine, reverses depressive-like behavior without altering learning deficit in olfactory bulbectomized mice. J Ethnopharmacol 2012; 143(1): 158-69.
[http://dx.doi.org/10.1016/j.jep.2012.06.017] [PMID: 22721880]

[69]   El-Hilaly J, Tahraoui A, Israili ZH, Lyoussi B. Acute hypoglycemic, hypocholesterolemic and hypotriglyceridemic effects of continuous intravenous infusion of a lyophilised aqueous extract of Ajuga iva L. Schreber whole plant in streptozotocin-induced diabetic rats. Pak J Pharm Sci 2007; 20(4): 261-8.
[PMID: 17604246]

[70]   Hussain Z, Waheed A, Qureshi R, *et al.* 303 of Pakistanon Insulin Secretion from INS-1 Cell's. J Phytother Res 2004; 18: 73-7.
[http://dx.doi.org/10.1002/ptr.1372] [PMID: 14750205]

[71]   Wargovich MJ, Woods C, Hollis DM, Zander ME. Herbals, cancer prevention and health. J Nutr 2001; 131(11) (Suppl.): 3034S-6S.
[http://dx.doi.org/10.1093/jn/131.11.3034S] [PMID: 11694643]

[72]   Ramiah SK, Zulkifli I, Rahim NA, Ebrahimi M, Meng GY. Effects of two herbal extracts and virginiamycin supplementation on growth performance, intestinal microflora population and Fatty Acid composition in broiler chickens. Asian-Australas J Anim Sci 2014; 27(3): 375-82.
[http://dx.doi.org/10.5713/ajas.2013.13030] [PMID: 25049964]

[73]   Demir E, Sarica S, Ozcan MA, Suicmez M. The use of natural feed additives as alternatives for an antibiotic growth promoter in broiler diet. Br Poult Sci 2003; 44: 44-5.
[http://dx.doi.org/10.1080/713655288]

[74]   Ademola SG, Farinu GO, Ajayi-Obe AO, Babatunde GM. Growth, haematological and biochemical studies on garlic and ginger fed broiler chicken. Moor J Agric Res 2004; 5(2): 122-8.

[75]   Ademola SG, Farinu GO, Babatunde GM. Serum Lipid, Growth and Hematological parameters of Broilers Fed Garlic, Ginger and their mixtures J. Agr Sci Res 2009; 5(1): 99-04.

[76]   Ziton AA. Response of broiler chicks to diets containing different mixture levels of garlic and ginger powder as natural feed additives. IJPRAS 2009; 3(4): 27-35.

[77]   Kumar S, Sharadamma KC, Radhakrishna PM. Effects of a garlic active based growth promoter on growth performance and specific pathogenic intestinal microbial counts of broiler chicks. Int J Poult Sci 2010; 9: 244-6.
[http://dx.doi.org/10.3923/ijps.2010.244.246]

[78]   Lewis MR, Rose SP, Mackenzie AM, Tuker LA. Effect of plant extracts on growth performance of male broiler chickens. Br Poult Sci 2003; 44(1): 43-4.
[http://dx.doi.org/10.1080/713655281]

[79]   Aji SB, Ignatius K, Adatu A, *et al.* Effect of feeding onion (*Allium cepa*) and garlic (*Allium sativum*) on some performance characteristics of broiler chickens. Res J Poult Sci 2011; 4: 22-7.
[http://dx.doi.org/10.3923/rjpscience.2011.22.27]

[80]   Issa KJ, Abo Omar JM. Effect of garlic powder on performance and lipid profile of broilers. Open J Anim Sci 2012; 2(2): 62-8.
[http://dx.doi.org/10.4236/ojas.2012.22010]

[81]   Fayed RH, Razek AHA, Jehan MO. Effect of dietary garlic supplementation on performance, carcass traits and meat quality in broiler chickens. In: Proceedings of the XVth International Congress of the International Society for Animal Hygiene Vienna, Austria 2011; 471-4.

[82]   Elagib HAA, Elamin WIA, Elamin KM, Malic HEE. Effect of dietary garlic (*Allium sativum*) supplementation as feed additive on broiler performance and blood profileJ. Anim Sci Adv 2013; 3(2): 58-64.
[http://dx.doi.org/10.5455/jasa.20130219104029]

[83]   Karan RK, Soujanya S. Effect of garlic and neem leaf powder supplementation on growth performance and carcass traits in broilers. Vet World 2014; 7(10): 799-02.
[http://dx.doi.org/10.14202/vetworld.2014.799-802]

[84]   Safa MA, Mohamed KA, Mukhtar MA. Effect of using garlic powder as natural feed additive on performance and carcass quality of broiler chicks. Vet Med J 2014; 60: 141.

[85]   Noman ZA, Hasan MM, Talukder S, *et al.* Effects of garlic extract on growth, carcass characteristics and haematological parameters in broiler. Vet 2015; 32(1): 1.

[86]   Puvača N, Lukač D, Stanaćev V, *et al.* Effects of dietary garlic addition on productive performance and blood lipid profile of broiler chickens. Bio Ani Husb 2014; 30(4): 669-76.
[http://dx.doi.org/10.2298/BAH1404669P]

[87]   Elkatcha MI, Sharaf MA, Soltan MA. Growth performance, immune response, blood serum parameters, nutrient digestibility and carcass traits of broiler chicken as affected by dietary supplementation of garlic extract (Allicin). AJVS 2016; 49(2): 50-64.
[http://dx.doi.org/10.5455/ajvs.219261]

[88]   Ismail IE , Alagawany M , Taha AE , Puvača N , Laudadio V , Tufarelli V . Effect of dietary supplementation of garlic powder and phenyl acetic acid on productive performance, blood haematology, immunity and antioxidant status of broiler chickens. Asian-Australas J Anim Sci 2020.
[http://dx.doi.org/10.5713/ajas.20.0140]

[89]   Tollba AAH, Hassan MSH. Using some natural additives to improve physiological and productive performance of broiler chicks under high temperature conditions. Black cumin (*Nigella sativa*) or Garlic (*Allium sativum*). Poult Sci 2003; 23: 327-40.

[90]   Ashayerizadeh OB, Daster M, Shams SE, *et al.* Use of garlic (*Allium sativum*), black cumin seeds (*Nigella sativa* L.) and wild mint (*Menthe longifolia*) in broiler chicken diets. J Anim Vet 2009; 8(9): 1860-3.

[91]   Ghasemi R, Zarei M, Torki M. Adding medicinal herbs including garlic (*Allium sativum*) and thyme (*Thyme vulgaris*) to diet of laying hens and evaluating productive performance and egg quality characteristics. Am J Anim Sci 2010; 5: 151-4.
[http://dx.doi.org/10.3844/ajavsp.2010.151.154]

[92]   Pourali M, Mirghelenj SA, Kermanshahi H. Effects of garlic on productive performance and immune response of broiler chickens challenged with newcastle disease virus. Glob Vet 2010; 4(6): 616-21.

[93]   Racesi MSA. Effect of periodically use of garlic (*Allium sativum*) powder on performance and carcass characteristics in broiler chickens. World Acad Sci Eng Technol 2010; 68: 1213-9.

[94]   Javandel F, Navidshad B, Seifdavati J, Pourrahimi GH, Baniyaghoub S. The favorite dosage of garlic meal as a feed additive in broiler chickens ratios. Pak J Biol Sci 2008; 11(13): 1746-9.
[http://dx.doi.org/10.3923/pjbs.2008.1746.1749] [PMID: 18819631]

[95]   Onu P. Evaluation of two herbal spices as feed additives for finisher broilers. Biotechnol Anim Husb 2010; 26: 383-92.
[http://dx.doi.org/10.2298/BAH1006383O]

[96]   Adjei MB, Atuahene CC, Attoh-Kotoku V. The response of broiler chickens to dietary inclusion of allicin, effects on growth performance and carcass traits. J Anim Sci Adv 2015; 5(5): 1295-301.

[http://dx.doi.org/10.5455/jasa.20150513121216]

[97]   Rahimi S, Zadeh Z, Torshizi MA, *et al.* Effect of the three Herbal extracts on growth performance, Immune system, blood factors and intestinal selected bacterial population in broiler chickens. J Agric Sci Technol 2011; 13: 527-39.

[98]   Sameh G, Ramadan A. Behavior, welfare and performance of broiler chicks fed dietary essential oils as growth promoter. Assiut Vet Med J 2013; 59: 137.

[99]   Yang WZ, Benchaar C, Ametaj BN, Chaves AV, He ML, McAllister TA. Effects of garlic and juniper berry essential oils on ruminal fermentation and on the site and extent of digestion in lactating cows. J Dairy Sci 2007; 90(12): 5671-81.
        [http://dx.doi.org/10.3168/jds.2007-0369] [PMID: 18024759]

[100]   Mohebbifar A, Torki M. Growth performance and humoral response of broiler chicks fed diet containing graded levels of ground date pits and garlic and thyme. Glob Vet 2011; 6: 389-98.

[101]   Motamedi SM, Taklim SMM. Investigating the effect of fenugreek seed powder and garlic powder in the diet on immune response of commerciallayinghens' egg. Indian J Soc Res 2014; 3(1): 277-83.

[102]   Amin A, Hamza AA. Hepatoprotective effects of Hibiscus, Rosmarinus and Salvia on azathioprine-induced toxicity in rats. Life Sci 2005; 77(3): 266-78.
        [http://dx.doi.org/10.1016/j.lfs.2004.09.048] [PMID: 15878355]

[103]   Babu US, Wiesenfeld PL, Jenkins MY. Effect of dietary rosemary extract on cell-mediated immunity of young rats. Plant Foods Hum Nutr 1999; 53(2): 169-74.
        [http://dx.doi.org/10.1023/A:1008040324935] [PMID: 10472794]

[104]   Martinez J, Tomas G, Merino S, Arriero E, Moreno J. Detection of serum immunoglobulins in wild birds by direct ELISA: a methodological study to validate the technique in different species using antichicken antibodies. Funct Ecol 2003; 17: 700-6.
        [http://dx.doi.org/10.1046/j.1365-2435.2003.00771.x]

[105]   Smits JEG, Baos R. Evaluation of the antibody mediated immune response in nestling American kestrels (*Falco sparverius*). Dev Comp Immunol 2005; 29(2): 161-70
        [http://dx.doi.org/10.1016/j.dci.2004.06.007] [PMID: 15450756]

[106]   Hou FX, Yang HF, Yu T, Chen W. The immunosuppressive effects of 10mg/kg cyclophosphamide in Wistar rats. Environ Toxicol Pharmacol 2007; 24(1): 30-6.
        [http://dx.doi.org/10.1016/j.etap.2007.01.004] [PMID: 21783786]

[107]   Wen XM, Zhang YL, Liu XM, Guo SX, Wang H. Immune responses in mice to arecoline mediated by lymphocyte muscarinic acetylcholine receptor. Cell Biol Int 2006; 30(12): 1048-53.
        [http://dx.doi.org/10.1016/j.cellbi.2006.09.015] [PMID: 17084646]

[108]   Lo Ai-Hsiang Y-CL, Lin-Shiau S-Y, *et al.* Carnosol, an antioxidant in rosemary, suppresses inducible nitric oxide synthase through down-regulating nuclear factor-κB in mouse macrophages. Carcinogenesis 2002; 23: 98391.
        [http://dx.doi.org/10.1093/carcin/23.6.983]

[109]   Dorman HJD, Peltoketo A, Hiltunen R, Tikkanen MJ. Characterization of the antioxidant properties of de-odorized aqueous extracts from selected Lamiaceae herbs. Food Chem 2003; 83: 255-62.
        [http://dx.doi.org/10.1016/S0308-8146(03)00088-8]

[110]   Abd El-Hakim AS, Cherian G. Ali1 MN. Use of organic acid, herbs and their combination to improve the utilization of commercial low protein broiler diets. Int J Poult Sci 2009; 8(1): 14-20.
        [http://dx.doi.org/10.3923/ijps.2009.14.20]

[111]   Oleforuh-Okoleh. Evaluation of growth performance, haematological and serum biochemical response of broiler chickens to aqueous extract of ginger and garlic. J Agric Sci 2015; 7: 167-73.

[112]   Lee KW, Kim GH, Kim JH, *et al.* Effects of dietary fermented garlic on the growth performance, relative organ weights, intestinal morphology, cecalMicroflora and serum characteristics of broiler

chickens. J Poult Sci 2016; 18(3): 511-8.

[113] Mahdi A, Ibrahim EI, Mohammad TN. Effect of dietary herbal plants supplement in turkey diet on performance and some blood biochemical parameters. GJBB 2015; 4: 153-7.

[114] Mohamed I, El-katcha M, Mohamed M. Growth performance, immune response, blood serum parameters, nutrient digestibility and carcass traits of broiler chicken as affected by dietary supplementation of garlic extract (allicin). Alex J Vet Sci 2016; 49(2): 50-64.
[http://dx.doi.org/10.5455/ajvs.219261]

[115] Kitagishi Y, Kobayashi M, Matsuda S. Protection against cancer with medicinal herbs *via* activation of tumor suppressor. J Oncol 2012; 2012: 236530.
[http://dx.doi.org/10.1155/2012/236530] [PMID: 23213333]

[116] El Deeb KS. Investigation of tannin in some labiatae species. Bull FacPharma 1993; 31: 237-41.

[117] Herrero M, Plaza M, Cifuentes A, Ibáñez E. Green processes for the extraction of bioactives from Rosemary: Chemical and functional characterization *via* ultra-performance liquid chromatography-tandem mass spectrometry and *in-vitro* assays. J Chromatogr A 2010; 1217(16): 2512-20.
[http://dx.doi.org/10.1016/j.chroma.2009.11.032] [PMID: 19945706]

[118] Saito Y, Shiga A, Yoshida Y, Furuhashi T, Fujita Y, Niki E. Effects of a novel gaseous antioxidative system containing a rosemary extract on the oxidation induced by nitrogen dioxide and ultraviolet radiation. Biosci Biotechnol Biochem 2004; 68(4): 781-6.
[http://dx.doi.org/10.1271/bbb.68.781] [PMID: 15118303]

[119] Matkowski A. Plant phenolic metabolites as antioxidants and antimutagens. In: Yaroslav B, Durzan DJ, Petro S, Eds. Cell Biology and Instrumentation: UV Radiation, Nitric Oxide and Cell Death in Plants. Amsterdam: IOS Press 2006; pp. 129-48.

[120] Zhang X. Traditional medicine and WHO world health. Magazine of World Health Organization. 2: 4-5.

[121] Saber AS, Hawazen AL. Protective effect of rosemary (*Rosmarinus officinalis*) leaves extract on carbon tetrachloride-induced nephrotoxicity in albino rats. Life Sci 2012; 9: 779-85.

[122] Sakr SS, Amin AY. EL-Mewafy EA, Eid NM. *In vitro* comparative study on *Rosmarinus officinalis* L. cultivars. Middle East J Agric Res 2018; 7(3): 703-15.

[123] Zheng W, Wang SY. Antioxidant activity and phenolic compounds in selected herbs. J Agric Food Chem 2001; 49(11): 5165-70.
[http://dx.doi.org/10.1021/jf010697n] [PMID: 11714298]

[124] Jimoh AA, Olorede BR, Abubakar A, *et al.* Lipids profile and haematological indices of broiler chickens fed garlic (*Allium sativum*) - supplemented diets. J Vet Adv 2012; 2(10): 474-80.

[125] Dearlove RP, Greenspan P, Hartle DK, Swanson RB, Hargrove JL. Inhibition of protein glycation by extracts of culinary herbs and spices. J Med Food 2008; 11(2): 275-81.
[http://dx.doi.org/10.1089/jmf.2007.536] [PMID: 18598169]

[126] Nabekura T, Yamaki T, Hiroi T, Ueno K, Kitagawa S. Inhibition of anticancer drug efflux transporter P-glycoprotein by rosemary phytochemicals. Pharmacol Res 2010; 61(3): 259-63.
[http://dx.doi.org/10.1016/j.phrs.2009.11.010] [PMID: 19944162]

[127] Fecka I, Raj D, Krauze-Baranowska M. Quantitative determination of four water-soluble compounds in herbal drug from lamiaceae using different chromatographic techniques. Chromatographia 2007; 66: 87-93.
[http://dx.doi.org/10.1365/s10337-007-0233-7]

[128] Labban L, El-Sayed Mustafa U, Ibrahim YM. The effects of rosemary (*Rosmarinus officinalis*) leaves powder on glucose level, lipid profile and lipid perodoxation. Int J Clin Med 2014; 5(6): 297-04.
[http://dx.doi.org/10.4236/ijcm.2014.56044]

[129] Berrougui H, Ettaib A, Herrera Gonzalez MD, Alvarez de Sotomayor M, Bennani-Kabchi N,

Hmamouchi M. Hypolipidemic and hypocholesterolemic effect of argan oil (*Argania spinosa* L.) in Meriones shawi rats. J Ethnopharmacol 2003; 89(1): 15-8.
[http://dx.doi.org/10.1016/S0378-8741(03)00176-4] [PMID: 14522427]

[130] Lee J, Chae K, Ha J, *et al.* Regulation of obesity and lipid disorders by herbal extracts from Morus alba, Melissa officinalis, and Artemisia capillaris in high-fat diet-induced obese mice. J Ethnopharmacol 2008; 115(2): 263-70.
[http://dx.doi.org/10.1016/j.jep.2007.09.029] [PMID: 18023310]

[131] Kaliora AC, Andrikopoulos NK. Effect of Alkanna albugam root on LDL oxidation. A comparative study with species of the Lamiaceae family. Phytother Res 2005; 19(12): 1077-9.
[http://dx.doi.org/10.1002/ptr.1774] [PMID: 16372379]

[132] Albu S, Joyce E, Paniwnyk L, Lorimer JP, Mason TJ. Potential for the use of ultrasound in the extraction of antioxidants from *Rosmarinus officinalis* for the food and pharmaceutical industry. Ultrason Sonochem 2004; 11(3-4): 261-5.
[http://dx.doi.org/10.1016/j.ultsonch.2004.01.015] [PMID: 15081992]

[133] Bragagnolo N, Danielsen B, Skibsted LH. Rosemary as antioxidant in pressure processed chicken during subsequent cooking as evaluated by electron spin resonance spectroscopy. Innov Food Sci Emerg Technol 2007; 8: 24-9.
[http://dx.doi.org/10.1016/j.ifset.2006.04.005]

[134] Elwan HAM, Elnesr SS, Mohany M, Al-Rejaie SS. The effects of dietary tomato powder (*Solanum lycopersicum* L.) supplementation on the haematological, immunological, serum biochemical and antioxidant parameters of growing rabbits. J Anim Physiol Anim Nutr (Berl) 2019; 103(2): 534-46.
[http://dx.doi.org/10.1111/jpn.13054] [PMID: 30597625]

[135] Capasso A. Antioxidant action and therapeutic efficacy of *Allium sativum* L. Molecules 2013; 18(1): 690-700.
[http://dx.doi.org/10.3390/molecules18010690] [PMID: 23292331]

[136] Chen S, Shen X, Cheng S, *et al.* Evaluation of garlic cultivars for polyphenolic content and antioxidant properties. PLoS One 2013; 8(11): e79730.
[http://dx.doi.org/10.1371/journal.pone.0079730] [PMID: 24232741]

[137] Borlinghaus J, Albrecht F, Gruhlke MC, Nwachukwu ID, Slusarenko AJ. Allicin: chemistry and biological properties. Molecules 2014; 19(8): 12591-618.
[http://dx.doi.org/10.3390/molecules190812591] [PMID: 25153873]

[138] Sotelo-Félix JI, Martinez-Fong D, Muriel P, Santillán RL, Castillo D, Yahuaca P. Evaluation of the effectiveness of *Rosmarinus officinalis* (Lamiaceae) in the alleviation of carbon tetrachloride-induced acute hepatotoxicity in the rat. J Ethnopharmacol 2002; 81(2): 145-54.
[http://dx.doi.org/10.1016/S0378-8741(02)00090-9] [PMID: 12065145]

[139] Wellwood CRL, Cole RA. Relevance of carnosic acid concentrations to the selection of rosemary, *Rosmarinus officinalis* (L.), accessions for optimization of antioxidant yield. J Agric Food Chem 2004; 52(20): 6101-7.
[http://dx.doi.org/10.1021/jf035335p] [PMID: 15453673]

[140] Perez RM, Gonzales FV. UV-B radiation effects on foliar concentrations of rosmarinic and carnosic acids in rosemary plants. Food Chem 2007; 101: 1211-5.
[http://dx.doi.org/10.1016/j.foodchem.2006.03.023]

[141] Tawaha K, Alali FQ, Gharaibeh M, Mohammad M, El-Elimat T. Antioxidant activity and total phenolic content of selected Jordanian plant species. Food Chem 2007; 104: 1372-8.
[http://dx.doi.org/10.1016/j.foodchem.2007.01.064]

[142] Block E, Naganathan S, Putman D, Zhao SH. Organo-sulfur chemistry of garlic and onion. Pure Appl Chem 1993; 65: 625-32.
[http://dx.doi.org/10.1351/pac199365040625]

[143] Quintero-Fabián S, Ortuño-Sahagún D, Vázquez-Carrera M, López-Roa RI. Alliin, a garlic (*Allium sativum*) compound, prevents LPS-induced inflammation in 3T3-L1 adipocytes. Mediators Inflamm 2013; 2013: 381815.
[http://dx.doi.org/10.1155/2013/381815] [PMID: 24453416]

[144] Kopeć A, Piątkowska E, Leszczyńska T, Elżbieta S. Healthy properties of garlic. Curr Nutr Food Sci 2013; 9: 59-64.

[145] Lanzotti V, Scala F, Bonanomi G. Compounds from Allium species with cytotoxic and antimicrobial activity. Phytochem Rev 2014; 13: 769-91.
[http://dx.doi.org/10.1007/s11101-014-9366-0]

[146] Marzouk Z, Mansour HB, Chraief I, *et al.* Chemical composition, antibacterial and antimutagenic activities of four populations of *Rosmarinus officinalis* L. oils from Tunisia. J Food Agric Environ 2006; 4(2): 89-94.

[147] Weckesser S, Engel K, Simon-Haarhaus B, Wittmer A, Pelz K, Schempp CM. Screening of plant extracts for antimicrobial activity against bacteria and yeasts with dermatological relevance. Phytomedicine 2007; 14(7-8): 508-16.
[http://dx.doi.org/10.1016/j.phymed.2006.12.013] [PMID: 17291738]

[148] Zaouali Y, Boussaid M. Isozyme markers and volatiles in Tunisian *Rosmarinus officinalis* L. (Lamiaceae): A comparative analysis of population structure. Biochem Syst Ecol 2008; 36: 11-21.
[http://dx.doi.org/10.1016/j.bse.2007.08.005]

[149] Bloem E, Haneklaus S, Schnug E. Influence of fertilizer practices on S-containing metabolites in garlic (*Allium sativum* L.) under field conditions. J Agric Food Chem 2010; 58(19): 10690-6.
[http://dx.doi.org/10.1021/jf102009j] [PMID: 20828155]

[150] Mena P, Cirlini M, Tassotti M, Herrlinger KA, Dall'Asta C, Del Rio D. Phytochemical profiling of flavonoids, phenolic acids, terpenoids, and volatile fraction of a rosemary (*Rosmarinus officinalis* L.) extract. Molecules 2016; 21(11): 1576.
[http://dx.doi.org/10.3390/molecules21111576] [PMID: 27869784]

[151] Birtić S, Dussort P, Pierre FX, Bily AC, Roller M. Carnosic acid. Phytochemistry 2015; 115: 9-19.
[http://dx.doi.org/10.1016/j.phytochem.2014.12.026] [PMID: 25639596]

[152] Petersen M, Simmonds MS. Rosmarinic acid. Phytochemistry 2003; 62(2): 121-5.
[http://dx.doi.org/10.1016/S0031-9422(02)00513-7] [PMID: 12482446]

CHAPTER 4

Nigella sativa Seeds and their Derivatives in Poultry Feed

Mohamed E. Abd El-Hack[1,*], **Sameh A. Abdelnour**[2], **Husein Ohran**[3], **Ayman E. Taha**[4] and **Mahmoud Alagawany**[1,*]

[1] *Department of Poultry, Faculty of Agriculture, Zagazig University, Zagazig 44511, Egypt*

[2] *Department of Animal Production, Faculty of Agriculture, Zagazig University, Zagazig 44511, Egypt*

[3] *Department of Physiology, University of Sarajevo, Veterinary Faculty, Zmaja od Bosne 90, 71 000 Sarajevo, Bosnia and Herzegovina*

[4] *Department of Animal Husbandry and Animal Wealth Development, Faculty of Veterinary Medicine, Alexandria University, Edfina 22578, Egypt*

Abstract: The addition of antibiotics to poultry diets caused many cases of antibiotic residues and a large number of pathogens that are resistant to drugs. So there was an urgent need to use alternative medicine. Many studies have assured that *Nigella sativa* (black cumin) seeds might be an adequate replacement for standard therapeutic procedures like antibiotics in poultry. *Nigella sativa* plays a significant role in promoting the bird's health and productivity, besides acting as a natural immuno-stimulant and antioxidant. The black seed oil contains high amounts of polyunsaturated fatty acids, and in this way, it lowers the total cholesterol content. Due to the high content of bioactive compounds, black cumin is proven to have anticancer effects. The present paper enumerates the natural benefits of *Nigella sativa* on nutritional and health aspects for poultry.

Keywords: Health, *Nigella sativa*, Poultry, Production, Seeds.

INTRODUCTION

Antibiotics and other food supplements have been used in large amounts for a long time in the poultry industry. Fortunately, the global awareness about antibiotic residues and diseases that are related to the resistance to antibiotics has risen [1 - 3]. Banning of antibiotics as dietary additives resulted in increased usage of various supplements, which has resulted in more studies regarding animal production using natural additives [4, 5].

* Corresponding authors Mohamed E. Abd El-Hack and Mahmoud Alagawany: Department of Poultry, Faculty of Agriculture, Zagazig University, Zagazig-44511, Egypt; E-mails: m.ezzat@zu.edu.eg and mmalagwany@zu.edu.eg

Aromatic herbs and their extracts could be such additives, like rosemary, thyme, and *Yucca schidigera* [6 - 8]. The seed of black cumin, which comes from the family of *Ranunculacease,* belongs to the hcrbs that could be used for such purpose. It is known under many names, like black cumin, black caraway, habbatul barakah, Qazhe shuniz, and probably some other. Black cumin is an herb that has been used as a therapeutic for over 2000 years for various diseases. It has also been mentioned in prophetic medicine, which has been practiced by the **Prophet Mohammad [PBUH].**

Furthermore, Abu Hurayrah [RA] PBUH narrated "use black seed regularly because it is a cure for every disease, except death [9, 10]. Moreover, the Holy Bible characterized the black seed as the curative "black cumin", Hippocrates and Dioscorides interpreted this herb as Melanthion, while Gith described it as Pliny [11]. This herb originates from Asia, South Europe, East Mediterranean, and is cultivated, especially in Turkey [12]. Regarding the composition, black cumin seed contains proteins [210 g kg^{-1}], oil [350-380 g kg^{-1}], and carbohydrates [g kg^{-1}]. One thousand seeds averagely weigh about 2-3 g. Seed efficiency alters between 75-150 kg/day, depending on various factors, like soil, climate, and cultivation conditions [12]. The primary purpose of black cumin seeds is medical, but it is also used as spice and supplement in food [13]. Lately, researchers determined that the black cumin seed has various positive effects in the organism, such as antibacterial, bronchodilatation, regulating blood pressure, and stimulating the bile flow. The goal of this chapter is to accentuate the significance of *Nigella sativa* seeds in poultry nutrition, as well as to give information on the pharmaceutical effects of this herb.

MORPHOLOGY OF *NIGELLA SATIVA* AND CHEMICAL COMPOSITION

Black cumin is an annual plant, height approximately 45 cm and 2-4 cm on average, with 2-3 narrow pinnatisect leaves (Fig. **1**). It has relatively blue flowers on long single pedicles. The seeds have a triangular cross-section and are black. With a rather stiff and branching stem, the black cumin plant has greyish-blue flowers and greyish-green leaves. Its small and compressed seeds, which mostly have three corners, are found in seed vessels, usually found in odd numbers. The seed vessels of black cumin have two flat sides and one convex side, and they are black or brown and have a strong odor, very aromatic – like the odor of nutmegs, while its taste is very spicy. *Nigella sativa* usually has blue and white flowers, with several petals in the range 5-10. Its fruit can be described as a large capsule, fairly inflated, and it contains single follicles [mostly 3-7] that provide a great amount of seed. It has a sharp and bitter taste, a faint strawberry aroma [14].

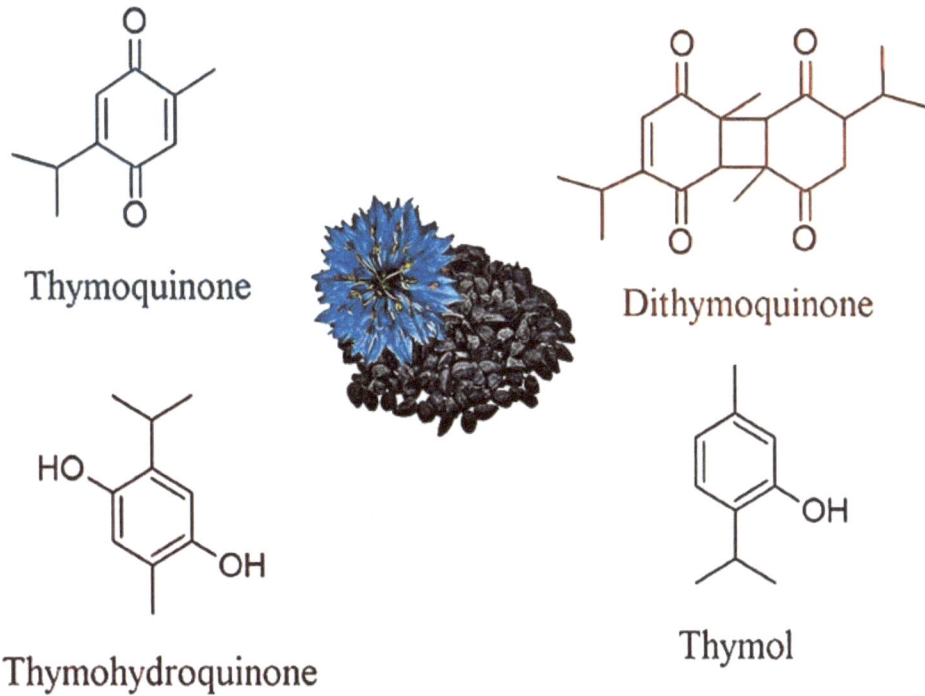

Fig. (1). Active chemical constituents in *Nigella sativa*.

PHARMACEUTICAL ACTIVITIES OF *NIGELLA SATIVA*

Antioxidant Effects

In streptozotocin-induced diabetic rats [60 mg/kg], the black cumin extracts proved to have a protective effect against oxidative stress [15]. Dietary concentrations of *Nigella sativa* [200 mg/kg] magnified the intensity of thiol in the hippocampus, in comparison to the control group of rats [15]. While using extracts of *Nigella sativa*, malondialdehyde [MDA] concentrations decreased in the hippocampus [200, 400 mg/kg] of diabetic rats compared to the control group [15]. Abbasnezhad *et al.* [15] showed that the black cumin applied to rats [200 mg/kg] had beneficial outcomes in minimizing oxidative stress in the hippocampus. Hosseinzadeh *et al.* [16] conducted a study, where they first inducted ischemia and afterward injected intraperitoneally the extract of *Nigella sativa* [0.048, 0.192 and 0.384 mg/kg] every 24 hours to 72 hours, which led to a significant decrease in levels of MDA in comparison to the ischemic group. Vafaee *et al.* [17] studied the remedial effects of the hydroalcoholic black cumin extract on the oxidative damage in the brain in PTZ-induced repeated seizures. The authors found that dietary levels of black cumin [200 and 400 mg/kg] reduced the levels of MDA in the hippocampus, simultaneously improving the total thiol concentration in comparison to the PTZ group.

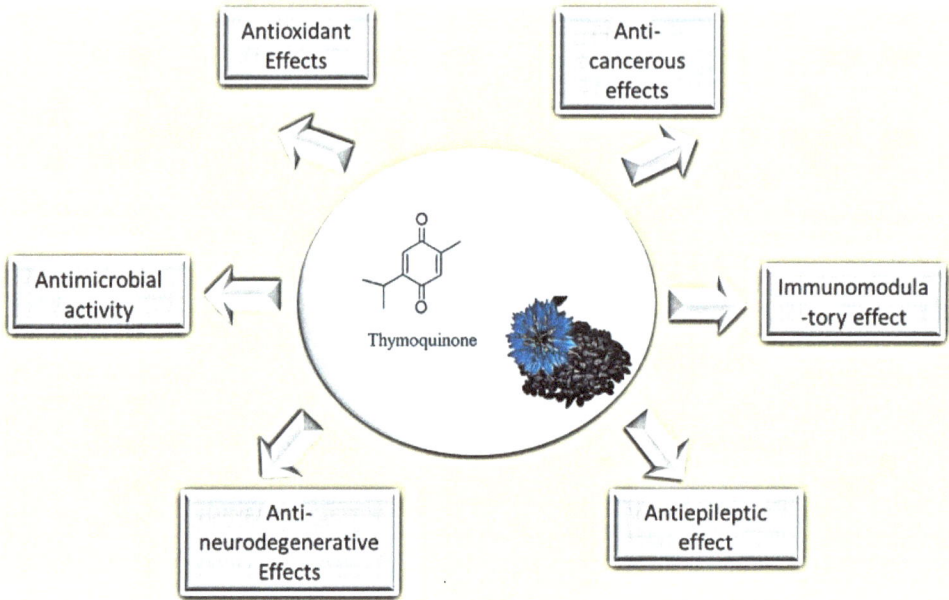

Fig. (2). The beneficial pharmaceutical activities of *Nigella sativa*.

Badary *et al*. [18] found that black cumin is an excellent superoxide anion scavenger. Bassim-Atta and Imaizumi [19] showed that adding black cumin extracts to corn oil protects triglycerides from oxidative damage. Through impeding 5-lipoxygenase and cyclooxygenase, black cumin has vital antioxidative effects *via* inhibiting thromboxane B_2, leukotriene B_4 and eicosanoids. Ilhan *et al*. [20] conducted an experiment in mice with pentylenetetrazol induced seizures. Black cumin oil was applied to the mice, and by detecting free radicals, the authors investigated the antioxidant activity. Such effects of black cumin seeds can be related to the significant components of this herb, such as anethole, carvacrol, thymoquinone, 4- and terpineol [21]. Mariod *et al*. [23] observed that dietary supplementation with 0.5 - 1% of seeds led to a decrease in MDA concentration in erythrocytes and lipid peroxidases in chicken, while the concentrations of glutathione [GSH] increased. The same researchers agreed that black cumin inhibits the production of free radicals and has a regulating role in glutathione activity, which inhibits oxidative stress. Tuluce *et al*. [24] determined that the seeds of black cumin can lower the concentrations of free radicals, such as hydroxyl [OH], hydrogen peroxide [H_2O_2], and superoxide [O_2]. Furthermore, Ilhan *et al.* [20] observed that *Nigella sativa* oil applied to rats significantly raised the levels of GSH and decreased the levels of MDA.

Antimicrobial Activity

Black cumin has an excellent antimicrobial effect on bacteria like *Pseudomonas aeruginosa* and *Salmonella typhi.* Multiple studies have reported that the oil of *Nigella sativa* has shown antimicrobial effects on Gram-negative and Gram-positive bacteria [25]. Furthermore, results showed that black cumin has better effects on Gram-positive bacteria, like *Vibrio cholerae* and *Staphylococcus aureus.* El-Kamali *et al.* [26] reported that *Nigella sativa* has been very effective against *S. viridans, S. aureus,* and *S. pyogenes.* In a research conducted by Ferdous *et al.* [27], it was shown that the activity of black cumin oil is very similar to ampicillin and synergistic with gentamycin and streptomycin, also showing positive results on antibiotic-resistant strains of *E. coli, Shigella* and *Vibrio cholerae.*

Immunomodulatory Effect

Several researchers have proved that *Nigella sativa* could be an adequate replacement for vaccines and antibiotics, as an immunity enhancer in poultry. Akhtar *et al.* [28] showed that adding 1.5% of black cumin to the diet significantly decreased the mortality rate from 16.67 to 4.17%. Mansour *et al.* [29] reported that broilers that were fed with diets that contain 1% of black cumin seeds showed an increased viability rate by 50% in comparison to the control group. Al-Jabre *et al.* [30] claim that extracts derived from black cumin contain 67 different ingredients that have beneficial effects on various bacteria, like *Staphylococcus* and *E. coli.* The active ingredients of black cumin seed showed important antioxidative, antimicrobial, and anti-inflammatory effects, and in this way, represent a successful immunomodulatory factor [31].

Toghyani *et al.* [32] reported that the substitution of dietary bacitracin with black cumin seeds in broilers, Infectious Bursal Disease [IBD] and Newcastle Disease [ND] antibody titer increased significantly. Such results are due to the components as carvacrol, thymol, thymoquinone, nigellimine, and nigellicine [33, 34]. Furthermore, Toghyani *et al.* [32] noticed a weight gain of the lymphoid organs in broilers that were fed with diets that contain black cumin seeds [0.2 – 0.4%]. However, it was found that dietary black cumin seeds did not have any impact on the antibody titers of the ND and Influenza virus in the age group of 18 and 28 days. The same results were determined for rations like A/G and heterophil to lymphocyte.

Anti-Cancerous Effects

Various studies have investigated the anti-cancerous impact of black cumin. El-Kadi and Kandil [35] reported a 200-300% rise in the activity of natural killer cells [NK] in advanced-stage cancer patients receiving a therapy that included black cumin seeds. Salomi *et al.* [36] showed that in mice, black cumin oil impeded skin induced carcinogenesis with dimethylbenz[α]anthracene/croton oil and decreased the amount and delayed the onset of papillomas. Iddamaldeniya *et al.* [37] claimed that black cumin suppressed the maturation of cell lines of solid tumors and leukemia. *Nigella sativa* extracts found to be effective in reducing cell amount in Ehrlich ascites tumor growth [38]. Multiple extracts produced from black cumin seeds express various levels of cytotoxicity on cell lines. For instance, essential oils had the most substantial influence on the cell lines of P815 in comparison with butanolic and ethanol acetate extracts. In contrast, ethyl acetate extracts demonstrated the best cytotoxic effects in BSR cell lines. Furthermore, Mbarek *et al.* [39] reported that essential oil that was applied in the tumors extended the life span in mice, also inhibiting the prevalence of metastasis in the liver.

Nigella Sativa Effect on Poultry Performance

The supplementation of *Nigella sativa* and its extracts into diets has proved to be beneficial to poultry performance [25, 40]. Meanwhile, Guler *et al.* [22] observed that the dietary addition of black cumin and antibiotics did not have any influence on the intake of feed in broilers. Regarding this fact, Durrani *et al.* [41] reported that in comparison to the control group, diets that contained 4% ground black cumin showed a decrease in feed consumption. However, a rise in feed efficiency was noticed. Other authors reported similar results that feed use of laying hens remained the same after adding dietary *Nigella sativa* oil [1, 2 and 3 ml/kg] and seeds [1, 2 and 3%] in 27 weeks of age [42].

El-Ghammry *et al.* [43] and Hassan *et al.* [44] determined that dietary supplementation with black cumin seeds resulted in body weight gain. Many authors, including Guler *et al.* [22] and Durrani *et al.* [41], founded that adding 1% black cumin into broiler diets raised the average daily weight gain and improved the feed conversion ratio [FCR]. In four week old broilers, FCR was enhanced by adding black seed in the following concentrations: 1.5% [45] 4 g/kg [32] and 1.5% [46]. The basis of such a positive influence on the performance of poultry could be the excellent nutritive value of black cumin seeds, as well as the presence of some active compounds. Black cumin seeds contain some compounds that the body cannot synthesize on its own, such as linoleic, linolenic and oleic acids. Black cumin proteins have fifteen amino acids; eight of them are indispensable [47]. Black cumin stimulates the absorption in the digestive system, which results in better performance [48]. Another beneficial effect of dietary supplementation with black cumin is the increase of bile flow, which consequently enhances the emulsification, stimulates lipases from the pancreas, and promotes the digestion of fats and absorption of liposoluble vitamins. Black seed oil, especially the component thymoquinone, is proven to have protective effects on the liver [29, 49], which resulted in great use for digestive disorders in traditional medicine [50]. Gilani *et al.* [51] theorized that beneficial effects on the performance of poultry might be attributed to the antimicrobial characteristics of black cumin seed. Black cumin was confirmed to be effective against the following microorganisms: *Bacillus pumilus, Bacillus suptilus, Escherichia coli, Pseudomonas aeruginos, Shigella sonne, Shigella dysenteriae, Shigella flrxneri, Staphylococcus aureus, Staphylococcus lutea, Vibrio cholera* [26, 27, 52]. Furthermore, it was reported that black cumin is potent in *Candida albicans* infections [53].

CONCLUDING REMARKS

This chapter summarized many studies to point out the beneficial effects of black cumin regarding health and nutritional issues. It can be stated that black cumin seeds and its multiple extracts exert significant antioxidant, antifungal, antibacterial, and immune-modulatory effects. It can enhance the healing process of serious diseases. Regarding poultry performance, the addition of black cumin seeds or their extracts into diets could increase feed efficiency and general performance traits. Another very significant conclusion is that black cumin could partially or fully substitute antibiotics in poultry diets.

CONSENT FOR PUBLICATION

Not Applicable.

CONFLICT OF INTEREST

The author confirms that this chapter contents have no conflict of interest.

ACKNOWLEDGEMENTS

Declared none.

REFERENCES

[1]   Jang IS, Ko YH, Kang SY, Lee CY. Effect of a commercial essential oil on growth performance, digestive enzyme activity and intestinal microflora population in broiler chickens. Anim Feed Sci Technol 2007; 134: 304-15.
[http://dx.doi.org/10.1016/j.anifeedsci.2006.06.009]

[2]   Abd El-Hack ME, Mahgoub SA, Hussein MMA, Saadeldin IM. Improving growth performance and health status of meat-type quail by supplementing the diet with black cumin cold-pressed oil as a natural alternative for antibiotics. Environ Sci Pollut Res Int 2018; 25(2): 1157-67. a
[http://dx.doi.org/10.1007/s11356-017-0514-0] [PMID: 29079983]

[3]   Abd El-Hack ME, Attia AI, Arif M, Soomro RN, Arain MA. The impacts of dietary *Nigella sativa* meal and Avizyme on growth, nutrient digestibility and blood metabolites of meat-type quail. Anim Prod Sci 2018; 58: 291-8. b
[http://dx.doi.org/10.1071/AN16226]

[4]   Arif M, Hayat Z, Abd El-Hack ME, *et al.* Growth, carcass traits, cecal microbiota, blood chemistry, and oxidative status of broilers fed diets enriched with a powder mixture of black cumin, moringa, and chicory seeds. S Afr J Anim Sci 2019; 49(3): 564-7.
[http://dx.doi.org/10.4314/sajas.v49i3.17]

[5]   Arif M, Rehman A, Abd El-Hack ME, *et al.* Growth, carcass traits, cecal microbial counts, and blood chemistry of meat-type quail fed diets supplemented with humic acid and black cumin seeds. Asian-Australas J Anim Sci 2018; 31(12): 1930-8.
[http://dx.doi.org/10.5713/ajas.18.0148] [PMID: 29879835]

[6]   Abd El-Hack ME, Alagawany M. Performance, egg quality, blood profile, immune function, and antioxidant enzyme activities in laying hens fed diets with thyme powder. J Anim Feed Sci 2015; 24: 127-33.
[http://dx.doi.org/10.22358/jafs/65638/2015]

[7]   Alagawany M, Abd El-Hack ME. The effect of rosemary herb as a dietary supplement on performance, egg quality, serum biochemical parameters, and oxidative status in laying hens. J Anim Feed Sci 2015; 24: 341-7.
[http://dx.doi.org/10.22358/jafs/65617/2015]

[8]   Alagawany M, Abd El-Hack ME, El-Kholy MS. Productive performance, egg quality, blood constituents, immune functions, and antioxidant parameters in laying hens fed diets with different levels of Yucca schidigera extract. Environ Sci Pollut Res Int 2016; 23(7): 6774-82. a
[http://dx.doi.org/10.1007/s11356-015-5919-z] [PMID: 26662788]

[9]   Al-Bukhari MI. The Collection of Authentic Sayings of Prophet Mohammad [Peace be Upon Him], Division 71 on Medicine. 2nd ed., Ankara, Turkey: Hilal Yayinlari 1976.

[10]   Rahmani AH, Aly SM. *Nigella sativa* and its active constituents thymoquinone shows pivotal role in the diseases prevention and treatment. Asian J Pharm Clin Res 2015; 8: 48-53.

[11]   Worthen DR, Ghosheh OA, Crooks PA. The *in vitro* anti-tumor activity of some crude and purified components of blackseed, *Nigella sativa* L. Anticancer Res 1998; 18(3A): 1527-32.
[PMID: 9673365]

[12]   Baydar H. Science and technology of medicinal and aromatic plants. 3rd ed. Isparta, Turkey: Süleyman Demirel University 2009; 51: pp. 227-8.

[13]   Kar Y. The Investigation of Black Cumin [*Nigella sativa* L.] Seed as the Resource of Natural Antioxidant and Alternative Energy. Selçuk University Graduate School of Natural and Applied Sciences, Department of Chemistry, PhD Thesis, Konya, Turkey 2008. p210.

[14]   Dwivedi SN. Ethnobotanical studies and conservational strategies of wild and naturnal resources of Rewa district of Madhya Pradesh. J Econ Taxon Bot 2003; 27: 233-4.

[15]   Abbasnezhad A, Hayatdavoudi P, Niazmand S, Mahmoudabady M. The effects of hydroalcoholic extract of *Nigella sativa* seed on oxidative stress in hippocampus of STZ-induced diabetic rats. Avicenna J Phytomed 2015; 5(4): 333-40.
[PMID: 26445713]

[16]   Hosseinzadeh H, Parvardeh S, Asl MN, Sadeghnia HR, Ziaee T. Effect of thymoquinone and *Nigella sativa* seeds oil on lipid peroxidation level during global cerebral ischemia-reperfusion injury in rat hippocampus. Phytomedicine 2007; 14(9): 621-7.
[http://dx.doi.org/10.1016/j.phymed.2006.12.005] [PMID: 17291733]

[17]   Vafaee F, Hosseini M, Hassanzadeh Z, *et al.* [] The effects of *Nigella sativa* hydro-alcoholic extract on memory and brain tissues oxidative damage after repeated seizures in rats. Iran J Pharm Res 2015; 14(2): 547-57.
[PMID: 25901163]

[18]   Badary OA, Taha RA, Gamal el-Din AM, Abdel-Wahab MH. Thymoquinone is a potent superoxide anion scavenger. Drug Chem Toxicol 2003; 26(2): 87-98.
[http://dx.doi.org/10.1081/DCT-120020404] [PMID: 12816394]

[19]   Bassim-Atta M, Imaizumi K. Antioxidant activity of Nigella [*Nigella sativa* L.] seeds extracts. Journal of Japanese Oil Chemists'. Society 1998; 47: 475-80.

[20]   Ilhan A, Gurel A, Armutcu F, Kamisli S, Iraz M. Antiepileptogenic and antioxidant effects of *Nigella sativa* oil against pentylenetetrazol-induced kindling in mice. Neuropharmacology 2005; 49(4): 456-64.
[http://dx.doi.org/10.1016/j.neuropharm.2005.04.004] [PMID: 15913671]

[21]   Guler T, Ertas ON, Kizil M, Dalkilic B, Ciftci M. Effect of dietary supplemental black cumin seeds on antioxidant activity in broilers. Med Weter 2007; 63: 1060-3.

[22]   Guler T, Dalkilic B, Ertas ON, Ciftci M. The effect of dietary black cumin seeds [*Nigella sativa* L.] on the performance of broilers. Asian-Australas J Anim Sci 2006; 19: 425-30.
[http://dx.doi.org/10.5713/ajas.2006.425]

[23]   Mariod AA, Ibrahim RM, Ismail M, Ismail N. Antioxidant activity and phenolic content of phenolic rich fractions obtained from cumin [*Nigella sativa*] seed cake. Food Chem 2009; 116: 306-12.
[http://dx.doi.org/10.1016/j.foodchem.2009.02.051]

[24]   Tuluce Y, Ozkol H, Sogut B, Celik I. Effects of *Nigella sativa* on lipid peroxidation and reduced glutathione levels in erythrocytes of broiler chickens. Cell Memb Free Rad Res 2009; 1: 1-3.

[25]   Abd El-Hack ME, Mahgoub SA, Alagawany M, Dhama K. Influences of dietary supplementation of antimicrobial cold-pressed oils mixture on growth performance and intestinal microflora of growing Japanese quails. Int J Pharmacol 2015; 11: 689-96.
[http://dx.doi.org/10.3923/ijp.2015.689.696]

[26]   El-Kamali HH, Ahmed AH, Mohamed AS, Yahia AAM, Eltayeb IH. ALI AA. Antibacterial properties of essential oils from *Nigella sativa* seeds, Cymbopogon citratus leaves and Pulicaria undulata aerial parts. Fitoterapia 1998; 69: 77-8.

[27]   Ferdous AJ, Islam SN, Ahsan M, Hasan CM, Ahmad ZU. *In vitro* antibacterial activity of the volatile oil of *Nigella sativa* seeds against multiple drug-resistant isolates of Shigella species and isolates of Vibrio cholerae and *Escherichia coli*. Phytother Res 1992; 6: 137-40.
[http://dx.doi.org/10.1002/ptr.2650060307]

[28]   Akhtar MS, Nasir Z, Abid AR. Effect of feeding powdered *Nigella sativa* L. seeds on poultry egg production and their suitability for human consumption. Vet Arh 2003; 73: 181-90.

[29]   Mansour MA, Nagi MN, El-Khatib AS, Al-Bekairi AM. Effects of thymoquinone on antioxidant enzyme activities, lipid peroxidation and DT-diaphorase in different tissues of mice: a possible mechanism of action. Cell Biochem Funct 2002; 20(2): 143-51.
[http://dx.doi.org/10.1002/cbf.968] [PMID: 11979510]

[30]   Al-Jabre S, Al-Akloby O. AL-Qurashi A, Akhatar NA, AL-Dossary MA, Rankawa S. Thymoquinone: an active principle of *Nigella sativa*, inhibited *Aspargillus niger.* Pak J Med Res 2003; 42: 102-4.

[31]   Al-Saleh IA, Billedo G, Inam IE. Level of selenium, DL-α-tocopgerol, DL-γ-tocopherol, all-trans retinol, thymoquinone and thymol in different brands of *Nigella sativa* seeds. J Food Compos Anal 2006; 19: 167-75.
[http://dx.doi.org/10.1016/j.jfca.2005.04.011]

[32]   Toghyani MA, Geisari G, Ghalamkari M, Mohammad R. Growth performance, serum biochemistry and blood hematology of broiler chicks fed different levels of black seed [*Nigella sativa* L.] and peppermint. Livest Sci 2010; 129: 173-8. [Mentha piperita].
[http://dx.doi.org/10.1016/j.livsci.2010.01.021]

[33]   El-Ghousein SS, Nofal AH. Replacing bacitracin methylene disalicylate by crushed *Nigella sativa* seeds in broiler rations and its effects on growth, blood constituents and immunity. Livest Sci 2009; 125: 304-7.
[http://dx.doi.org/10.1016/j.livsci.2009.03.012]

[34]   Alagawany M, Abd El-Hack ME, Farag MR, Tiwari R, Dhama K. Biological effects and modes of action of carvacrol in animal and poultry production and health - A review. Adv Anim Vet Sci 2015; 3: 73-84. b
[http://dx.doi.org/10.14737/journal.aavs/2015/3.2s.73.84]

[35]   El-Kadi A, Kandil O. Effect of *Nigella sativa* [the black seed] on immunity. In: Proceedings of the Fourth International Conference on Islamic Medicine 4 November Kuwait 1986; 344-8.

[36]   Salomi MJ, Nair SC, Panikkar KR. Inhibitory effects of *Nigella sativa* and saffron (*Crocus sativus*) on chemical carcinogenesis in mice. Nutr Cancer 1991; 16(1): 67-72.
[http://dx.doi.org/10.1080/01635589109514142] [PMID: 1923908]

[37]   Iddamaldeniya SS, Wickramasinghe N, Thabrew I, Ratnatunge N, Thammitiyagodage MG. Protection against diethylnitrosoamine-induced hepatocarcinogenesis by an indigenous medicine comprised of *Nigella sativa*, Hemidesmus indicus and Smilax glabra: a preliminary study. J Carcinog 2003; 2(1): 6.
[http://dx.doi.org/10.1186/1477-3163-2-6] [PMID: 14613573]

[38]   Musa D, Dilsiz N, Gumushan H, Ulakoglu G, Bitiren M. n M. Antitumor activity of an ethanol extract of *Nigella sativa* seeds. Bratislava 2004; 59: 735-40.

[39]   Ait Mbarek L, Ait Mouse H, Elabbadi N, *et al.* Anti-tumor properties of blackseed (*Nigella sativa* L.) extracts. Braz J Med Biol Res 2007; 40(6): 839-47.
[http://dx.doi.org/10.1590/S0100-879X2006005000108] [PMID: 17581684]

[40]   Al-Homidan A, Al-Qarawi AA, Al-Waily SA, Adam SEI. Response of broiler chicks to dietary *Rhazya stricta* and *Nigella sativa.* Br Poult Sci 2002; 43(2): 291-6.
[http://dx.doi.org/10.1080/00071660120121526] [PMID: 12047095]

[41]   Durrani FR, Chand N, Zaka K, Sultan A, Khattak FM, Durrani Z. Effect of different levels of feed added black seed (*Nigella sativa* L.) on the performance of broiler chicks. Pak J Biol Sci 2007; 10(22): 4164-7.
[http://dx.doi.org/10.3923/pjbs.2007.4164.4167] [PMID: 19090301]

[42]   Bolukbasi SC, Kaynar O, Erhan MK, Uruthan H. Effect of feeding *Nigella sativa* oil on laying hen performance, cholesterol and some proteins ratio of egg yolk and *Escherichia coli* count in faeces. Arch Geflugelkd 2009; 73: 167-72.

[43]   EL-Mallah GM, EL-Yamny AT. The effect of incorporation yeast culture, *Nigella sativa* seeds and fresh garlic in broiler diets on their performance. Egypt Poult Sci 2002; 22: 445-59.

[44]   Hassan II, Askar AA, Gehan A. EL-Shourbagy A. Influence of some medicinal plants on performances; physiological and meat quality traits of broiler chicks. Egypt Poult Sci 2004; 24: 247-66.

[45] Ziad HM. Abu-Dieyeh, Abu-Darwish MS. Effect of feeding powdered black cumin seeds [*Nigella sativa* L.] on growth performance of 4-8 week-old broilers. J Anim Vet Adv 2008; 7: 286-90.

[46] Hermes IH, Faten AM, Attia KA. Ibrahim, EL-Nesr SS. Effect of dietary *Nigella sativa* l. On productive performance and nutrients utilization of broiler chicks raised under summer conditions of Egypt. Egypt Poult Sci 2009; 29: 145-72.

[47] Takruri HRH, Dameh MAF. Study of the national value of black cumin seeds. J Sci Food Agric 1998; 76: 404-10. [*Nigella sativa* L].
[http://dx.doi.org/10.1002/(SICI)1097-0010(199803)76:3<404::AID-JSFA964>3.0.CO;2-L]

[48] Jamroz D, Kamel C. Plant extracts enhance broiler performance. In non-ruminant nutrition; antimicrobial agents and plant extracts on immunity, health and performance. J Anim Sci 2002; 80: 41.

[49] Mahmoud MR, El-Abhar HS, Saleh S. The effect of *Nigella sativa* oil against the liver damage induced by Schistosoma mansoni infection in mice. J Ethnopharmacol 2002; 79(1): 1-11.
[http://dx.doi.org/10.1016/S0378-8741(01)00310-5] [PMID: 11744288]

[50] El-Abhar HS, Abdallah DM, Saleh S. Gastroprotective activity of *Nigella sativa* oil and its constituent, thymoquinone, against gastric mucosal injury induced by ischaemia/reperfusion in rats. J Ethnopharmacol 2003; 84(2-3): 251-8.
[http://dx.doi.org/10.1016/S0378-8741(02)00324-0] [PMID: 12648823]

[51] Gilani AH, Jabeen Q, Khan MAU. A review of medicinal uses and pharmacological activities of *Nigella sativa.* Pak J Biol Sci 2004; 7: 441-51.
[http://dx.doi.org/10.3923/pjbs.2004.441.451]

[52] Chowdhury AKA, Islam A, Rashid A, Ferdous A. Therapeutic potential of the volatile oil of *Nigella sativa* seeds in monkey model with experimental shigellosis. Phytother Res 1998; 12: 361-3.
[http://dx.doi.org/10.1002/(SICI)1099-1573(199808)12:5<361::AID-PTR302>3.0.CO;2-1]

[53] Hanafy MS, Hatem ME. Studies on the antimicrobial activity of *Nigella sativa* seed (black cumin). J Ethnopharmacol 1991; 34(2-3): 275-8. [Black cumin].
[http://dx.doi.org/10.1016/0378-8741(91)90047-H] [PMID: 1795532]

CHAPTER 5

Beneficial Impacts of Licorice (*Glycyrrhiza glabra*) Herb to Promote Poultry Health and Production

Mohamed E. Abd El-Hack[1,*], **Sameh A. Abdelnour**[2], **Asmaa F. Khafaga**[3], **Ayman A. Swelum**[4] and **Mahmoud Alagawany**[1,*]

[1] *Department of Poultry, Faculty of Agriculture, Zagazig University, Zagazig 44511, Egypt*

[2] *Department of Animal Production, Faculty of Agriculture, Zagazig University, Zagazig 44511, Egypt*

[3] *Department of Pathology, Faculty of Veterinary Medicine, Alexandria University, Edfina 22758, Egypt*

[4] *Department of Theriogenology, Faculty of Veterinary Medicine, Zagazig University, Zagazig 44511, Egypt*

Abstract: Supplementations of livestock diets with herbs that have many active constituents revealed favourable effects as natural feed additives. These compounds could stimulate nutrient digestion, growth performance, food utilization, enhance immunological sides and antioxidant status and decrease health disorders. Various previous reports have employed mixture formulas of herbal with partial enclosure of licorice. However, the data about using licorice independently is very scared. The poultry industry faces many epidemiological syndromes; principally, those are confined to digestive, respiratory and immune system syndromes. Flavonoids and glycyrrhizin are the main bioactive components in Licorice. The roots of this herb contain 1-9% glycyrrhizin, which has several pharmacological actions such as anti-oxidant, antimicrobial, anti-heat stress, and anti-infective antiviral and anti-inflammatory activities. Licorice extracts (LE) have affirmative impacts on the management of high incidence ailments, such as the immune system, lung, and liver disease. Licochalcone A (2-8µg/mL) inhibits cancer cell proliferation by reducing DNA synthesis in these cells . Moreover, the hepatoprotective effect of LE (100-300 mg) against CCI_4-induced hepatic injury in rats has been observed. Studies suggested the potential role of LE (0.1, 0.2, or 0.3 g/L of drinking water) in reducing serum total cholesterol of broiler chicken significantly. Also, the presence of licorice root extract (0.1 g/d) in the patient diet for 1 mo led to a decrease in plasma triglyceride (by about 14%) and cholesterol (by about 5%) levels.

* **Corresponding authors Magmoud Alagawany and Mohamed E. Abd El-Hack:** Poultry Department, Faculty of Agriculture, Zagazig University, Zagazig, Egypt; E-mails: mmalagwany@zu.edu.eg and m.ezzat@zu.edu.eg

Moreover, dietary supplementation of LE plays a substantial role in the productive performance of poultry owing to the improvement of organ development and stimulating influence on digestion and appetite. Along with its growth promoting properties, licorice has antioxidant, detoxifying, anti-inflammatory, antimicrobial, and many more health benefits as enclosed in the current chapter. This chapter highlights the favourable applications and modern features of *Glycyrrhiza glabra* (licorice) herb, including its chemical composition and maintenance of the health status of poultry. Hence, it will be highly useful for nutritionists, physiologists, pharmacists, veterinarians, and poultry producers.

Keywords: Health, Licorice, Pharmacological, Poultry, Production.

INTRODUCTION

Herbs have gained great attention for their many favorable uses in humans and animal studies, and their importance is realized over the world [1]. Nowadays, the addition of feed additives and nutritional supplements in diets of birds, including growth promoters, nutraceuticals, herbs, and probiotics, is gaining significant attention due to their multiple constructive practices while improving the production and growth performances as well as maintaining the health status of poultry [2 - 7]. This chapter is focusing on one such medicinal plant known as licorice (*Glycyrrhiza glabra*). Licorice, a common medicinal plant that belongs to the legume family (Fabaceae), has been widely employed in traditional medicine for more than thousands of years [8, 9]. Not only humans consume licorice, but it is also the most extensively used herb in animal and poultry diet [10]. It is mainly employed as a food preservative agent, for commercial purposes and in the medicine sector [11]. It is derived from the sweet root of different kinds of Glycyrrhiza; however, cultivation and harvesting pursuits alter the ingredients of different biologically significant constituents of the *Glycyrrhiza* plant [12, 13]. Licorice appears a replacement candidate, described as beneficial for its antimicrobial, radical scavenging, antiatherosclerotic, antioxidative, anti-inflammatory, and antifungal estrogen-like, antiviral, anti-infective, and antinephritic activities [14].

Considering phytochemical screening, the main fraction of licorice extract (LE) contains flavonoids (*e.g.*, liquidity, isoflavonoids and formononetin), and triterpene saponins (*e.g.*, glycyrrhizin, glycyrrhetinic acid and licorice acid), phytosterols, coumarins, amino acids, choline, sugars, starch, ascorbic acid and some other bitter principles [15]. Notably, many pharmacological impacts have been termed for LE and its derived bioactive components in animals. Liquorice lollipops were found effective in reducing *S. mutans* counts from dental caries cases in children [16, 17] and recommended to be used as growth promoters in poultry diet as a supplement. Therefore, the extracts are used as a remedy for the treatment of different ailments and disorders such as hypocortisolism, bronchitis, cough, arthritis, rheumatism, hypoglycemia, dental caries, inflammatory and allergic conditions, gastric ulcer, and chronic hepatitis B and C [18, 19].

Aoki *et al.* [20] concluded a significant decrease in body weight gain and abdominal fat pad with an increase in lean body mass as a physiological effect of LFO inclusion in mice diet (1 & 2%, for eight weeks) that stimulates lipid breakdown in adipocytes; these findings have been confirmed in another study conducted by Armanini *et al.* [21], where they concluded significant decrease in body fat mass (from 12.0 to 10.8 in male, and from 24. 9 to 22.1 in female) after 2 months of dietary inclusion of 3.5 g a day of licorice, several studies confirmed similar finding later [22, 23].

This chapter defines the beneficial uses and modern features of licorice herb containing chemical components, valuable applications, health welfares, which will be extremely convenient for nutritionists, pharmacists, scientists, poultry breeders, veterinarians, and pharmaceutical industries. So, we can end up with a safe validation and get a new apparition to promote the exploration of licorice profits in the poultry industry.

CHEMICAL COMPOSITION AND STRUCTURE

Liquorice is also identified as Liquiritiae radix or Radix Glycyrrhizae. It is the root part of *Glycyrrhiza glabra* L., or *Glycyrrhiza uralensis* Fisch or *Glycyrrhiza inflate* Bat., Leguminosae [24]. Roots of *Glycyrrhiza glabra* are broadly employed in preparing numerous pharmaceutical purposes (Fig. **1**).

Based on that, phytochemical inquiry of licorice root extract revealed that it comprises flavonoids (formononetin, liquiritin and isoflavonoids), saponin triterpenes (liquirtic acid and glycyrrhizin), and other bioactive constituents such as tannins, phytosterols, coumarins, sugars, starch, amino acids, and vitamins as ascorbic acid [15, 25 - 28]. Documents showed that more than 300 flavonoids and 20 triterpenoids had been screened in licorice [29]. As per literature, *Glycyrrhizae radix et rhizoma* is broadly used in traditional Chinese medicine for curing various diseases. However, the bioavailability of various components after absorption from the intestinal tract varies. Due to transformation within the body, some structural modifications occur, which affect their uptake through the cells within the body. This variation in absorption has been deliberated using the human Caco-2 monolayer cell line model to assess the intestinal absorption of flavonoids and triterpenoids obtained from Glycyrrhizae radix rhizoma plant as it can alter the oral dosage of various components used in clinical applications or as nutritional supplements. Results projected that licochalcone B, licochalcone C, glycyrrhetinic acid, echinatin and liquiritigenin were very nicely absorbed among major triterpenoids. Glycyrrhetic acid-3-*O*-mono-β-d-glucuronide and licochalcone A were fairly absorbed and glycyrrhizin, isoliquiriti apioside and liquiritin apioside were poorly absorbed components in the Caco-2 cell monolayer [30]. Fiore *et al.* [31] suggested that the roots of the herb comprise 1-9% glycyrrhizin, while Sohail *et al.* [32] indicated that glycyrrhizin constitutes 10-25% of the root extract. Glycyrrhizin contains several bioactive agents as glycyrrhetinic acid (one molecule) and glucuronic acid (two molecules) [33]. The licorice root color is yellow due to its flavonoid constituents as glabridin and hispaglabridins [34]. Besides, the dried aqueous extracts of licorice have about 4-25% glycyrrhizinic acid [35]. Glychionide A (5, 8-dihydroxy-flavone-7-O-beta-D-glucuronide) and glychionide B (5-hydroxy-8-methoxyl-flavone-7-O-beta-D-glucuronide) are two new flavonosides recently derived from the roots of *Glychirriza glabra* [36].

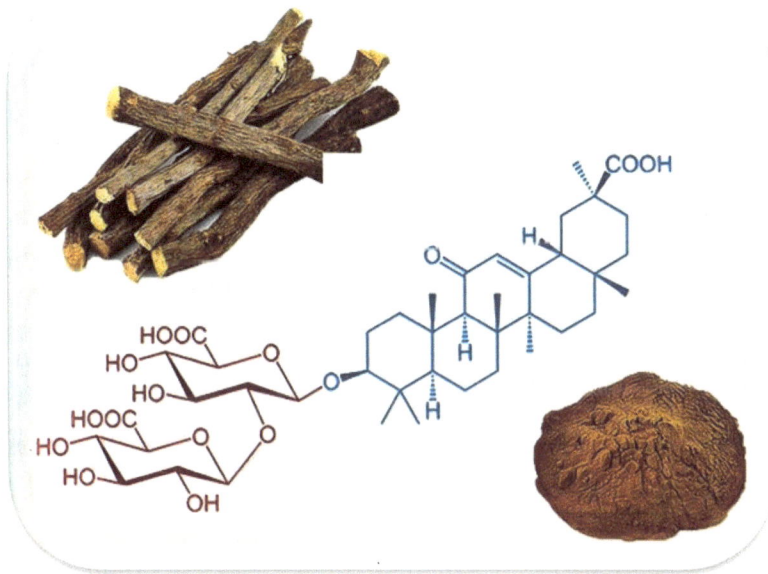

Fig. (1). Chemical composition of Glycyrrhizic acid ($C_{42}H_{62}O_{16}$).

Licorice is rich in flavonoids abscisic, syringic, trans ferulic, 2,5-dihydroxy benzoic, and salicylic acids [37]. Both Asl and Hosseinzadeh [38] and Ohno *et al.* [39] described that the principal active components of LE are liquiritin, liquiritigenin, isoliquiritigenin, and glycyrrhetinic acid.

BENEFICIAL HEALTH ROLE OF LICORICE

For thousands of years, *Glycyrrhiza glabra* was utilized as a flavoring agent and medicinal purposes. Additionally, it is a calming herb that safeguards the liver and is used in different states as mouth ulcers, arthritis, as it is a powerful anti-inflammatory agent. Likewise, the herb extracts are used as an expectorant in cough provisions and some preparations to conceal bitter taste (Fig. **2**). Also, it has curative benefits against some viruses and is used to treat chronic hepatitis. Glycyrrhiza polysaccharide enhances body function, decreases cancer cell production, and is used as anti-tumor and anti-aging [40, 41]. The use of the root extract of licorice is very old. It was commonly used in Egyptian, Greek, in Roman times in the West and during earlier times of the Han era (the 2nd, 3rd century B.C.) in ancient China in the Eastside. In conventional Chinese drug preparation, licorice was among the most commonly applied for pharmaceutical uses. Japan still has stored the oldest specimen of licorice received from China in the middle of the 8th century in the Japanese Imperial Storehouse, in Nara. Licorice extract preparations such as Carbenoxolon sodium, hemisuccinate Na, glycyrrhetinic acid (GA), and glycyrrhizin (GL) as Stronger Neo-Minophagen C (SNMC) were used for treating ulcers and as antiallergic and anti-hepatitis agent in UK, Japan and in the Netherlands in 1946 [42]. In Japan, SNMC has also been used in clinics for the treatment of allergy and hepatitis.

Licorice has many pharmacological activities such as antioxidant; where glycyrrhizin at levels 25 to 50 µg/ml interferes replication of highly pathogenic influenza A H_5N_1 virus by inhibition of ROS regeneration [43], anti-inflammatory activity; *via* upregulation of IL10 and downregulation of TNF-α in mice [44], antiatherosclerotic; where inclusion of licorice root extract (0.1 g/d) in the patient diet for one month led to a reduction in plasma cholesterol (by about 5%) and triglyceride (by about 14%) levels [45], antifungal (in tea beverage products, with a minimum inhibitory concentration between 62.5 and 125 microg/ml) [46], anti-helicobacter [47], antiviral [31], estrogen-like [48, 49], anti-infective [50], anti-cancer and hepatoprotective effects [38], radical scavenging activities and antinephritic [14], and also as a remedy for intestine and stomach problems and adrenal insufficiency [51]. The alcoholic root extract of *Glycyrrhiza glabra* against *Streptococcus mutans* and *Lactobacillus acidophilus* was found superior compared to aqueous licorice root extract and chlorhexidine (CHX) [52]. Moreover, LE is used in treating hypocortisolism and Addison's disease (daily intake of 600-800 mg glycyrrhizic acid) [53], arthritis, bronchitis, hypoglycemia, rheumatism [19], allergic conditions [18], chronic hepatitis (B and C) [54] and collagen-induced arthritis [55]. Additionally, licorice was used to treat cardiovascular disease or/and hypertension through glycyrrhizin acid affinity to a mineralocorticoid receptors, which resulted in edema and hypertension [56]. As well, glycyrrhizin leads to hypertension and other indicators of mineralocorticoid excess [57], due to glycyrrhetinic acid (the metabolism product of glycyrrhizin by microorganisms of the gut), which is an inhibitor of 11β-hydroxysteroid dehydrogenase [58].

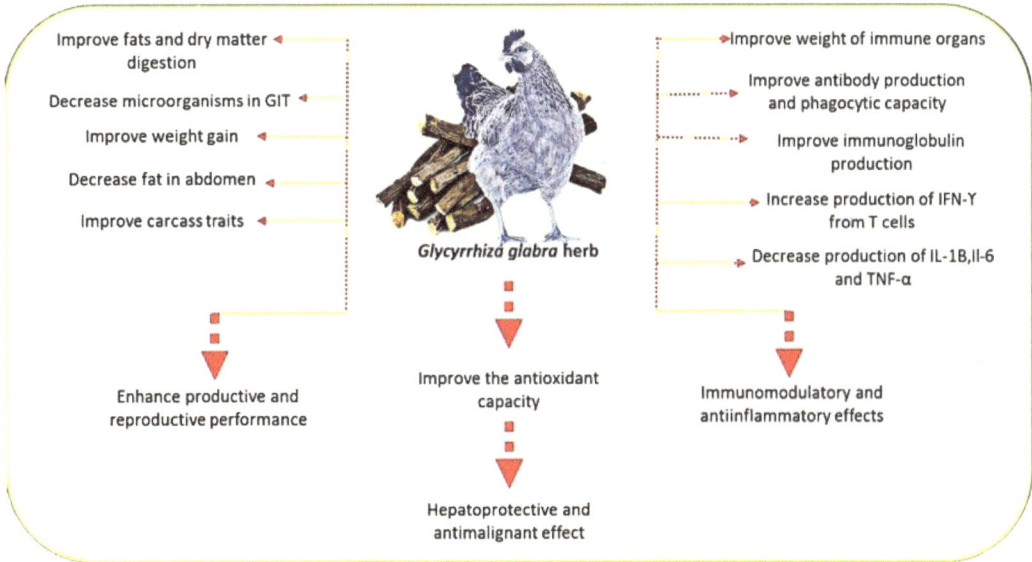

Fig. (2). Beneficial effects of *Glycyrrhiza glabra* herb.

Regarding mechanisms of licorice action, Zadeh *et al.* [59] stated that the beneficial impacts of *Glycyrrhiza glabra* might be attributed to several effects as follows: firstly, glycyrrhizin has been revealed to inhibit cytopathology and growth of several DNA and RNA viruses. Secondly, glycyrrhizin and its metabolites suppress 5-ßreductase and prevent the hepatic metabolism of aldosterone. Thirdly, licorice constituents exhibit anti-inflammatory action, like the hydrocortisone action, owing to hindering phospholipase A2 as a critical enzyme to different inflammatory development pathways. Finally, glycyrrhizic acid directly inhibits cyclooxygenase activity and formation of prostaglandin E2 and indirectly impedes platelet aggregation and any factor in the process of the inflammation. The licorice plant has biological activities, as will follow through the presentation of all updated information.

HEPATOPROTECTIVE, ANTI-MALIGNANT AND DETOXIFYING ACTIVITIES

The liver is the central organ in the detoxification of xenobiotics and the metabolism in the body, and its ailment is one of the causes leading to death in the poultry industry. Detoxification occurs *via* various mechanisms. Detoxification usually takes place due to certain chemical reactions through precipitation and by chelation reactions by which the concentration of toxin can be diminished to reduce their effects [60]. Similarly, some studies advocated that in another mode of action either by down- or up-regulating the hepatic cytochrome enzyme system P450, because of phytochemicals present in liquorice such as Cytochrome P450 3A4 (CYP3A) enzyme, they particularly stimulate the metabolism and elimination of toxins from the body [61, 62].

Licorice offers some of the bioactive components as glycyrrhizin for the medication of liver syndromes; Huo *et al*. [63] illustrated the hepatoprotective effect of licorice extract (100, 150, and 300 mg/kg against CCI_4-induced hepatic damage in rats). Besides, it has been shown that daily intake of Glycyrrhizic acid, as a constituent of licorice, for six months decreases the activity score of nonalcoholic fatty liver disease from 4.18 to 0.54 points compared to control [64]. Glycyrrhizic acid increases body excretion from potassium and augmented blood pressure with subsequent worsen effect on the heart [65]. Likewise, licorice can decrease liver injury by enhancing the anti-inflammatory and antioxidant capacity [66]. Pre-treatment with licorice extract (LE) ameliorated the acute hepatic damage and improved the biological parameters for hepatotoxicity. Moreover, the administration of LE prohibited CCI_4-induced hepatotoxicity by stimulating the antioxidant enzyme activity and declining production of TNF-α [63]. Jeong *et al*. [67] studied the hepatoprotective properties of 18β-glycyrrhetinic acid, one of LE's active components. They concluded that this component's treatment downregulates the rise in hepatic lipid peroxidation and serum ALT and AST activities in dose dependant manners. Also, this component is significantly protected from the depletion of glutathione (GSH). So, we think that LE may play a significant role in medicine by stimulating antioxidant enzymes, discontinuing inflammatory cytokine production, and scavenging free radicals. The anti malignant activities of licorice ingredients may attribute to its general antioxidant effects. Chen *et al*. [68] stated that licochalcone A (2-8μg/mL) overturns the cells' oxidation and prevents cancer cell proliferation by decreasing DNA synthesis in these cells.

ANTIOXIDANT AND ANTI-INFLAMMATORY ACTIVITIES

Antioxidant and anti-inflammatory agents play a pivotal role in rendering protection from many ailments [69 - 71]. Screening the phytochemical activity examines the bioactive ingredients of licorice root as a source of flavonoids (isoflavonoids and liquiritin), triterpenes (glycyrrhizin) and saponins, along with their antioxidant and anti-inflammatory properties [72, 73]. In several studies, extracts of *Glycyrrhiza glabra* were used in *in vitro* models because it possesses the antioxidant property, this extract inhibits lipid peroxidation of mitochondrial fractions. It reduces the oxidative frequency and reactive substance formation of thiobarbituric acid (with antioxidative activity equal to 24.25±0.52) [74]. Haraguchi *et al.* [75] reported that licorice contains Isoflavones, which protect the mitochondrial function against any oxidative stress, and also promote estradiol synthesis as concluded by Takeuchi *et al.* [76]. Visavadiya *et al.* [77] illustrated that LE possesses antioxidant activity and defensive effect against the lipoprotein oxidative system (the concentration which inhibits 50% of nitric oxide was 72 microg/ml (for aqueous) and 62.1 microg/ml (for ethanolic) extract. However, glycyrrhetinic acid may lead to a decrease in the synthesis of cortisol with subsequent great altitudes of oxidation that increased the weight of the heart [78].

Inflammatory responses play a significant role in many highly prevalent diseases such as lung [79] and liver [80] diseases, and herbs have been reported to be protective in countering several inflammatory diseases and disorders [71]. Glycyrrhizin inhibits the complement-mediated lytic pathway to reduce the inflammatory influence on liver cells in cases of chronic viral hepatitis [81]. Licochalcone A (Lico A) inhibited the lipopolysaccharide-induced inflammatory responses in a dose-dependent manner in *in vitro* and *in vivo* studies by decreasing the activation of NF-κB and p38/ERK MAPK signaling in mice model with acute lung injury and confirmed the potent anti-inflammatory activity of Lico A of licorice root [82]. Treatment with licorice flavonoids discontinues the brain's pro-inflammatory action, abrogate neuronal death [83], and declines the main inflammatory markers in the liver [84]. Accordingly, and based on traditional herbal medicine, LE can stimulate T cells, therefore, it may be used to protect the animal from inflammatory and autoimmune ailments [85]. Yu *et al.* [86] showed that active components of LE as glycyrrhizic acid, liquiritigenin and liquiritin reduced the transcripts levels of pro-inflammatory cytokines (IL-1β, IL-6 and TNF-α) in the liver. In addition, they suggested that these ingredients block the synthesis of numerous inflammatory mediators produced by activated macrophages, and so LE could inhibit inflammation in the liver. Moreover, flavonoids in the licorice plant possess remarkable antioxidant and anti-inflammatory actions [87, 88].

Additionally, Liu *et al.* [89] assumed that licorice flavonoids might target the pathway of NF-κB signal to inhibit the secretion of the inflammatory cytokine. Previous *in vitro* and *in vivo* study was conducted by Chu *et al.* [82]; they showed that licochalcone A found in the licorice has significant anti-inflammatory actions by inhibiting NF-κB activation. Similarly, licorice is used for a long time to treat gastric ulcers and inflammation as traditional herbal medicine [47, 90]. Also, LE may be favorable in avoiding and inhibiting chronic and acute inflammatory conditions [55].

IMMUNOMODULATOR AND ANTIVIRAL EFFECTS

Documents revealed that several phytogenic compounds had proven persuasive immunomodulatory and antiviral activities [1, 13]. LE has an affirmative effect on the immune system, birds' immune status and, therefore, enhances product performance. Some earlier studies showed that dietary inclusion of 0.1% LE enhanced the humoral immunity responses by promoting antibody titers' synthesis against non-specific and specific antigens in broilers. In many commercial broiler chicks breeds, studies were carried out to evaluate the influence of dietary inclusion of licorice root extracts over the immune profile. Comparison with 1% *G. glabra* crude extract powder in chick diets, the 0.1% *G. glabra* extract powder presented significant enhancement in immune responses [91]. Besides, licorice is used as an immunity enhancer because it increases white blood cells (WBCs) and finally increases interferon levels [92]. Moreover, LE's inclusion at level 50 microg/mL in laying hens diet had certain supportive immunological impressions on cellular immunity through increasing the phagocytic capacity of granulocytes and mononuclear cells [93].

As glycyrrhiza polysaccharide has a robust immune action and is broadly used in some functions of immune regulation [41, 94], glycyrrhizin can stimulate T cells to create gamma interferon (IFN-γ) [95]. Furthermore, IgM$^+$ B cells (%) were increased in the pigeons administered LE than in the control pigeons. As well, LE has immunomodulatory features and can be used to avoid viral diseases (VD), improve immunity and treat many VD in pigeons [96]. While Moradi *et al.* [97] described that AI viruses and antibody titers against ND and lymphoid (thymus, spleen and bursa of Fabricius) and liver organs weights are not influenced by the LE addition in broiler drinking water.

In an experimental study, results suggested that glycyrrhizin (GL) inhibited the expression of hepatitis C virus (HCV) 3a core gene both at mRNA and protein levels, means inhibition of HCV full-length viral particles as well as HCV core gene expression in a dose-dependent manner and also had synergistic action along with interferon and proposed an alternate therapeutic choice for the treatment of

HCV infection [98]. Along with *Glycyrrhiza glabra*, methanol extract of *G. uralensis* roots and its chloroform fraction also exhibited anti-hepatitis C virus (anti-HCV) activity. It is observed that glabridin from *G. glabra* and glycyrrhizin, licochalcone A, glycycoumarin, glycyrin, glycyrol, isoliquiritigenin and liquiritigenin obtained from *G. uralensis* showed anti-HCV activity, hence can be explored to develop as antiviral drugs against hepatitis C virus [99].

Notably, incorporation of licorice in broiler diets enhanced the weight of immune organs as bursa and spleen, leading to promoting the immune efficacy and situation of liveability and health [100]. Similarly, glycyrrhizic acid increased immune organ weights in broiler chicks [101]. Glycyrrhetinic acid possesses several favorable pharmacological actions, such as immunomodulation and synthesis of interleukin (1, 2 and 12) with following synthesis of antibodies [102, 103], IFN-γ, and T-cells that show its antiviral properties. Additionally, glycyrrhizin regulates the expression of inducible and synthase nitric oxide (NO) in macrophage [104]. On the other hand, Hosseini *et al.* [105] indicated that the addition of LE (2.5 and 5 g/kg diet) in the broiler diet did not influence immune organs' weight, T3 and T4 cells. Furthermore, LE exerts several types of antiviral activity; it inhibits virus-related replication by becoming linked to the membrane of the cell and compromising the ability of cells to undergo endocytosis, which inhibits the virus from cells penetration [106], and also by activation of NF-κB protein complex which stimulates IL-8 secretion and regulates the immune response to infections [107]. Omer *et al.* [108] reported that phytogenic feed additive as LE (60 mg/100 ml Glycyrrhiza extract) had antiviral activity against Newcastle Disease Virus (NDV). Furthermore, glycyrrhizic acid (GRA) treated broilers at the level of (60 μg of GRA/mL of water) resulted in greater antibody titers against ND virus as well as boosted cellular immune response with the increase in blood lymphocyte and thrombocyte counts [109]. In addition, Dziewulska *et al.* [96] itemized that dietary LE (0.3-.5g/Kg body weight) prevents the replication of paramyxovirus type 1 in pigeons, and also the viral RNA copy number in the liver and kidney of pigeons fed with LE was around 4-fold inferior compared with that in the control pigeons. Accordingly, they proposed that LE has antiviral activity.

Also, glycyrrhizin inhibited the cytopathic impact of DHV, leading to antiviral effect [110] by an interaction with the membrane of the cell, which results in the reduction of endocytotic activity and decreases virus uptake [106]. Regarding the protection role of licorice, the inclusion in the broiler diet against aflatoxins, Al–Daraji *et al.* [111], stated that licorice supplemented at (150, 300 or 450 mg licorice/kg of diet) to the aflatoxicosis contaminated diet of broiler had significantly recovered the negative influences of aflatoxicosis on the majority of carcass variables. Finally, scientists have approved the positive impression of licorice on the immune potential; further explorations are mentioned to boost presence levels of LE in poultry diets and to decide their possible interfering physiological effects and economic value. A recent medical study displays that the bioactive constituents of licorice have anti-inflammatory, antioxidants, and immunomodulatory and antiviral properties, enhancing the immunity status of the bird body.

IMPACTS OF LICORICE ON SOME BLOOD COMPONENTS

The addition of LE (0.1, 0.2, or 0.3 g/L) in the drinking water of broiler chickens reduced serum glucose, total cholesterol and Low-density lipoprotein (LDL) ($P <$ 0.05) [112]. Inclusion of *Glycyrrhiza glabra* in broiler diets (0.5%) induced globulin concentration in the serum, these high levels of the globulin lead to best humoral immune status [113]. However, white blood cell (WBCs) count augmented (P <0.05) in broiler fed 0.5 and 1 g licorice/kg in the growth stages compared to the control. Also, licorice root encloses phytoestrogens that decrease the number of erythrocytes and boost erythrocyte sedimentation [114]. Additionally, injected LE stimulates activity in lymphocytes and cell cycle [115]. Sedghi *et al.* [116] suggested that serum LDL and cholesterol significantly reduced in birds given diets comprising licorice (0.5, 1, 2 g/kg) compared to the untreated group. Sharifi *et al.* [117] clarified that supplementation of roots of licorice in broiler diets (2 mg/kg diet) decreased blood constituents as LDL, cholesterol, and triglycerides and augmented the levels of high-density lipoprotein (HDL) in the serum. This may attribute to suppression of lipid peroxidation, lipoxygenase and cyclooxygenase enzymes, and reduction of LDL oxidation by licorice [118]. Besides, licorice (saponin) molecules are capable of decreasing LDL accompanying carotenoids and inhibit the lipid peroxide formation in birds fed licorice [119]. This significant reduction in LDL levels is linked with a hepatic clearance of LDL from the bloodstream and enhancement of cholesterol transformation rate to acids of bile by saponin [120, 121]. Notably, cholesterol-lowering influences of LE are accredited to the high synthesis of cholesterol, neutral sterols, bile acid, and enhancement in hepatic bile acid content [122]. In the other study, Al-Daraji [123] found an increase of glucose in the serum as affected by high levels of LE (150 to 450 mg/L of water) in the heat-stressed broiler.

On the other hand, Sedghi *et al.* [116] clarified that inclusion of licorice at level (0.5, 1, 2 g/kg) did not exert significant impacts on the differential of white blood cell such percentages of monocyte, heterophil (H), lymphocyte (L), H/L ratio and red blood cell proliferation. Besides, the levels of H and L and H/L ratio were not influenced by the supplementation of LE to drinking water at levels 0.1- 0.3 mg of

LE/L [97]. But the feeding on licorice (0.5, 1, 2 g/kg) in the study by Sedghi *et al.* [116] did not have a significant influence on triglyceride, HDL, very-low-density lipoprotein (VLDL) and glucose contents in blood serum of broiler. Also, Nakagawa *et al.* [22] found that dietary supplementation of LFO (2 g/kg) decreased serum glucose levels. LE's dietary inclusion augmented the levels of HDL and HDL/LDL ratio in serum due to flavonoids and ascorbic acid contained in LE [112]. Moreover, the inclusion of 0.4% licorice extracts in the drinking water of broilers augmented the content of HDL in the serum with the lowest ($P<0.05$) activity of alanine transaminase (ALT) [124]. However, Shahryar *et al.* [125] revealed no statistical impact of dietary inclusion of licorice powder (0.5, 1.0, 1.5 and 2.0%) on the serum blood components of the laying hens.

After considering that, the attendance of phytosterols and saponins in LE could be indispensable in cholesterol-lowering and improved the hepatic bile acid content in animals given LE. These compounds may replace cholesterol from the micelles in the intestinal lumen, lowering cholesterol absorption in the intestine, then reducing blood cholesterol [126]. Also, ascorbic acid and flavonoids were revealed to synergistically increase lipid profile and decline lipid peroxidation [127]. In this context, Fuhrman *et al.* [45] mentioned that LE has *in vitro* antioxidant activity. At the same time, Vaya *et al.* [128] and Fukai *et al.* [129] illustrated that the glabridin is one of the potent antioxidants able to prevent LDL oxidation.

IMPACT OF LICORICE ON GROWTH PERFORMANCE

Presently, significant multiple research recognized that growth parameter and laying production indices of poultry are generally enhanced *via* growth promoters or feed additives, which have a constructive effect on overall growth performance and health status [130]. Salary *et al.* [124] alarmed that the addition of 0.4% licorice extracts in drinking water of broilers augmented ($P<0.05$) feed consumption at 21 and 42 days and feed conversion ratio at 21 days of age but not affected body weight at different ages.

Both body weight and feed conversion rates have been improved as affected by the supplementation of LE at level 1% to the broiler chickens [131]. In a study on Japanese quails, Myandoab and Mansoub [132] described that a mixture of Liquorice root extract (200 ppm) and probiotic (1%) to the quail diet increased the body weight gain and daily feed intake significantly. Liquorice extract has affirmative properties on heat-stressed broiler chickens [133, 134].

Researchers have demonstrated the impacts of Glycyrrhizin on the growth parameters of broilers [135]. Regarding the application of glycyrrhizic acid

(GRA), broilers enriched with GRA (60 μg of GRA/mL of drinking water) had greater body weight and feed efficiency. The lowest mortality rate was compared with the controls [109]. Some of the previous investigations demonstrated that licorice powder's inclusion had no effects on the growth stimulation in broilers [97, 116, 125]. The previous study showed no significant difference in the feed consumption of laying hens fed with 0.5, 1.0, 1.5 and 2.0% of licorice powder [125]. Instantaneously, Hosseini *et al.* [105] point out that licorice at the level of 5 g/Kg in broiler diet had no significant impact on body weight, feed efficiency, and production index as livability. Furthermore, Moradi *et al.* [97] determined that the addition of a different level of LE into the drinking water of broiler (0.1, 0.2 and 0.3 mg of LE/L) exhibited no significant impacts on the growth performance variables compared with that in control. Likewise, the dietary addition of 0.5, 1, or 2g licorice extract/kg into broilers diet did not affect broiler's growth performance [116].

The improvement of productivity and the poultry's growth performance has been achieved by adding licorice with different levels and given in combination. The dietary inclusion of 1% mixture of licorice powder and garlic had improved the production performance of broiler birds [136 - 138]. Another study was conducted over broiler chicks (one day old, male, Ross 308) to explore the potential impacts of 1% licorice extract (*Glycyrrhiza glabra* L.) on growth performance, blood variables and immune state of broilers mixed with other plants, Yarrow, garlic, Eucalyptus, German chamomile, Iranian caraway and one antibiotic virginiamycin [139]. It has been reported that the LE can be able to decrease the abdominal fat of chicks without demonstrating any negative influences on the growth and immune responses of broilers when given along with drinking water for 42 days [140].

Efforts were achieved to debit the influence of dietary inclusion of peppermint, green tea, thyme and licorice in broiler chickens for improving their growth indices, carcass features, immune response and lipid profile. Results illustrated an overall improvement in the performance of chicks at level (200 and 1000 ppm) compared to the control and a noteworthy enhancement in humoral immunity compared to the positive control. Results suggested including LE blend at the 200 ppm in poultry nutrition to promote the immune profile and performance and as an alternative to antibiotics as a growth promoter [141]. The licorice root (*Glycyrrhiza glabra*) extract given in the diet of laying hens also improved the production of functional eggs and modulated the performance, lower cholesterol in the egg, and LDL with a rise in plasma HDL and total antioxidant capacity of plasma-based on a study performed over one hundred 40-week old laying hens [142]. Literature perceived the global impression of this phytogenic on performance, immune state, haematological and biochemical components and other carcass criteria and meat quality when liquorice (*Glycyrrhiza glabra*) is supplemented in poultry diet either in feed and/or with drinking water [10].

CONCLUDING REMARKS

In this chapter, it has been hypothesized that the extract of *Glycyrrhiza glabra* may play a great part in the preparation of many pharmaceutical components for promoting its employ in poultry nutrition. Licorice comprises many bioactive compounds such as glycyrrhizin, saponins, tannis and flavonoids, which possess many pharmacological activities and medicinal approaches. The major advantage of licorice extract can be described in the possibility of given throughout poultry rearing without any harmful effects. It is a valuable herb for the poultry sector as its extracts have potent immunogenic and antioxidant activity, besides its capacity to treat health problems in poultry farms due to its effectiveness against respiratory, digestive and immune problems. Also, licorice extract inclusion in poultry diets has a beneficial effect on productive performance, food intake, blood haematological and biochemical indices and carcass traits. Nevertheless, we recommend more researches to investigate other beneficial properties of this multipurpose medicinal plant. Exploring more researches on licorice and its bioactive compounds, conducting appropriate validation and clinical trials as well as exploiting the recent advances in biotechnology, nanotechnology and pharmacology would promote the nutritional and medicinal values of this important herb for enhancing productivity and protecting the health of poultry. Great efforts need to be made to improve the distribution of this significant herb in poultry by exploring the practices of nanodelivery and *in ovo* delivery of supplements for powerfully improving the production and boosting the health profile of birds in a better way.

CONSENT FOR PUBLICATION

Not Applicable.

CONFLICT OF INTEREST

The author confirms that this chapter contents have no conflict of interest.

ACKNOWLEDGEMENTS

Declared none.

REFERENCES

[1]   Dhama K, Karthik K, Khandia R, *et al.* Medicinal and therapeutic potential of herbs and plant metabolites/extracts countering viral pathogens-current knowledge and future prospects. Curr Drug Metab 2018; 19(3): 236-63.

[http://dx.doi.org/10.2174/1389200219666180129145252] [PMID: 29380697]

[2]   Dhama K, Tiwari R, Chakraborty S, *et al.* Evidence based antibacterial potentials of medicinal plants and herbs countering bacterial pathogens especially in the era of emerging drug resistance: An integrated update. Int J Pharmacol 2014; 10(1): 1-43.
[http://dx.doi.org/10.3923/ijp.2014.1.43]

[3]   Laudadio V, Lorusso V, Lastella NMB, *et al.* Enhancement of nutraceutical value of table eggs through poultry feeding strategies. Int J Pharmacol 2015; 11(3): 201-12.
[http://dx.doi.org/10.3923/ijp.2015.201.212]

[4]   Yadav AS, Kolluri G, Gopi M, Karthik K, Malik YS, Dhama K. Exploring alternatives to antibiotics as health promoting agents in poultry- a review. J Exp Biol Agric Sci 2016; 4(3s): 368-83.
[http://dx.doi.org/10.18006/2016.4(3S).368.383]

[5]   Alagawany M, Abd El-Hack ME, Farag MR, Sachan S, Karthik K, Dhama K. The use of probiotics as eco-friendly alternatives for antibiotics in poultry nutrition. Environ Sci Pollut Res Int 2018; 25(11): 10611-8.
[http://dx.doi.org/10.1007/s11356-018-1687-x] [PMID: 29532377]

[6]   Arif M, Hayat Z, Abd El-Hack ME, *et al.* Impacts of supplementing broiler diets with a powder mixture of black cumin, Moringa and chicory seeds. S Afr J Anim Sci 2019; 49(3): 564-72.
[http://dx.doi.org/10.4314/sajas.v49i3.17]

[7]   Ashour EA, El-Kholy MS, Alagawany M, *et al.* Effect of dietary supplementation with *Moringa oleifera* leaves and/or seeds powder on production, egg characteristics, hatchability and blood chemistry of laying japanese quails. Sustainability 2020; 12(6): 2463.
[http://dx.doi.org/10.3390/su12062463]

[8]   Shebl RI, Amin MA, Emad-Eldin A, *et al.* Antiviral activity of liquorice powder extract against varicella zoster virus isolated from Egyptian patients. Chang Gung Med J 2012; 35(3): 231-9.
[PMID: 22735054]

[9]   Alagawany M, Elnesr SS, Farag MR, *et al.* Use of licorice (*Glycyrrhiza glabra*) herb as a feed additive in poultry: Current knowledge and prospects. Animals (Basel) 2019; 9(8): 536. a
[http://dx.doi.org/10.3390/ani9080536] [PMID: 31394812]

[10]   Alagawany M, Elnesr SS, Farag MR. Use of liquorice (*Glycyrrhiza glabra*) in poultry nutrition: Global impacts on performance, carcass and meat quality. Worlds Poult Sci J 2019; 75(2): 293-304.
[http://dx.doi.org/10.1017/S0043933919000059]

[11]   Quirós-Sauceda AE, Ovando-Martínez M, Velderrain-Rodríguez GR, González-Aguilar GA, Ayala-Zavala JF. Essential Oils in Food Preservation, Flavor and Safety. Licorice (*Glycyrrhiza glabra* Linn.) oils. Academic Press 2016; pp. 523-30.
[http://dx.doi.org/10.1016/B978-0-12-416641-7.00060-2]

[12]   Karkanis A, Martins N, Petropoulos SA, Ferreira ICFR. Phytochemical composition, health effects, and crop management of liquorice (*Glycyrrhiza. glabra* L.): A medicinal plant. Food Rev Int 2016; 34(2): 1-22.

[13]   Tiwari R, Latheef SK, Ahmed I, *et al.* Herbal immunomodulators, a remedial panacea for the designing and developing effective drugs and medicines: Current scenario and future prospects. Curr Drug Metab 2018; 19(3): 264-301.
[http://dx.doi.org/10.2174/1389200219666180129125436] [PMID: 29380694]

[14]   Mukhopadhyay M, Panja P. A novel process for extraction of natural sweetener from licorice (*Glycyrrhiza glabra*) roots Separation and Purification. Technol 2008; 63: 539-45.

[15]   Shalaby MA, Ibrahim HS, Mahmoud EM, Mahmoud AF. Some effects of *Glycyrrhiza glabra* (liquorice) roots extract on male rats. Egyptian J Nat Toxins 2004; 1: 83-94.

[16]   Peters MC, Tallman JA, Braun TM, Jacobson JJ. Clinical reduction of S. mutans in pre-school children using a novel liquorice root extract lollipop: a pilot study. Eur Arch Paediatr Dent 2010;

11(6): 274e8.

[17] Krishnakumar G, Gaviappa D, Guruswamy S. Anticaries efficacy of liquorice lollipop: an *ex vivo* study. J Contemp Dent Pract 2018; 19(8): 937-42.
[http://dx.doi.org/10.5005/jp-journals-10024-2361] [PMID: 30150493]

[18] Racková L, Jancinová V, Petríková M, *et al.* Mechanism of anti-inflammatory action of liquorice extract and glycyrrhizin. Nat Prod Res 2007; 21(14): 1234-41.
[http://dx.doi.org/10.1080/14786410701371280] [PMID: 18075885]

[19] Suchitra G, Shakunthala V. Effect of *Glycyrrhiza glabra* root extract on behaviour and fitness of drosophila melanogaster and vestigial wing mutant. Int J Curr Microbiol Appl Sci 2014; 3(7): 1047-54.

[20] Aoki F, Honda S, Kishida H, *et al.* Suppression by licorice flavonoids of abdominal fat accumulation and body weight gain in high-fat diet-induced obese C57BL/6J mice. Biosci Biotechnol Biochem 2007; 71(1): 206-14.
[http://dx.doi.org/10.1271/bbb.60463] [PMID: 17213668]

[21] Armanini D, De Palo CB, Mattarello MJ, *et al.* Effect of licorice on the reduction of body fat mass in healthy subjects. J Endocrinol Invest 2003; 26(7): 646-50.
[http://dx.doi.org/10.1007/BF03347023] [PMID: 14594116]

[22] Nakagawa K, Kishida H, Arai N, Nishiyama T, Mae T. Licorice flavonoids suppress abdominal fat accumulation and increase in blood glucose level in obese diabetic KK-A(y) mice. Biol Pharm Bull 2004; 27(11): 1775-8.
[http://dx.doi.org/10.1248/bpb.27.1775] [PMID: 15516721]

[23] Parvaiz M, Hussain K, Khalid S, *et al.* A review: Medicinal importance of *Glycyrrhiza glabra* L. (Fabaceace Family). Glob J Pharmacol 2014; 8: 8-13.

[24] He Y, Ci X, Xie Y, *et al.* Potential detoxification effect of active ingredients in liquorice by upregulating efflux transporter. Phytomedicine 2019; 56: 175-82.
[http://dx.doi.org/10.1016/j.phymed.2018.10.033] [PMID: 30668338]

[25] Snow J. *Glycyrrhiza glabra* monograph. J Bot Med 1996; 1: 9-14.

[26] Fukai J, Baosheng C, Marun K, *et al.* An isopernylated flavonone from *Glycyrrhiza glabra* and re-assay of liquorice phenols. Phytochemistry 1998; 49(18): 2005-13.
[http://dx.doi.org/10.1016/S0031-9422(98)00389-6]

[27] Arystanova TP, Irismetov MP, Sopbekova AO. Chromatographic determination of glycyrrhizinic acid in *Glycyrrhiza glabra* preparation. Chem Nat Compd 2001; 1(37): 89-90.
[http://dx.doi.org/10.1023/A:1017675115337]

[28] Badr SE, Sakr DM, Mahfouz SA, Abdelfattah MS. Licorice (*Glycyrrhiza glabra* L.): Chemical composition and biological impacts. Res J Pharm Biol Chem Sci 2013; 4: 606-21.

[29] Li W, Asada Y, Yoshikawa T. Flavonoid constituents from *Glycyrrhiza glabra* hairy root cultures. Phytochemistry 2000; 55(5): 447-56.
[http://dx.doi.org/10.1016/S0031-9422(00)00337-X] [PMID: 11140606]

[30] Zhang LQ, Yang XW. Intestinal permeability of liquiritin and isoliquiritin in the Caco-2 cell monolayer model. J Chin Pharm Sci 2010; 19: 451-8.
[http://dx.doi.org/10.5246/jcps.2010.06.060]

[31] Fiore C, Eisenhut M, Krausse R, *et al.* Antiviral effects of Glycyrrhiza species. Phytother Res 2008; 22(2): 141-8.
[http://dx.doi.org/10.1002/ptr.2295] [PMID: 17886224]

[32] Sohail M, Rakha A, Butt MS, Asghar M. Investigating the antioxidant potential of licorice extracts obtained through different extraction modes. J Food Biochem 2018; 42(2): e12466.
[http://dx.doi.org/10.1111/jfbc.12466] ·

[33]   Mao SJ, Hou SX, He R, *et al.* Uptake of albumin nanoparticle surface modified with glycyrrhizin by primary cultured rat hepatocytes. World J Gastroenterol 2005; 11(20): 3075-9.
[http://dx.doi.org/10.3748/wjg.v11.i20.3075] [PMID: 15918193]

[34]   Shabani L, Ehsanpour AA, Asghari G, Emami J. Glycyrrhizin production by *in vitro* cultured *Glycyrrhiza glabra* elicited by methyl jasmonate and salicylic acid. Russ J Plant Physiol 2009; 56(5): 621-6.
[http://dx.doi.org/10.1134/S1021443709050069]

[35]   Dastagir G, Rizvi MA. *Glycyrrhiza glabra* L. (Liquorice). Pak J Pharm Sci 2016; 29(5): 1727-33.
[PMID: 27731836]

[36]   Li JR, Wang YQ, Deng ZZ. Two new compounds from *Glycyrrhiza glabra*. J Asian Nat Prod Res 2005; 7(4): 677-80.
[http://dx.doi.org/10.1080/10286020310001625067] [PMID: 16087644]

[37]   Erdoğan Z, Erdoğan S, Doğanlar ZB, Doğanlar O, Canoğulları S. *Glycyrrhiza glabra* protects the liver hepatocytes from the volatile organic compounds. Toxicol Lett 2016; (258): S180.
[http://dx.doi.org/10.1016/j.toxlet.2016.06.1668]

[38]   Asl MN, Hosseinzadeh H. Review of pharmacological effects of Glycyrrhiza sp. and its bioactive compounds. Phytother Res 2008; 22(6): 709-24.
[http://dx.doi.org/10.1002/ptr.2362] [PMID: 18446848]

[39]   Ohno H, Araho D, Uesawa Y, *et al.* Evaluation of cytotoxiciy and tumor-specificity of licorice flavonoids based on chemical structure. Anticancer Res 2013; 33(8): 3061-8.
[PMID: 23898061]

[40]   Martins N, Barros L, Duenas M, Santos-Buelga C, Ferreira IC. Characterization of phenolic compounds and antioxidant properties of *Glycyrrhiza glabra* L. rhizomes and roots. RSC Adv 2015; 5(34): 26991-7.
[http://dx.doi.org/10.1039/C5RA03963K]

[41]   Hosseinzadeh H, Nassiri-Asl M. Pharmacological effects of *Glycyrrhiza spp.* and its bioactive constituents: update and review. Phytother Res 2015; 29(12): 1868-86.
[http://dx.doi.org/10.1002/ptr.5487] [PMID: 26462981]

[42]   Shibata S. A drug over the millennia: pharmacognosy, chemistry, and pharmacology of licorice. Yakugaku Zasshi 2000; 120(10): 849-62.
[http://dx.doi.org/10.1248/yakushi1947.120.10_849] [PMID: 11082698]

[43]   Michaelis M, Geiler J, Naczk P, *et al.* Glycyrrhizin exerts antioxidative effects in H_5N_1 influenza A virus-infected cells and inhibits virus replication and pro-inflammatory gene expression. PLoS One 2001; 6.
[PMID: 21611183]

[44]   Shi JR, Mao LG, Jiang RA, Qian Y, Tang HF, Chen JQ. Monoammonium glycyrrhizinate inhibited the inflammation of LPS-induced acute lung injury in mice. Int Immunopharmacol 2010; 10(10): 1235-41.
[http://dx.doi.org/10.1016/j.intimp.2010.07.004] [PMID: 20637836]

[45]   Fuhrman B, Volkova N, Kaplan M, *et al.* Antiatherosclerotic effects of licorice extract supplementation on hypercholesterolemic patients: increased resistance of LDL to atherogenic modifications, reduced plasma lipid levels, and decreased systolic blood pressure. Nutrition 2002; 18(3): 268-73.
[http://dx.doi.org/10.1016/S0899-9007(01)00753-5] [PMID: 11882402]

[46]   Sato J, Goto K, Nanjo F, Kawai S, Murata K. Antifungal activity of plant extracts against *Arthrinium sacchari* and *Chaetomium funicola*. J Biosci Bioeng 2000; 90(4): 442-6.
[http://dx.doi.org/10.1016/S1389-1723(01)80016-5] [PMID: 16232887]

[47]   Fukai T, Marumo A, Kaitou K, Kanda T, Terada S, Nomura T. Anti-*Helicobacter pylori* flavonoids

from licorice extract. Life Sci 2002; 71(12): 1449-63.
[http://dx.doi.org/10.1016/S0024-3205(02)01864-7] [PMID: 12127165]

[48]   Tamir S, Eizenberg M, Somjen D, Izrael S, Vaya J. Estrogen-like activity of glabrene and other constituents isolated from licorice root. J Steroid Biochem Mol Biol 2001; 78(3): 291-8.
[http://dx.doi.org/10.1016/S0960-0760(01)00093-0] [PMID: 11595510]

[49]   Somjen D, Knoll E, Vaya J, Stern N, Tamir S. Estrogen-like activity of licorice root constituents: glabridin and glabrene, in vascular tissues *in vitro* and *in vivo*. J Steroid Biochem Mol Biol 2004; 91(3): 147-55.
[http://dx.doi.org/10.1016/j.jsbmb.2004.04.003] [PMID: 15276622]

[50]   Nowakowska Z. A review of anti-infective and anti-inflammatory chalcones. Eur J Med Chem 2007; 42(2): 125-37.
[http://dx.doi.org/10.1016/j.ejmech.2006.09.019] [PMID: 17112640]

[51]   Arora P, Wani ZA, Nalli Y, Ali A, Riyaz-Ul-Hassan S. Antimicrobial potential of thiodiketopiperazine derivatives produced by *Phoma sp.*, an Endophyte of *Glycyrrhiza glabra* Linn. Microb Ecol 2016; 72(4): 802-12.
[http://dx.doi.org/10.1007/s00248-016-0805-x] [PMID: 27357141]

[52]   Ajagannanavar SL, Battur H, Shamarao S, Sivakumar V, Patil PU, Shanavas P. Effect of aqueous and alcoholic licorice (*Glycyrrhiza glabra*) root extract against streptococcus mutans and lactobacillus acidophilus in comparison to chlorhexidine: an *in vitro* study. J Int Oral Health 2014; 6(4): 29-34.
[PMID: 25214729]

[53]   Doeker BM, Andler W. Liquorice, growth retardation and Addison's disease. Horm Res 1999; 52(5): 253-5.
[PMID: 10844416]

[54]   Al-Qarawi AA, Abdel-Rahman HA, El-Mougy SA. Hepatoprotective activity of licorice in rat liver injury models. J Herbs Spices Med Plants 2001; 8(1): 7-14.
[http://dx.doi.org/10.1300/J044v08n01_02]

[55]   Kim KR, Jeong CK, Park KK, *et al.* Anti-inflammatory effects of licorice and roasted licorice extracts on TPA-induced acute inflammation and collagen-induced arthritis in mice. J Biomed Biotechnol 2010; 2010: 709378.
[http://dx.doi.org/10.1155/2010/709378] [PMID: 20300198]

[56]   Ottenbacher R, Blehm J. An unusual case of licorice-induced hypertensive crisis. S D Med 2015; 68(8): 346-347, 349.
[PMID: 26380428]

[57]   Heikens J, Fliers E, Endert E, Ackermans M, van Montfrans G. Liquorice-induced hypertension--a new understanding of an old disease: case report and brief review. Neth J Med 1995; 47(5): 230-4.
[http://dx.doi.org/10.1016/0300-2977(95)00015-5] [PMID: 8544895]

[58]   Sardi A, Geda C, Nerici L, Bertello P. [Rhabdomyolysis and arterial hypertension caused by apparent excess of mineralocorticoids: a case report]. Ann Ital Med Int 2002; 17(2): 126-9.
[http://dx.doi.org/10.1016/0300-2977(95)00015-5] [PMID: 12150047]

[59]   Zadeh JB, Kor ZM, Goftar MK. Licorice (*Glycyrrhiza glabra* Linn) as a valuable medicinal plant. Int J Adv Biol Biomed Res 2013; 1(10): 1281-8.

[60]   Cho HJ, Lim SS, Lee YS, *et al.* Hexane/ethanol extract of Glycyrrhiza uralensis licorice exerts potent anti-inflammatory effects in murine macrophages and in mouse skin. Food Chem 2010; 121(4): 959-66.
[http://dx.doi.org/10.1016/j.foodchem.2010.01.027]

[61]   Xiao-Hong MA, Peng ZH, Han FM, Chen Y. Inhibitory effects of triptolide on rat CYP450 enzymes and the metabolic interaction with glycyrrhetinic acid *in vitro*. China Acad J 2013; 28: 691-4.

[62]   He W, Ning J, Wu JJ, *et al.* Research progress in interaction between chemical components of

Glycyrrhizae Radix and cytochrome P450 enzyme. Chin Tradit Herbal Drugs 2016; 47: 1974-81.

[63]   Huo HZ, Wang B, Liang YK, Bao YY, Gu Y. Hepatoprotective and antioxidant effects of licorice extract against CCI$_4$-induced oxidative damage in rats. Int J Mol Sci 2011; 12(10): 6529-43.
[http://dx.doi.org/10.3390/ijms12106529] [PMID: 22072903]

[64]   Vilar Gomez E, Rodriguez De Miranda A, Gra Oramas B, *et al.* Clinical trial: a nutritional supplement Viusid, in combination with diet and exercise, in patients with nonalcoholic fatty liver disease. Aliment pharmacol Therap 2009; 30(10): 999-1009.
[http://dx.doi.org/10.1111/j.1365-2036.2009.04122.x]

[65]   Omar HR, Komarova I, El-Ghonemi M, *et al.* Licorice abuse: time to send a warning message. Ther Adv Endocrinol Metab 2012; 3(4): 125-38.
[http://dx.doi.org/10.1177/2042018812454322] [PMID: 23185686]

[66]   Fu Y, Chen J, Li YJ, Zheng YF, Li P. Antioxidant and anti-inflammatory activities of six flavonoids separated from licorice. Food Chem 2013; 141(2): 1063-71.
[http://dx.doi.org/10.1016/j.foodchem.2013.03.089] [PMID: 23790887]

[67]   Jeong HG, You HJ, Park SJ, *et al.* Hepatoprotective effects of 18β-glycyrrhetinic acid on carbon tetrachloride-induced liver injury: inhibition of cytochrome P450 2E1 expression. Pharmacol Res 2002; 46(3): 221-7.
[http://dx.doi.org/10.1016/S1043-6618(02)00121-4] [PMID: 12220964]

[68]   Chen X, Liu Z, Meng R, Shi C, Guo N. Antioxidative and anticancer properties of Licochalcone A from licorice. J Ethnopharmacol 2017; 198: 331-7.
[http://dx.doi.org/10.1016/j.jep.2017.01.028] [PMID: 28111219]

[69]   Rahal A, Kumar A, Singh V, *et al.* Oxidative stress, prooxidants, and antioxidants: the interplay. BioMed Res Int 2014; 2014: 761264.
[http://dx.doi.org/10.1155/2014/761264] [PMID: 24587990]

[70]   Vlaisavljević S, Šibul F, Sinka I, Zupko I, Ocsovszki I, Jovanović-Šanta S. Chemical composition, antioxidant and anticancer activity of licorice from Fruska Gora locality. Ind Crops Prod 2018; 112: 217-24.
[http://dx.doi.org/10.1016/j.indcrop.2017.11.050]

[71]   Yatoo MI, Gopalakrishnan A, Saxena A, *et al.* Anti-inflammatory drugs and herbs with special emphasis on herbal medicines for countering inflammatory diseases and disorders - a review. Recent Pat Inflamm Allergy Drug Discov 2018; 12(1): 39-58.
[http://dx.doi.org/10.2174/1872213X12666180115153635] [PMID: 29336271]

[72]   Asan-Ozusaglam M, Karakoca K. Evaluation of biological activity and antioxidant capacity of Turkish licorice root extracts. Rom Biotechnol Lett 2014; 19(1): 8994.

[73]   Zhou H, Wang C, Ye J, Chen H, Tao R. Effects of dietary supplementation of fermented Ginkgo biloba L. residues on growth performance, nutrient digestibility, serum biochemical parameters and immune function in weaned piglets. Anim Sci J 2015; 86(8): 790-9.
[http://dx.doi.org/10.1111/asj.12361] [PMID: 25827443]

[74]   Ashawat MS, Shailendra S, Swarnlata S. *In vitro* antioxidant activity of ethanolic extracts of Centella asiatica, Punica granatum, *Glycyrrhiza glabra* and *Areca catechu.* Res J Med Plant 2007; 1(1): 13-6.
[http://dx.doi.org/10.3923/rjmp.2007.13.16]

[75]   Haraguchi H, Yoshida N, Ishikawa H, Tamura Y, Mizutani K, Kinoshita T. Protection of mitochondrial functions against oxidative stresses by isoflavans from *Glycyrrhiza glabra.* J Pharm Pharmacol 2000; 52(2): 219-23.
[http://dx.doi.org/10.1211/0022357001773724] [PMID: 10714953]

[76]   Takeuchi T, Nishii O, Okamura T, Yaginuma T. Effect of paeoniflorin, glycyrrhizin and glycyrrhetic acid on ovarian androgen production. Am J Chin Med 1991; 19(1): 73-8.
[http://dx.doi.org/10.1142/S0192415X91000119] [PMID: 1897494]

[77]   Visavadiya NP, Soni B, Dalwadi N. Evaluation of antioxidant and anti-atherogenic properties of *Glycyrrhiza glabra* root using *in vitro* models. Int J Food Sci Nut 2009; 60(sup2): 49-135.

[78]   Awadein NB, Eid YZ, Abd El-Ghany FA. Effect of dietary supplementation with phytoestrogens sources before sexual maturity on productive performance of mandarah hens. Egypt Poult Sci 2010; 30(3): 829-46.

[79]   Yang CL, Or TC, Ho MH, Lau AS. Scientific basis of botanical medicine as alternative remedies for rheumatoid arthritis. Clin Rev Allergy Immunol 2013; 44(3): 284-300.
       [http://dx.doi.org/10.1007/s12016-012-8329-8] [PMID: 22700248]

[80]   Matsuzaki K, Murata M, Yoshida K, *et al.* Chronic inflammation associated with hepatitis C virus infection perturbs hepatic transforming growth factor beta signaling, promoting cirrhosis and hepatocellular carcinoma. Hepatology 2007; 46(1): 48-57.
       [http://dx.doi.org/10.1002/hep.21672] [PMID: 17596875]

[81]   Fujisawa Y, Sakamoto M, Matsushita M, Fujita T, Nishioka K. Glycyrrhizin inhibits the lytic pathway of complement--possible mechanism of its anti-inflammatory effect on liver cells in viral hepatitis. Microbiol Immunol 2000; 44(9): 799-804.
       [http://dx.doi.org/10.1111/j.1348-0421.2000.tb02566.x] [PMID: 11092245]

[82]   Chu X, Ci X, Wei M, *et al.* Licochalcone a inhibits lipopolysaccharide-induced inflammatory response *in vitro* and *in vivo*. J Agric Food Chem 2012; 60(15): 3947-54.
       [http://dx.doi.org/10.1021/jf2051587] [PMID: 22400806]

[83]   Kim J, Kim J, Shim J, *et al.* Licorice-derived dehydroglyasperin C increases MKP-1 expression and suppresses inflammation-mediated neurodegeneration. Neurochem Int 2013; 63(8): 732-40.
       [http://dx.doi.org/10.1016/j.neuint.2013.09.013] [PMID: 24083986]

[84]   Jung JC, Lee YH, Kim SH, *et al.* Hepatoprotective effect of licorice, the root of Glycyrrhiza uralensis Fischer, in alcohol-induced fatty liver disease. BMC Complement Altern Med 2016; 16: 19.
       [http://dx.doi.org/10.1186/s12906-016-0997-0] [PMID: 26801973]

[85]   Guo A, He D, Xu HB, Geng CA, Zhao J. Promotion of regulatory T cell induction by immunomodulatory herbal medicine licorice and its two constituents. Sci Rep 2015; 5: 14046.
       [http://dx.doi.org/10.1038/srep14046] [PMID: 26370586]

[86]   Yu JY, Ha JY, Kim KM, Jung YS, Jung JC, Oh S. Anti-Inflammatory activities of licorice extract and its active compounds, glycyrrhizic acid, liquiritin and liquiritigenin, in BV2 cells and mice liver. Molecules 2015; 20(7): 13041-54.
       [http://dx.doi.org/10.3390/molecules200713041] [PMID: 26205049]

[87]   Simmler C, Pauli GF, Chen SN. Phytochemistry and biological properties of glabridin. Fitoterapia 2013; 90: 160-84.
       [http://dx.doi.org/10.1016/j.fitote.2013.07.003] [PMID: 23850540]

[88]   Song NR, Kim JE, Park JS, *et al.* Licochalcone A, a polyphenol present in licorice, suppresses UV-induced COX-2 expression by targeting PI3K, MEK1, and B-Raf. Int J Mol Sci 2015; 16(3): 4453-70.
       [http://dx.doi.org/10.3390/ijms16034453] [PMID: 25710724]

[89]   Liu DY, Gao L, Zhang J, Huo XW, Ni H, Cao L. Anti-inflammatory and Anti-oxidant Effects of Licorice Flavonoids on Ulcerative Colitis in Mouse Model. Chin Herb Med 2017; 9: 358-68.
       [http://dx.doi.org/10.1016/S1674-6384(17)60116-3]

[90]   Alkofahi A, Atta AH. Pharmacological screening of the anti-ulcerogenic effects of some Jordanian medicinal plants in rats. J Ethnopharmacol 1999; 67(3): 341-5.
       [http://dx.doi.org/10.1016/S0378-8741(98)00126-3] [PMID: 10617070]

[91]   Jagadeeswaran A, Selvasubramanian S. Effect of supplementation of licorice root (*Glycyrrhiza glabra* L.) extracts on immune status in commercial broilers. Int J Adv Vet Sci Technol 2014; 3: 88-92.
       [http://dx.doi.org/10.23953/cloud.ijavst.190]

[92]   Gilani SM, Zehra S, Galani S, Ashraf A. Effect of natural growth promoters on immunity, and biochemical and haematological parameters of broiler chickens. Trop J Pharm Res 2018; 17(4): 627-33.
[http://dx.doi.org/10.4314/tjpr.v17i4.9]

[93]   Dorhoi A, Dobrean V, Zăhan M, Virag P. Modulatory effects of several herbal extracts on avian peripheral blood cell immune responses. Phytother Res 2006; 20(5): 8-352. 20:352–8.
[http://dx.doi.org/10.1002/ptr.1859]

[94]   Jassal PS, Kaur G, Kaur L. Synergistic effect of *Curcuma longa* and *Glycyrrhiza glabra* extracts with copper ions on food spoilage bacteria. Int J Pharm Pharm Sci 2015; 7: 371-5.

[95]   Utsunomiya T, Kobayashi M, Pollard RB, Suzuki F. Glycyrrhizin, an active component of licorice roots, reduces morbidity and mortality of mice infected with lethal doses of influenza virus. Antimicrob Agents Chemother 1997; 41(3): 551-6.
[http://dx.doi.org/10.1128/AAC.41.3.551] [PMID: 9055991]

[96]   Dziewulska D, Stenzel T, Śmiałek M, Tykałowski B, Koncicki A. The impact of Aloe vera and licorice extracts on selected mechanisms of humoral and cell-mediated immunity in pigeons experimentally infected with PPMV-1. BMC Vet Res 2018; 14(1): 148.
[http://dx.doi.org/10.1186/s12917-018-1467-3] [PMID: 29716604]

[97]   Moradi N, Ghazi S, Amjadian T, Khamisabadi H, Habibian M. Performance and some immunological parameter responses of broiler chickens to licorice (*Glycyrrhiza glabra*) extract administration in the drinking water. Annu Res Rev Biol 2014; 4: 675-83.
[http://dx.doi.org/10.9734/ARRB/2014/5277]

[98]   Ashfaq UA, Masoud MS, Nawaz Z, Riazuddin S. Glycyrrhizin as antiviral agent against Hepatitis C Virus. J Transl Med 2011; 9(1): 112.
[http://dx.doi.org/10.1186/1479-5876-9-112] [PMID: 21762538]

[99]   Adianti M, Aoki C, Komoto M, *et al.* Anti-hepatitis C virus compounds obtained from Glycyrrhiza uralensis and other Glycyrrhiza species. Microbiol Immunol 2014; 58(3): 180-7.
[http://dx.doi.org/10.1111/1348-0421.12127] [PMID: 24397541]

[100]   Kalantar M, Hosseini SM, Yang L, *et al.* Performance, immune, and carcass characteristics of broiler chickens as affected by thyme and licorice or enzyme supplemented. Open J Anim Sci 2017; 7: 105-9.
[http://dx.doi.org/10.4236/ojas.2017.72009]

[101]   Toghyani M, Tohidi M, Gheisari AB, Tabeidian SA. Performance, immunity, serum biochemical and hematological parameters in broiler chicks fed dietary thyme as alternative for an antibiotic growth promoter. Afr J Biotechnol 2010; 9: 6819-25.

[102]   Zhang YH, Isobe K, Nagase F, *et al.* Glycyrrhizin as a promoter of the late signal transduction for interleukin-2 production by splenic lymphocytes. Immunology 1993; 79(4): 528-34.
[PMID: 8406577]

[103]   Dai JH, Iwatani Y, Ishida T, *et al.* Glycyrrhizin enhances interleukin-12 production in peritoneal macrophages. Immunology 2001; 103(2): 235-43.
[http://dx.doi.org/10.1046/j.1365-2567.2001.01224.x] [PMID: 11412311]

[104]   Crance JM, Scaramozzino N, Jouan A, Garin D. Interferon, ribavirin, 6-azauridine and glycyrrhizin: antiviral compounds active against pathogenic flaviviruses. Antiviral Res 2003; 58(1): 73-9.
[http://dx.doi.org/10.1016/S0166-3542(02)00185-7] [PMID: 12719009]

[105]   Hosseini SA, Goudarzi M, Zarei A, Meimandipour A, Sadeghipanah A. The effects of funnel and licorice on immune response, blood parameter and gastrointestinal organs in broiler chicks. Iran J Med Arom Plants 2014; 30: 583-90.
[http://dx.doi.org/10.22092/ijmapr.2014.9837]

[106]   Wolkerstorfer A, Kurz H, Bachhofner N, Szolar OH. Glycyrrhizin inhibits influenza A virus uptake into the cell. Antiviral Res 2009; 83(2): 171-8.

[http://dx.doi.org/10.1016/j.antiviral.2009.04.012] [PMID: 19416738]

[107] Shaneyfelt ME, Burke AD, Graff JW, Jutila MA, Hardy ME. Natural products that reduce rotavirus infectivity identified by a cell-based moderate-throughput screening assay. Virol J 2006; 3(1): 68.
[http://dx.doi.org/10.1186/1743-422X-3-68] [PMID: 16948846]

[108] Omer MO, Almalki WH, Shahid I, Khuram S, Altaf I, Imran S. Comparative study to evaluate the anti-viral efficacy of *Glycyrrhiza glabra* extract and ribavirin against the Newcastle disease virus. Pharmacognosy Res 2014; 6(1): 6-11.
[http://dx.doi.org/10.4103/0974-8490.122911] [PMID: 24497736]

[109] Ocampo CL, Gómez-Verduzco G, Tapia-Perez G, Gutierrez OL, Sumano LH. Effects of glycyrrhizic acid on productive and immune parameters of broilers. Braz J Poult Sci 2016; 18: 435-42.
[http://dx.doi.org/10.1590/1806-9061-2015-0135]

[110] Soufy H, Yassein S, Ahmed AR, *et al.* Antiviral and immune stimulant activities of glycyrrhizin against duck hepatitis virus. Afr J Tradit Complement Altern Med 2012; 9(3): 389-95.
[http://dx.doi.org/10.4314/ajtcam.v9i3.14] [PMID: 23983372]

[111] Al-Daraji HJ, Taha AK. A study on herbal protection of aflatoxicosis in broiler chickens by dietary addition of licorice extract. Iraqi Poult Sci J 2006; 1(1): 129-44.

[112] Naser M, Shahab G, Mahmood H. Drinking water supplementation of licorice (*Glycyrrhiza glabra* L. root) extract as an alternative to in-feed antibiotic growth promoter in broiler chickens GSC. Biol Pharm Bull 2017; 1(3): 20-8.

[113] Rezaei M, Kalantar M, Nasr J. Thymus vulgaris L., *Glycyrrhiza glabra* and combo enzyme in corn or barley-basal diets in broiler chickens. Int J Plant Anim Environ Sci 2014; 4: 418-23.

[114] Huang CF, Lin SS, Liao PH, Young SC, Yang CC. The immunopharmaceutical effects and mechanisms of herb medicine. Cell Mol Immunol 2008; 5(1): 23-31.
[http://dx.doi.org/10.1038/cmi.2008.3] [PMID: 18318991]

[115] Isbrucker RA, Burdock GA. Risk and safety assessment on the consumption of Licorice root (Glycyrrhiza sp.), its extract and powder as a food ingredient, with emphasis on the pharmacology and toxicology of glycyrrhizin. Regul Toxicol Pharmacol 2006; 46(3): 167-92.
[http://dx.doi.org/10.1016/j.yrtph.2006.06.002] [PMID: 16884839]

[116] Sedghi M, Golian A, Kermanshahi H, Ahmadi H. Effect of dietary supplementation of licorice extract and a prebiotic on performance and blood metabolites of broilers. S Afr J Anim Sci 2010; 40: 371-80.

[117] Sharifi SD, Khorsandi SH, Khadem AA, Salehi A, Moslehi H. The effect of four medicinal plants on the performance, blood biochemical traits and ileal microflora of broiler chicks. Vet Arh 2013; 83(1): 69-80.

[118] Craig WJ. Health-promoting properties of common herbs. Am J Clin Nutr 1999; 70(3) (Suppl.): 491S-9S.
[http://dx.doi.org/10.1093/ajcn/70.3.491s] [PMID: 10479221]

[119] Belinky PA, Aviram M, Fuhrman B, Rosenblat M, Vaya J. The antioxidative effects of the isoflavan glabridin on endogenous constituents of LDL during its oxidation. Atherosclerosis 1998; 137(1): 49-61.
[http://dx.doi.org/10.1016/S0021-9150(97)00251-7] [PMID: 9568736]

[120] Harwood HJ Jr, Chandler CE, Pellarin LD, *et al.* Pharmacologic consequences of cholesterol absorption inhibition: alteration in cholesterol metabolism and reduction in plasma cholesterol concentration induced by the synthetic saponin beta-tigogenin cellobioside (CP-88818; tiqueside). J Lipid Res 1993; 34(3): 377-95.
[PMID: 8468523]

[121] Venkatesan N, Devaraj SN, Devaraj H. Increased binding of LDL and VLDL to apo B,E receptors of hepatic plasma membrane of rats treated with Fibernat. Eur J Nutr 2003; 42(5): 262-71.
[http://dx.doi.org/10.1007/s00394-003-0420-8] [PMID: 14569407]

[122] Visavadiya NP, Narasimhacharya AV. Hypocholesterolaemic and antioxidant effects of *Glycyrrhiza glabra* (Linn) in rats. Mol Nutr Food Res 2006; 50(11): 1080-6.
[http://dx.doi.org/10.1002/mnfr.200600063] [PMID: 17054099]

[123] Al-Daraji HJ. Influence of drinking water supplementation with licorice extract on certain blood traits of broiler chickens during heat stress. Pharmacogn Commun 2012; 2(4): 29-33.

[124] Salary J, Kalantar M, Ala MS, Ranjbar K, Matin HH. Drinking water supplementation of licorice and aloe vera extracts in broiler chickens. Scient J Anim Sci 2014; 3(2): 41-8.

[125] Shahryar AM, Ahmadzadeh A, Nobakht A. Effects of different levels of Licorice (*Glycyrrhiza glabra*) medicinal plant powder on performance, egg quality and some of serum biochemical parameters in laying hens. Iran J Appl Anim Sci 2018; 8(1): 119-24.

[126] Ostlund RE Jr. Phytosterols and cholesterol metabolism. Curr Opin Lipidol 2004; 15(1): 37-41.
[http://dx.doi.org/10.1097/00041433-200402000-00008] [PMID: 15166807]

[127] Vinson JA, Hu SJ, Jung S, Stanski AM. A citrus extract plus ascorbic acid decreases lipids, lipid peroxides, lipoprotein oxidative susceptibility, and atherosclerosis in hypercholesterolemic hamsters. J Agric Food Chem 1998; 46(4): 1453-9.
[http://dx.doi.org/10.1021/jf970801u]

[128] Vaya J, Belinky PA, Aviram M. Antioxidant constituents from licorice roots: isolation, structure elucidation and antioxidative capacity toward LDL oxidation. Free Radic Biol Med 1997; 23(2): 302-13.
[http://dx.doi.org/10.1016/S0891-5849(97)00089-0] [PMID: 9199893]

[129] Fukai T, Satoh K, Nomura T, Sakagami H. Antinephritis and radical scavenging activity of prenylflavonoids. Fitoterapia 2003; 74(7-8): 720-4.
[http://dx.doi.org/10.1016/j.fitote.2003.07.004] [PMID: 14630182]

[130] Shewita RS, Taha AE. Influence of dietary supplementation of ginger powder at different levels on growth performance, haematological profiles, slaughter traits and gut morphometry of broiler chickens. S Afr J Anim Sci 2018; 48: 997-1008.

[131] Jagadeeswaran A, Selvasubramanian S. Growth promoting potentials of indigenous drugs in broiler chicken. Int J Adv Vet Sci Technol 2014; 3: 93-8. b
[http://dx.doi.org/10.23953/cloud.ijavst.191]

[132] Myandoab MP, Mansoub NCH. Comparative effect of liquorice root extract medicinal plants and probiotic in diets on performance, carcass traits and serum composition of japanese quails. Glob Vet 2012; 8: 39-42.

[133] Al-Daraji HJ. Effects of liquorice extract, probiotic, potassium chloride and sodium bicarbonate on productive performance of broiler chickens exposed to heat stress. Int J Adv Res (Indore) 2013; 1(4): 172-80.

[134] Lashin IA, Iborahem I, Ola FA, Talkhan F, Mohamed F. Influence of licorice extract on heat stress in broiler chickens. Anim Health Res J 2017; 5: 40-6.

[135] Wang LR, Zhang HT, Liu BG, *et al.* Extraction of Glycyrrhizin polysaccharide and its effects on growth performance of broilers. Chinese Feeds Ind 2004; 25: 44-5.

[136] Al-Zuhairy MA, Hashim ME. Influence of different levels of licorice (*Glycyrrhiza glabra* Inn.) and garlic (Alliumsativum) mixture powders supplemented diet on broiler Productive traits. Iraqi J Vet Med 2015; 39(1): 9-14.

[137] Abd El-Hack ME, Alagawany M, Farag MR, *et al.* Nutritional and pharmaceutical applications of nanotechnology: trends and advances. Int J Pharmacol 2017; 13(4): 340-50.
[http://dx.doi.org/10.3923/ijp.2017.340.350]

[138] Saeed M, Babazadeh D, Naveed M, *et al. In ovo* delivery of various biological supplements, vaccines and drugs in poultry: current knowledge. J Sci Food Agric 2019; 99(8): 3727-39.

[http://dx.doi.org/10.1002/jsfa.9593] [PMID: 30637739]

[139]   Karimi B, Rahimi SH, Karimi TMA. Comparing the effects of six herbal extracts and antibiotic virginiamycin on immune response and serum lipids in broiler chickens. Iranian J Med Arom Plants 2015; 31: 177-84.

[140]   Khamisabadi H, Pourhesabi G, Chaharaein B, Naseri HR. Comparison of the effects of licorice extract (*Glycyrrhiza glabra*) and lincomycine on abdominal fat biochemical blood parameter and immunity of broiler chickens. Anim Sci J 2015; 105: 229-44. [Pajouhesh and Sazandegi].

[141]   Attia G, Hassanein E, El-Eraky W, El-Gamal M, Farahat M, Hernandez-Santana A. Effect of dietary supplementation with a plant extract blend on the growth performance, lipid profile, immune response and carcass traits of broiler chickens. Int J Poult Sci 2017; 16: 248-56.
[http://dx.doi.org/10.3923/ijps.2017.248.256]

[142]   Dogan SC, Baylan M, Erdoğan Z, Küçükgül A, Bulancak A. The effects of Licorice (*Glycyrrhriza glabra*) root on performance, some serum parameters and antioxidant capacity of laying hens. Braz J Poult Sci 2018; 20(4): 699-706.
[http://dx.doi.org/10.1590/1806-9061-2018-0767]

CHAPTER 6

The Useful Applications of *Origanum Vulgare* in Poultry Nutrition

Mohamed E. Abd El-Hack[1,*], Sameh A. Abdelnour[2], Asmaa F. Khafaga[3], Gaber E. Batiha[4, 5] and Mahmoud Alagawany[1,*]

[1] *Department of Poultry, Faculty of Agriculture, Zagazig University, Zagazig 44511, Egypt*

[2] *Department of Animal Production, Faculty of Agriculture, Zagazig University, Zagazig 44511, Egypt*

[3] *Department of Pathology, Faculty of Veterinary Medicine, Alexandria University, Edfina 22758, Egypt*

[4] *National Research Center for Protozoan Diseases, Obihiro University of Agriculture and Veterinary Medicine, Nishi 2-13, Inada-cho, 080-8555, Obihiro, Hokkaido, Japan*

[5] *Department of Pharmacology and Therapeutics, Faculty of Veterinary Medicine, Damanhour University, Damanhour 22511, AlBeheira, Egypt*

Abstract: *Origanum Vulgare* (OV) is a member of the family Lamiaceae which grows naturally in the Mediterranean area. It is a less toxic, residue-free and standard natural feed additive for poultry. There were many promoting characteristics of oregano dependent on its bioactive constituents as carvacrol and thymol. It possesses many properties, including antimicrobial, antiviral, antioxidant, antiparasitic and immunomodulatory. The possible benefits of utilizing OV in the poultry sector include enhancement of the growth, feed utilization, feed efficiency and improvement of the absorption and digestion and consequently a better productive performance. On the other hand, OV can reduce the disease occurrence and economic losses. The inclusion of oregano essential oil [OEO] in broiler diets at levels of 0.6-1% enhanced the growth performance and reduced the mortality in the broiler herds. Remarkable enhancement on the intestinal microbiota, fewer fermentation products andenhanced intestinal mucus synthesis and intestinal cell functionality have been observed by 15 mg/kg of OEO, reflecting a whole better intestinal equilibrium in poultry. Dietary supplementation of OEO at 300-ppm displayed higher IgG titers and enhanced the immune responses in the broiler. Bioactive ingredients isolated from OV could be employed in poultry feeding. To acheive the best productivity of poultry, oregano feed supplements should be used as an alternative to antibiotics and drugs due to the absence of side effects and residual impacts. The present chapter provides evidence on the usage of OV and its products in poultry feeding besides their application as feed additives in the poultry industry.

* **Corresponding authors Mahmoud Alagawany and Mohamed E. Abd El-Hack:** Poultry Department, Faculty of Agriculture, Zagazig University, Zagazig, Egypt; E-mails: mmalagwany@zu.edu.eg and m.ezzat@zu.edu.eg

Keywords: Antioxidant, Health, Immunity, *Origanum vulgare*, Performance, Poultry.

INTRODUCTION

The inclusion of phytogenic feed additives may have several positive effects on poultry production. Generally, they could regulate the intestinal functions and improve the growth performances of birds in addition to supporting the general health of the animal and improving the storage safety and meat measurements [1, 2]. *Origanum vulgare* L. (OV) from Lamiaceae family is an aromatic herb, which grows easily in Mediterranean countries [3]. The pharmacodynamics properties of the OV extract may be due to its active components such as carvacrol and thymol which act synergistically as broad-spectrum antimicrobial (bactericidal, fungicidal, and viricidal), antispasmodic, antiparasitic, diuretic, stomachic and immunomodulation agent.

The previously declared results on the usefulness of the dietary application of OV and its extracts or essential oils as growth promoters are deliberated in the present chapter. However, the impacts of OV addition to poultry diets on some hematological variables are very rare [4]. In this chapter, we have described the chemical structure and ingredients, biological activities and favorable uses of OV in feeding and its impacts on health features of poultry. The evidence offered in this chapter would be valuable for the nutritionists, scientists, researchers, veterinarians, students, pharmacists and medical professionals and poultry producers.

SCIENTIFIC CLASSIFICATION AND ANATOMICAL STRUCTURE

The basic components of *Origanum vulgare* are presented in Fig. (1).

Biological Activities and Beneficial Aspects in Poultry

Enhanced Intestinal Functions, Growth Rate and Productivity

Natural feed additives have shown favorable impacts on intestinal functions, gastrointestinal cell wall, and whole productivity of birds, meat measurements and storage safety. Abdo *et al.* [5] studied the impacts of marjoram [1.5 and 3%] on broiler performance. Authors showed that marjoram at 1.5% gave the best body weight (BW) and body weight gain (BWG). Besides, Ali [6] evaluated the influences of three levels of marjoram [0.5, 1.0 and 1.5%] on the performance of broiler chicks. The author reported that supplementing the broiler diet with marjoram improved BW and BWG at 6 weeks of age. Moreover, the oregano

[15mg/kg diet] can make a noticeable enhancement on the ileal villus height and intestinal microbiota of broilers when mixed with attapulgite [2.4 g/kg diet] [7].

Also, Bozkurt *et al.* [8] assessed the influences of oregano essential oil (OEO) at the level of 1000 mg/kg diet, on the broilers performance, and they concluded that BWG was significantly improved at 3-6 weeks of age compared to the control group (no antibiotic of prebiotic feed additives). Additionally, a study conducted by Fotea *et al.* [9] showed better BWG with a diet containing 1% of the oregano oil. Moreover, BWG was improved significantly by the inclusion of OEO at a level of 0.6g/kg in the broiler diet compared with the unsupplemented group. Ghazi *et al.* [10] stated that feeding broiler with diet with OEO [250 mg/kg diet] improved BW and BWG compared with those in the control group. The addition of 0.005 and 0.010% of OEO enhanced the BWG in broiler chickens. While, at the marketing age, the upper dosage of OEO acheived the maximum BWG.

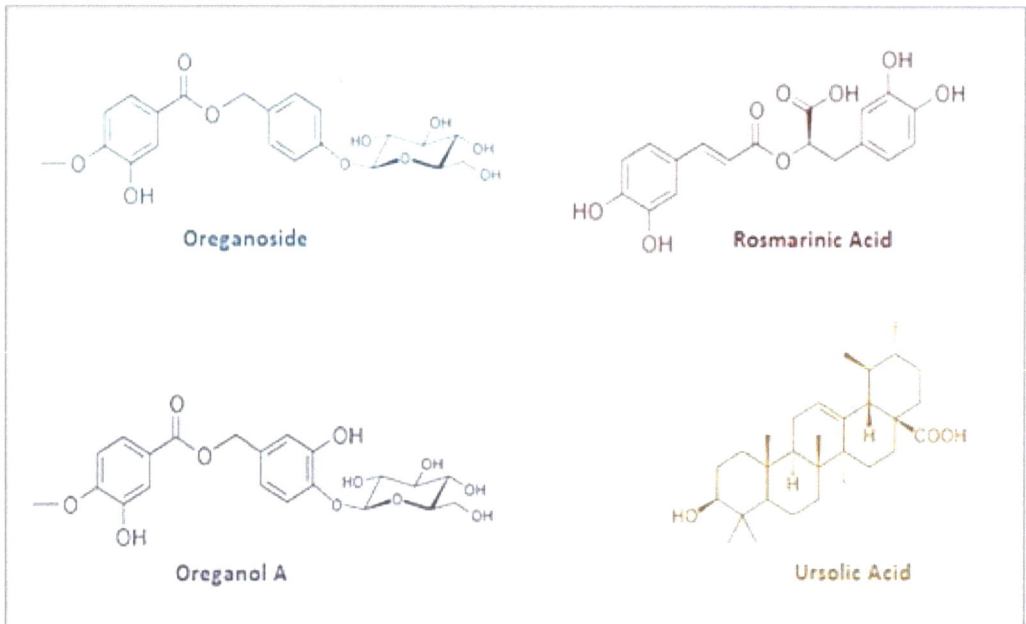

Fig. (1). The composition of the dried leaves of oregano.

Furthermore, several studies indicated that the inclusion of oregano oil [300ppm] in the poultry feed significantly enhanced the intestinal microbiota function [11, 12]. Broilers received a 0.3g/Kg diet of OEO which exhibited higher daily BWG compared with those receiving a higher level of OEO [0.5g/kg diet] or no treated group [4]. Badiri and Saber [13] recorded the effect of different levels of OEO [0, 50, 100, 200 and 400 mg/kg] on the growth criteria of Japanese quail. The consequences advised that the BW and BWG were noticeably augmented in the group that was treated with 50 mg/kg oil than other groups. These affirmative impacts of essential oil were revealed by Cowan [14], who suggested that herbs are containing primary metabolites such as terpenoids, which have antimicrobial properties and could protect against cancer and stimulate the immune system [15]. Besides, Triantaphyhou *et al.* [16] found that marjoram had antioxidant activity and could act as a digestibility booster, enhancethe gut microbial balance and enrich the secretion of digestive enzymes, thus improve the growth performance in poultry [17]. Recently, the use of Mexican OEO at 0.4 g/kg in broiler chickens diets could increase BW, feed utilization efficiency and high-density lipoprotein (HDL) (Méndez Zamora, Durán Meléndez [18]).

The improvement of production and growth measurements was clarified by Gilani, Howarth [19] who explored the impacts of OEO on the fasted broiler intestinal morphometry and detected the significant growth of villi height and crypt depth only in ileum after nine hours fasting that could be indirectly associated with the increase of intestinal permeability. Moreover, Çabuk, Eratak [20] investigated the effects of a combination of OEO with other herbal oil on the intestinal morphometric of quails. Results indicatedsignificant enhancement in the size and number of goblet cells by the dose of 48 mg/kg diet for 38 days without any influences on villi width and height and crypt depth. Besides, under the *Clostridium perfringens* challenge, OEO improved the villus height and width significantly so it could be supplemented in broiler chickens ration exposed to this bacteria [21]. The beneficial aspects of the oregano plant in poultry are described in Fig. (**2**).

Improved Nutrient Digestibility and Nutrient Utilization

Abdo *et al.* [5] indicated the effect of marjoram (1.5 and 3%) on broiler performance and the results showed that dietary marjoram at 1.5% gave the best feed conversion (FCR) but decreased feed intake. Supplementing the broiler diet with marjoram leaves powder improved feed conversion ratio and markedly reduced daily feed intake at six weeks of age [6]. Essential oils have a significant impact on FCR, through the improvement of poultry digestive tract. Since they help to improve the microorganisms' stability and enhance nutrients digestion and absorption. Besides, essential oils promote the secretions of digestive enzymes and boost the absorption of nutrients.

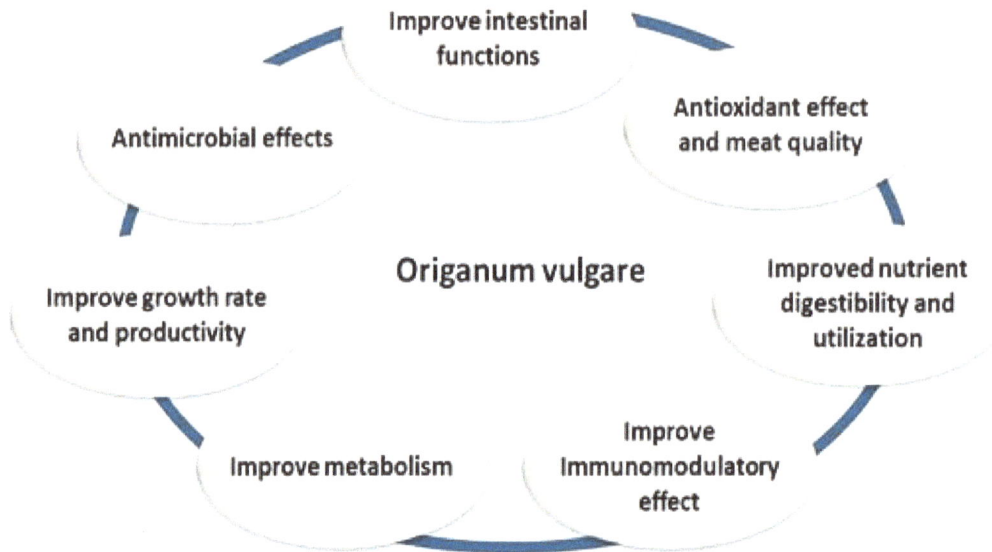

Fig. (2). The beneficial activity of the oregano plant in poultry.

It has been reported that the inclusion of 48 or 72mg of a combination essential oils/kg into the broiler diets exhibited significant improvement in feed intake (FI), BW and FCR at the period of 21-42 of age [22]. Furthermore, Lee *et al.* [23] presented that thymol and carvacrol enhanced FCR in broiler chickens. Also, basic oils assisted in better protein digestibility by lessening the hydrochloric acid (HCl) synthesis and pepsin secretion in the stomach [24, 25]. Fotea *et al.* [9] stated the effect of OEO at levels [0.3, 0.7 and 1%] on the performance of broiler chickens. The findings displayed that 1% oregano oil enhanced FCR. Moreover, Roofchaee *et al.* [26] indicated that broiler diets enriched with 0.6g/kg of OEO, decreased FI and improved FCR. Feeding broiler with OEO at 300 mg/kg improves FCR and FI from 21 to 42 [27].

Moreover, Esper *et al.* [28] performed gas chromatography/mass spectro photometer (GC/MS) analysis of OV essential oils constituents and showed that the OEO contained 4-terpineol which can inhibit aflatoxins production. Bodyweight was increased and feed efficiency was decreased due to essential oil (250 mg of OEO/kg of diet) supplementation alone or mixed with vitamin C (200 mg/kg of diet) when compared with that fed a basal diet [10]. Also, Vázquez, Meléndez [29] compared the impacts of 2 supplementations of Mexican OEO [the 1st; 60% carvacrol +4% thymol and the 2nd; 20% carvacrol +40% thymol] in broiler chicken diets on water intake and the growth indices (feed efficiency, FI, BW and BWG). The authors revealed that the mixture significantly enhanced the growth indices and water consumption in growing broiler chickens. Also, Abd Al Haleem *et al.* [30] found that a diet with 0.60g Orego-Stim/kg diet significantly improved the growth performance of broiler chicks. Mohiti-Asli and Ghanaatparast-Rashti [4] detected that feeding broilers diet enriched with OEO (0.3g/kg) enhanced the average FI than those fed with a high dose (0.5g/kg) at 3-4 weeks of age. Dietary supplementation of 300ppm OEO reduced FI in comparison with the control. Both levels of 0.3 or 0.5g OEO enriched in broiler diets did not affect FCR at the period of 4 and 5 weeks of the age. In Japanese quail, FI was evidently augmented in the quails that were given 50 mg/kg OEO compared with the other groups 0.1, 0.2 and 0.4g/kg diet and control group, but FCR was significantly reduced [13].

Antioxidant Effect on Meat Quality

Researchers have studied the potential effect of OV and its derived components on enhancing the antioxidative capacity of poultry meat. Abdo *et al.* [5] found that 1.5% marjoram significantly changed the percentage of heart, while carcass, liver and gizzard percentages were not affected by dietary marjoram levels [1.5 or 3%]. Soliman *et al.* [31] observed that using marjoram oil, at 1.5%, leads to decreased gizzard percentage, while liver and heart percentages were not affected by dietary marjoram. Bozkurt *et al.* [8] enriched the broiler diets with 1% of OEO and reported that carcass measurements (the weight of liver, carcass and slaughter) were not influenced by OEO supplementation. Similarly, dietary OEO at the level of 300 mg/kg did not affect pre-slaughter weight or carcass yield of broilers at seven weeks of age [27]. Corduk *et al.* [32] pointed out that supplementing OEO in broiler chicken diet had a change in the liver weight of birds. Kirkpinar *et al.* [33] studied the effect of OEO at the levels of 0.15g and 0.3 g/kg diet on the broiler carcass measurements and the authors suggested that carcass weight and yield were significantly influenced by the dietary OEO addition. Accordingly, the liver and heart weights of Japanese quail were markedly greater in the group that given 50 mg/kg OEO compared with other 0.1, 0.2 or 0.4g/kg and the control groups [13]. On the other side, the supplementation of OEO had no significant influence on liver, breast, heart, liver, and wings weights, but it significantly boosted neck and thigh weights [34].

Based on the chemical constitution, there was an antioxidative and antimicrobial effect of feed, particularly of herb essential oils containing phenolic active components that could ameliorate the shelf life. There was a comprehensive modification of the intestinal ecosystem performance, particularly as referred to the FCR due to essential oil. Additionally, antioxidative substances in herbal essential oils can advance oxidative firmness of the meat, fat, and the carcass in addition to the egg yolk [35].

A mixture of OEO in the levels of 50-100 mg/kg to chicken diets displayed an antioxidant effect in the animal cells. Such antioxidant impacts would be suggested to advance poultry livestock welfare [36]. The active phytogenic products may stabilize the antioxidative mechanism of broilers owing to the antioxidant outcome of carvacrol and thymol by raising the effectiveness of antioxidant enzymes [37]. The antioxidant impact of OEO was more significant than vitamin E as reflected by the quality of poultry meat produced from dietary OEO [38]. The study by Akbarian [39] revealed that phenolic compounds in dietary OEO could give a possibility for improving the antioxidant mechanism against heat stress induced changes in heat shock protein 70 mRNA, antioxidant enzyme and oxidative status system. Consequently, meat produced from broiler reared under heat stress can stand against oxidative changes. Ghazi *et al.* [10] reported that lower malondialdehyde (MDA) was significantly decreased using oregano oil (250 mg/kg of diet).

The MDA is the most significant indicator of lipid peroxidation in the liver or serum [40]. Besides, Ri, Jiang [41] revealed that dietary oregano in chicks diets increased the total antioxidant activity and lowered the level of serum MDA. On the other side, the carcass weight, pH value, meat color, dripping and cooking losses were not affected by the OEO addition in broiler diets. Synergistic effect of OEO and rosemary essential oil has been performed by 150 mg/kg which resulted in a perfect effect in inhibiting the lipid oxidation of broiler meat, thus preserves the meat quality for guaranteeing a long shelf life [42].

Based on the literature, dietary supplementation with OV and OEO has been evidenced to enhance the total antioxidant capacity of broilers. For this reason, OV and it extracts or active compounds are observed as natural sources of antioxidants to protect the oxidation in meat and prolong its storage time.

Antimicrobial and Immunomodulation Effects

Another approach and the well-accept mechanism that can clarify the growth-stimulating influence of OV, essential oils, or their extracts or bioactive compounds in diets of broiler chickens as phytobiotics is the equilibrium of the ecosystem of gut microbiota owing to their powerful antioxidants and antimicrobial activities. Phytogenic feed additives have a possible antimicrobial property contributed to reducing intestinal pathogens count through suppression of their attachment to the mucosa. Phytogenics had a significant part in the improvement of the secretion of digestive enzymes and absorption capacity and, thereby, growth stimulation. Roofchaee *et al.* [26] stated that dietary inclusion of

OV essential oil at 0.6 and 1.2g/kg exhibited a significant advance in FCR and higher antioxidant serum activity. Colonization of lactic acid bacteria continued in the same manner and reduced assemblage of cecal *E. coli* were noticed, followed by 0.3 and 0.6 g/kg OEO treatment. Hulánková and Bořilová [43] evaluated *in vitro* suppression of foodborne disease-producing microorganisms *via* the action of OEO [carvacrol content 72%]. Incorporation of OEO and citric or acetic acids appeared to be a potent mixture for depression of foodborne disease-producing microorganisms, particularly *L. monocytogenes*, and *Salmonella* spp. ubiquitous in slightly acidic foods. Mathlouthi *et al.* [25] showed that OEO had antimicrobial results on the *Bacillus subtilis Escherichia coli, Listeria innocua, Salmonella indiana*, and *Staphylococcus aureus*.

Additionally, Betancourt reported [44] OEO showed antibacterial activity and decreased the morality percentage from ascites by around 59% in treated groups than the unsupplemented group. Dietary administration of essential oils [25% carvacrol +25% thymol] at doses of 60, 120 and 240 mg/kg mitigated the intestinal scores, improved the intestinal characteristics, minimized the inflammatory responses and boosted the specific immunity in the *C. perfringens*-challenged broiler chickens. Giving to the information obtained, the 240 mg oregano supplementation/kg diet was the recommended level for protecting broiler chickens from *C. perfringens* hazards.The favorable impacts of oregano might be associated with their improvement consequences on the immunity status and intestinal characteristics [45]. Nowotarska *et al.* [46] mentioned that carvacrol and OEO could inhibit the growth of *Mycobacterium avium* subsp. paratuberculosis. The suppression of the pathogenic bacteria may be linked with the impairment of the bacterial cell membrane.

There are some data on the activity and mechanisms of OEO on viruses, however, have not been fully termed. Galal *et al.* [47] examined the effects of oral treatment with 0.005 and 0.01% OEO on chicken interferon-alpha (IFNα) signaling pathway post-New Castle Disease Virus (NDV) vaccination, and found that these OEO levels did not exhibit any noticeable positive immune-modulatory properties on Myxovirus resistance 1 transcripts level except at 29 days of age. On the other side, a dose-dependent up-regulation in both IFNα RNA and IFN regulatory factor-7 [IRF-7] values was detected. It has been indicated that both levels of OEO could safeguard the broilers from nervous symptoms causing by the challenge with the NDV vaccine.

Utilization of immune stimulants by using some herbal oils was one process to improve the immunity and vulnerability to infectious ailments in animals. Alagawany *et al.* [48] found that bursa was not affected by OEO. Acamovic and Brooker [49] reported the immune-stimulatory effect of oregano and thymol oils with respect to the mononuclear phagocytes system, in addition to both cell-mediated and humoral immunity. Perez-Roses [50] found that the organism's immunity including phagocytes, humoral and cellular immune responses could be enhanced by herbs or their extracts or essential oils, which improved the capability of the defense system to interrelate with infectious mediators. Although the dietary OEO significantly dropped the counts of excreta oocyst compared to those fed basal diet, its anticoccidial properties were significantly lower than the influences in broilers that received the diet with the anticoccidial drug .

Furthermore, chicks fed with OEO at level of 300-ppm in their diet presented greater IgG titers compared with those reared on the untreated diet [12]. The study conducted by Mohiti-Asli and Ghanaatparast-Rashti [51] declared that birds take 500-ppm OEO in their diets, which showed inferior coccidial infections score lesions in the middle and upper portions of the intestine, and consequently, inferior dropping marks and litter scores in respect to other unchallenged birds. Franciosini *et al*. [52] observed that the supplementation of aqueous oregano extract to broiler chickens and enhanced total serum IgG levels. Additionally, higher Lactobacilli counts in ileum and cecum and lower counts of *Staphylococcus* spp. were detected in all groups supplemented with aqueous extract. Scocco *et al*. [53] discovered that oregano aqueous extract treatment generally advanced goblet cell activity (glycoconjugates) more than vitamins E and C administration. The coliform population was decreased in the ileum of the oregano treated group at 21 and 42 days compared with other groups. *Escherichia coli* displayed the lowest marks in the caecum as affected by the oregano aqueous extract treatment. *Staphylococci, enterococci,* and *lactobacilli* counts exhibited no noticeable differences among the different experimental treatments in the caecum. In the ileum, the oregano aqueous extract group did not display the sharp fall in the lactic acid bacteria count observed in the other experimental groups [53].

Effect on Hematology and Biochemical Parameters

Feeding basal diets with marjoram supplementation did not adversely affect the hemoglobin concentration and hematocrit percent [54]. Ali [6] described that enriching the broiler diet with marjoram (5, 10, and 15mg/kg diet) significantly augmented globulin and reduced albumin and albumin/globulin ratio than the control group but no significant effect on hematocrit and hemoglobin was observed after six weeks of age.

Mohiti-Asli *et al*. [4] discovered the impacts of OEO at the level of (300 and 500 ppm) on the immunological variables of broilers. Authors presented that birds received OEO at 0.3g/kg diet had inferior counts of heterophils and heterophils to lymphocytes ratio. On the other side, there was no statistical difference between both OEO doses on the counts of white blood cells [WBCs], monocytes and lymphocytes count. Birds fed with Mexican OEO at 0.4 g/kg diet had slightly superior WBCs, erythrocytes, and hemoglobin. They reduced the values of mean corpuscular hemoglobin, mean corpuscular volume, monocytes and lymphocytes compared with the control diet with no additives [18].

Abdo *et al.* [5] found non-significant differences by 1.5% of marjoram on blood total protein and albumin. But, the level of A/G ratio and total lipids, as well as the activity of GOT and GPT were significantly increased by marjoram supplementation. Ali [6] reported that supplementing broiler diet with marjoram leaves powder significantly increased globulin than the basal diet, moreover the addition of marjoram reduced albumin and albumin/globulin ratio (A/G) significantly compared with the unsupplemented group. Plasma triglyceride was markedly decreased by the supplementation of OEO at 250.0 mg/kg diet in the broiler diets [10].

In another study conducted by Soliman *et al.* [55], there were no differences in the values of total proteins, albumin, globulin, A/G ratio, alanine aminotransferase (ALT) and aspartate aminotransferase (AST) between Inshas chickens strain fed diets containing OEO and those in the control group . However, Zamora *et al.* [18] described that birds' diets enriched with 0.4% OEO slightly augmented in hemoglobin and albumin.

Abdo *et al.* [5] demonstrated that supplementing broilers diet with 1.5% marjoram did not affect total lipids or cholesterol levels. Similarly, Soliman *et al.* [31] showed that the addition of marjoram at 1.5% led to a slight reduction in total protein and cholesterol values. In Japanese quail, high-density lipoprotein (HDL) and cholesterol levels were greater in-group that given 100 mg/kg OEO. In contrast, triglyceride level was greater in-group that received 50 mg/kg oil, but the values of low-density lipoprotein (LDL) and cholesterol were inferior in-group that received 200 mg/kg oil [13].

Ghazi *et al.* [10] stated that if OEO was mixed with vitamin C, they could have favorable influences on birds raised under hot environmental conditions by increasing the contents of glucose, MDA, triglycerides and corticosterone hormone in the broiler serum. Additionally, a study conducted by Zamora *et al.* [18] reported a significant augment of the levels of HDL and cholesterol with diets enriched with 400mg/kg of OEO. However, no differences were observed regarding triglycerides and LDL contents at eight weeks of age.

CONCLUDING REMARKS

The literature above and results pointed out that oregano feed supplement can be employed as a supportive growth promoter (non-therapeutic feed additive). Besides, this herb and its derivatives have antioxidant, antimicrobial, and immunostimulant properties in the poultry industry. The antioxidant results of oregano and its bioactive constituents could safeguard the quality of feed and poultry products. These impacts showed that oregano additives could correlate to the enhancement of poultry productivity and health.

CONSENT FOR PUBLICATION

Not Applicable.

CONFLICT OF INTEREST

The author confirms that this chapter contents have no conflict of interest.

ACKNOWLEDGEMENTS

Declared none.

REFERENCES

[1]   Abd El-Hack ME, Alagawany M, Ragab Farag M, *et al.* Beneficial impacts of thymol essential oil on health and production of animals, fish and poultry: a review. J Essent Oil Res 2016; 28(5): 365-82.
[http://dx.doi.org/10.1080/10412905.2016.1153002]

[2]   Alagawany M, Abd El-Hack ME, Arain M, Arif M. Effect of some phytogenic additives as dietary supplements on performance, egg quality, serum biochemical parameters and oxidative status in laying hens. Indian J Anim Sci 2017; 87: 103-8.

[3]   Onofrei V, Teliban G-C, Clinciu-Radu R-A, Teliban I-V, Robu T. *Ocimum basilicum* L.: presence, influence and evolution in human concerns ever. Agron Ser Sci Res 2015; 58: 6-161.

[4]   Mohiti-Asli M, Ghanaatparast-Rashti M. Comparison of the effect of two phytogenic compounds on growth performance and immune response of broilers. J Appl Anim Res 2017; 45(1): 603-8.
[http://dx.doi.org/10.1080/09712119.2016.1243119]

[5]   Abdo ZM, Soliman A, Barakat OS. Effect of hot pepper and marjoram as feed additives on the growth performance and the microbial population of the gastrointestinal tract of broilers. Egypt Poult Sci 2003; 23: 91-113.

[6]   Ali A. Productive performance and immune response of broiler chicks as affected by dietary thyme leaves powder. Egypt Poult Sci J 2014; 34(1): 71-84.
[http://dx.doi.org/10.21608/epsj.2014.5307]

[7]   Skoufos I, Giannenas I, Tontis D, *et al.* Effects of oregano essential oil and attapulgite on growth performance, intestinal microbiota and morphometry in broilers. S Afr J Anim Sci 2016; 46(1): 77-88.
[http://dx.doi.org/10.4314/sajas.v46i1.10]

[8]   Bozkurt M, Alçiçek A, Çabuk M, Küçükyilmaz K, Çatli AU. Effect of an herbal essential oil mixture on growth, laying traits, and egg hatching characteristics of broiler breeders. Poult Sci 2009; 88(11): 2368-74.
[http://dx.doi.org/10.3382/ps.2009-00048] [PMID: 19834088]

[9]   Fotea L, Costăchescu E, Hoha G, Leonte D. The effect of oregano essential oil [*Origanum vulgare* L] on broiler performance. Lucrări Ştiinţifice Seria Zootehnie 2010; 53: 253-6.

[10] Ghazi S, Amjadian T, Norouzi S. Single and combined effects of vitamin C and oregano essential oil in diet, on growth performance, and blood parameters of broiler chicks reared under heat stress condition. Int J Biometeorol 2015; 59(8): 1019-24.
[http://dx.doi.org/10.1007/s00484-014-0915-4] [PMID: 25336108]

[11] Fonseca-García I, Escalera-Valente F, Martínez-González S, Carmona-Gasca CA, Gutiérrez-Arenas DA, Ávila-Ramos F. Effect of oregano oil dietary supplementation on production parameters, height of intestinal villi and the antioxidant capacity in the breast of broiler. Austr J Vetern Sci 2017; 49(2): 9-83.
[http://dx.doi.org/10.4067/S0719-81322017000200083]

[12] Mohiti-Asli M, Ghanaatparast-Rashti M. Comparing the effects of a combined phytogenic feed additive with an individual essential oil of oregano on intestinal morphology and microflora in broilers. J Appl Anim Res 2018; 46(1): 184-9.
[http://dx.doi.org/10.1080/09712119.2017.1284074]

[13] Badiri R, Saber SN. Effects of Dietary Oregano Essential Oil on Growth Performance, Carcass Parameters and Some Blood Parameters in Japanese Male Quail. Int J Pure Appl Biosci 2016; 4(5): 17-22.
[http://dx.doi.org/10.18782/2320-7051.2397]

[14] Cowan MM. Plant products as antimicrobial agents. Clin Microbiol Rev 1999; 12(4): 564-82.
[http://dx.doi.org/10.1128/CMR.12.4.564] [PMID: 10515903]

[15] Craig WJ. Health-promoting properties of common herbs. Am J Clin Nutr 1999; 70(3) (Suppl.): 491S-9S.
[http://dx.doi.org/10.1093/ajcn/70.3.491s] [PMID: 10479221]

[16] Triantaphyllou K, Blekas G, Boskou D. Antioxidative properties of water extracts obtained from herbs of the species Lamiaceae. Int J Food Sci Nutr 2001; 52(4): 313-7.
[http://dx.doi.org/10.1080/09637480120057512] [PMID: 11474895]

[17] Cross DE, McDevitt RM, Hillman K, Acamovic T. The effect of herbs and their associated essential oils on performance, dietary digestibility and gut microflora in chickens from 7 to 28 days of age. Br Poult Sci 2007; 48(4): 496-506.
[http://dx.doi.org/10.1080/00071660701463221] [PMID: 17701503]

[18] Méndez Zamora G, Durán Meléndez LA, Hume ME, Silva Vázquez R. Performance, blood parameters, and carcass yield of broiler chickens supplemented with Mexican oregano oil. Rev Bras Zootec 2017; 46(6): 515-20.
[http://dx.doi.org/10.1590/s1806-92902017000600006]

[19] Gilani S, Howarth G, Nattrass G, et al. Gene expression and morphological changes in the intestinal mucosa associated with increased permeability induced by short-term fasting in chickens. J Anim Physiol Anim Nutr (Berl) 2017.
[PMID: 29034530]

[20] Çabuk M, Eratak S, Alçiçek A, Tuglu I. Effect of herbal essential oil mixture on intestinal mucosal development, growth performance, and weights of internal organs of quails. J Essen Oil Bear Plants 2014; 17(4): 599-606.
[http://dx.doi.org/10.1080/0972060X.2014.935025]

[21] Abudabos AM, Alyemni AH, Dafalla YM, Khan RU. The effect of phytogenics on growth traits, blood biochemical and intestinal histology in broiler chickens exposed to *Clostridium perfringens* challenge. J Appl Anim Res 2018; 46(1): 691-5.
[http://dx.doi.org/10.1080/09712119.2017.1383258]

[22] Alcicek A, Bozkurt M, Çabuk M. The effect of an essential oil combination derived from selected herbs growing wild in Turkey on broiler performance. S Afr J Anim Sci 2003; 33(2): 89-94.
[http://dx.doi.org/10.4314/sajas.v33i2.3761]

[23]   Lee K-W, Everts H, Kappert HJ, Frehner M, Losa R, Beynen AC. Effects of dietary essential oil components on growth performance, digestive enzymes and lipid metabolism in female broiler chickens. Br Poult Sci 2003; 44(3): 450-7.
[http://dx.doi.org/10.1080/0007166031000085508] [PMID: 12964629]

[24]   Gopi M, Karthik K, Manjunathachar HV, *et al.* Essential oils as a feed additive in poultry nutrition. Adv Anim Vet Sci 2014; 2(1): 1-7.
[http://dx.doi.org/10.14737/journal.aavs/2014.2.1.1.7]

[25]   Mathlouthi N, Bouzaienne T, Oueslati I, *et al.* Use of rosemary, oregano, and a commercial blend of essential oils in broiler chickens: *In vitro* antimicrobial activities and effects on growth performance. J Anim Sci 2012; 90(3): 813-23.
[http://dx.doi.org/10.2527/jas.2010-3646] [PMID: 22064737]

[26]   Roofchaee A, Irani M, Ebrahimzadeh MA, Akbari MR. Effect of dietary oregano [*Origanum vulgare* L.] essential oil on growth performance, cecal microflora and serum antioxidant activity of broiler chickens. Afr J Biotechnol 2011; 10(32): 6177-83.

[27]   Alp M, Midilli M, Kocabağlı N, *et al.* The effects of dietary oregano essential oil on live performance, carcass yield, serum immunoglobulin G level, and oocyst count in broilers. J Appl Poult Res 2012; 21(3): 630-6.
[http://dx.doi.org/10.3382/japr.2012-00551]

[28]   Esper RH, Gonçalez E, Marques MO, Felicio RC, Felicio JD. Potential of essential oils for protection of grains contaminated by aflatoxin produced by Aspergillus flavus. Front Microbiol 2014; 5: 269.
[http://dx.doi.org/10.3389/fmicb.2014.00269] [PMID: 24926289]

[29]   Vázquez RS, Meléndez LAD, Estrada ES, *et al.* Performance of broiler chickens supplemented with Mexican oregano oil. Rev Bras Zootec 2015; 44(8): 283-9. [Lippia berlandieri Schauer].
[http://dx.doi.org/10.1590/S1806-92902015000800003]

[30]   AbdAlHaleem HA. Elsayed OA, Fadl AA, AbdElto FA. Effect of dietary oregano supplementation on productive, physiological and immunological performance of broiler chicks. Egypt Poult Sci J 2020; 40: 507-24.
[http://dx.doi.org/10.21608/epsj.2020.96098]

[31]   Soliman A, Ali M, Abdo ZM. Effect of marjoram, bacitracin and active yeast as feed additives on the performance and the microbial content of the broiler's intestinal tract. Poult Sci 2003; 23(3): 445-67.

[32]   Corduk M, Sarica S, Yarim G. Effects of oregano or red pepper essential oil supplementation to diets for broiler chicks with delayed feeding after hatching. 1. Performance and microbial population. J Appl Poult Res 2013; 22(4): 738-49.
[http://dx.doi.org/10.3382/japr.2012-00672]

[33]   Kirkpinar F, Ünlü HB, Serdaroğlu M, Turp GY. Effects of dietary oregano and garlic essential oils on carcass characteristics, meat composition, colour, pH and sensory quality of broiler meat. Br Poult Sci 2014; 55(2): 157-66.
[http://dx.doi.org/10.1080/00071668.2013.879980] [PMID: 24404997]

[34]   Badiri R, Saber SN. Effects of dietary oregano essential oil on growth performance, carcass parameters and some blood parameters in japanese male quail. Int J Pure App Biosci 2016; 4(5): 17-22.
[http://dx.doi.org/10.18782/2320-7051.2397]

[35]   Franz C, Baser K, Windisch W. Essential oils and aromatic plants in animal feeding–a European perspective. A review. Flavour Fragrance J 2010; 25(5): 327-40.
[http://dx.doi.org/10.1002/ffj.1967]

[36]   Botsoglou NA, Florou-Paneri P, Christaki E, Fletouris DJ, Spais AB. Effect of dietary oregano essential oil on performance of chickens and on iron-induced lipid oxidation of breast, thigh and abdominal fat tissues. Br Poult Sci 2002; 43(2): 223-30.

[http://dx.doi.org/10.1080/00071660120121436] [PMID: 12047086]

[37] Hashemipour H, Kermanshahi H, Golian A, Veldkamp T. Effect of thymol and carvacrol feed supplementation on performance, antioxidant enzyme activities, fatty acid composition, digestive enzyme activities, and immune response in broiler chickens. Poult Sci 2013; 92(8): 2059-69.
[http://dx.doi.org/10.3382/ps.2012-02685] [PMID: 23873553]

[38] Avila-Ramos F, Pro-Martínez A, Sosa-Montes E, *et al.* Effects of dietary oregano essential oil and vitamin E on the lipid oxidation stability of cooked chicken breast meat. Poult Sci 2012; 91(2): 505-11.
[http://dx.doi.org/10.3382/ps.2011-01731] [PMID: 22252366]

[39] Akbarian A, Michiels J, Golian A, Buyse J, Wang Y, De Smet S. Gene expression of heat shock protein 70 and antioxidant enzymes, oxidative status, and meat oxidative stability of cyclically heat-challenged finishing broilers fed Origanum compactum and Curcuma xanthorrhiza essential oils. Poult Sci 2014; 93(8): 1930-41.
[http://dx.doi.org/10.3382/ps.2014-03896] [PMID: 24931966]

[40] Gumus R, Ercan N, Imik H. The effect of thyme essential oil [Thymus vulgaris] added to quail diets on performance, some blood parameters, and the antioxidative metabolism of the serum and liver tissues. Braz J Poult Sci 2017; 19(2): 297-304.
[http://dx.doi.org/10.1590/1806-9061-2016-0403]

[41] Ri C-S, Jiang X-R, Kim M-H, *et al.* Effects of dietary oregano powder supplementation on the growth performance, antioxidant status and meat quality of broiler chicks. Ital J Anim Sci 2017; 1-7.
[http://dx.doi.org/10.1080/1828051X.2016.1274243]

[42] Basmacioglu H, Tokusoglu Ö, Ergül M. The effect of oregano and rosemary essential oils or alpha-tocopheryl acetate on performance and lipid oxidation of meat enriched with n-3 PUFA's in broilers. S Afr J Anim Sci 2004; 34(3): 197-210.

[43] Hulánková R, Bořilová G. *In vitro* combined effect of oregano essential oil and caprylic acid against *Salmonella serovars*, *Escherichia coli* O_{157}: H_7, *Staphylococcus aureus* and *Listeria monocytogenes*. Acta Vet Brno 2012; 80(4): 343-8.
[http://dx.doi.org/10.2754/avb201180040343]

[44] Betancourt L, Rodriguez F, Phandanouvong V, *et al.* Effect of Origanum chemotypes on broiler intestinal bacteria. Poult Sci 2014; 93(10): 2526-35.
[http://dx.doi.org/10.3382/ps.2014-03944] [PMID: 25071230]

[45] Du E, Wang W, Gan L, Li Z, Guo S, Guo Y. Effects of thymol and carvacrol supplementation on intestinal integrity and immune responses of broiler chickens challenged with *Clostridium perfringens*. J Anim Sci Biotechnol 2016; 7(1): 19.
[http://dx.doi.org/10.1186/s40104-016-0079-7] [PMID: 27006768]

[46] Nowotarska SW, Nowotarski K, Grant IR, Elliott CT, Friedman M, Situ C. Mechanisms of Antimicrobial Action of Cinnamon and Oregano Oils, Cinnamaldehyde, Carvacrol, 2,5-Dihydroxybenzaldehyde, and 2-Hydroxy-5-Methoxybenzaldehyde against *Mycobacterium avium* subsp. paratuberculosis (Map). Foods 2017; 6(9): 72. [Map].
[http://dx.doi.org/10.3390/foods6090072] [PMID: 28837070]

[47] Galal A, El-Araby I, Hassanin O, El-Said Omar A. Positive impact of oregano essential oil on growth performance, humoral immune responses and chicken interferon alpha signalling pathway in broilers. Adv Anim Vet Sci 2016; 4(1): 57-65.
[http://dx.doi.org/10.14737/journal.aavs/2016/4.1.57.65]

[48] Alagawany M, El-Hack M, Farag MR, Tiwari R, Dhama K. Biological effects and modes of action of carvacrol in animal and poultry pro-duction and health-a review. Adv Anim Vetern Sci 2015; 3(2s): 73-84.
[http://dx.doi.org/10.14737/journal.aavs/2015/3.2s.73.84]

[49] Acamovic T, Brooker JD. Biochemistry of plant secondary metabolites and their effects in animals.

Proc Nutr Soc 2005; 64(3): 403-12.
[http://dx.doi.org/10.1079/PNS2005449] [PMID: 16048675]

[50] Pérez-Rosés R, Risco E, Vila R, Peñalver P, Cañigueral S. Effect of some essential oils on phagocytosis and complement system activity. J Agric Food Chem 2015; 63(5): 1496-504.
[http://dx.doi.org/10.1021/jf504761m] [PMID: 25599399]

[51] Mohiti-Asli M, Ghanaatparast-Rashti M. Dietary oregano essential oil alleviates experimentally induced coccidiosis in broilers. Prev Vet Med 2015; 120(2): 195-202.
[http://dx.doi.org/10.1016/j.prevetmed.2015.03.014] [PMID: 25864115]

[52] Franciosini MP, Casagrande-Proietti P, Forte C, *et al.* Effects of oregano [*Origanum vulgare* L.] and rosemary [*Rosmarinus officinalis* L.] aqueous extracts on broiler performance, immune function and intestinal microbial population. J Appl Anim Res 2016; 44(1): 474-9.
[http://dx.doi.org/10.1080/09712119.2015.1091322]

[53] Scocco P, Forte C, Franciosini MP, *et al.* Gut complex carbohydrates and intestinal microflora in broiler chickens fed with oregano (*Origanum vulgare* L.) aqueous extract and vitamin E. J Anim Physiol Anim Nutr (Berl) 2017; 101(4): 676-84. [Berl].
[http://dx.doi.org/10.1111/jpn.12588] [PMID: 27550621]

[54] Osman M, Yakout H, Motawe H, El-Arab WE. Productive, physiological, immunological and economic effects of supplementing natural feed additives to broiler diets. Egypt Poult Sci J 2010; 30(1): 25-53.

[55] Soliman MM, Abdo Nassan M, Ismail TA. *Origanum Majoranum* extract modulates gene expression, hepatic and renal changes in a rat model of type 2 diabetes. Iran J Pharm Res 2016; 15: 45-54.
[PMID: 28228803]

CHAPTER 7

Importance of Quinoa (*Chenopodium Quinoa*) in Poultry Nutrition

Muhammad Asif Arain[1,*], **Mahmoud Alagawany**[2,*], **Muhammad Saeed**[3], **Muhammad Umar**[1], **Nasrullah**[1], **Feroza Soomro**[4], **Mayada R. Farag**[5] and **Mohamed E. Abd El-Hack**[2]

[1] *Faculty of Veterinary and Animal Sciences, Lasbela University of Agriculture, Water and Marine Sciences, Uthal-3800, Balochistan, Pakistan*

[2] *Department of Poultry, Faculty of Agriculture, Zagazig University, Zagazig 44511, Egypt*

[3] *Department of Animal Nutrition, Cholistan University of Veterinary and Animal Sciences Bahawalpur, Pakistan*

[4] *Department of Veterinary Parasitology, Faculty of Animal Husbandry and Veterinary Sciences, Sindh Agriculture University, Tandojam, Pakistan*

[5] *Forensic Medicine and Toxicology Department, Veterinary Medicine Faculty, Zagazig University, Zagazig 44519, Egypt*

Abstract: Quinoa is a grain-like food crop with a higher nutritional value compared to other cereals. It has been reported to be an excellent source of fiber, protein, lipids, minerals, amino acids and vitamins. Quinoa represents a good source of fiber (10%), which is much higher than that of wheat 2.7%, corn 1.7%, and rice 0.4%. The quinoa seed comprises protein (120-180 g/kg), which contains a better-balanced amino acid composition than conventional crops such as cereals. Quinoa also contains several beneficial health compounds, including phytoecdysteroids, phytosterols, saponins, betalains, glycine and phenolics. Dietary supplementation of quinoa has shown significant effects on growth performance, public health and production performance of large and small animals. Birds fed diets supplemented with quinoa at a low level (50 g/kg) had achieved a better performance without any adverse effects. But the high level (150 g/kg diet) of quinoa reduced live body weight at 20 days of age from 627 to 601 g and at 39 days of age from 1760 to 1709 g, respectively, while feed conversion ratio was increased from 1437 to 1486 g feed kg^{-1} live body weight at 20 days of age. Birds fed a diet enriched with 30 g/100 Kg recorded higher body weight and feed intake compared to those fed on 10 g/100 Kg and the control group. Supplementation of 40 or 80 mg/kg of iso-flavones increased total antioxidant capacity in the blood of chickens.Hitherto, there is a gap in the knowledge base of quinoa as a feed additive, which is not widely considered in poultry feeds.

[*] **Corresponding authors Muhammad Asif Arain:** Faculty of Veterinary and Animal Sciences, Lasbela University of Agriculture, Water and Marine Sciences, Uthal-3800, Balochistan, Pakistan; E-mail: asifarain77@yahoo.com;

Mahmoud Alagawany: Department of Poultry, Faculty of Agriculture, Zagazig University, Zagazig 44511, Egypt; E-mail: mmalagwany@zu.edu.eg

Thus, this chapter aims to find the medicinal and nutritional importance of quinoa to boost the performance and health in poultry farming.

Keywords: Anti-oxidant, Feed additive, Health benefits, Poultry, Quinoa.

INTRODUCTION

Quinoa (*Chenopodium quinoa*) is one of the most famous medicinal plants that belong to the Chenopodiaceae family and was originally found in the Andean region in South America region. Quinoa has a broadleaf and its seeds are used as cereal-based foods. The seeds of quinoa crops have been known as pseudo-cereal gluten-free grains. They have gained attention in recent decades because of their extraordinary nutritional value and potential health benefits. The Food and Agriculture Organization of the United Nations (FAO) pays great attention to the promotion of planting, research and development on quinoa. Quinoa is cultivated in most of the world's arable regions and can adapt to the tropical climate under various harsh environmental conditions. Also, it is being used in foods and for pharmaceutical purposes [1].

The grain of this plant has been recognized as a rich source of good quality macro- and micro-nutrients such as proteins, carbohydrates, vitamins, fat and minerals, as compared to other cereal grains such as wheat, oats, maize and rice [2, 3]. Additionally, seeds of this plant are rich in vitamins such as vitamins B, C and E [4]. Biological compounds such as betanins, terpenoids, and phenolic compounds and their potential health benefits have been shown in many studies [5, 6]. The bioactive phytochemical compounds of quinoa grain have exhibited various therapeutic effects like anti-oxidant, anti-inflammatory, immuno-modulation and other health-promoting effects based on different *in vitro* and *in vivo* studies [1]. It should be pointed out that the mechanisms of action of these bioactive compounds individually or collectively contribute to the overall nutritional value, especially to the health benefits, which have not yet been fully explored. Commercial poultry farming derives its daily energy from cereal-based foods. Quinoa is a grain-like food that can provide nutrition and sustenance to animals and has recently attracted more attention in poultry diets. Previously published studies have proven several functions of quinoa seeds in livestock and poultry due to their high nutritional value, numerous biological activities and health benefits. The available literature regarding the use of quinoa seeds as a functional food and therapeutic application in poultry feed is relatively scarce. However, additional scientific investigations are needed to recognize further and promote the role of quinoa in the production performance of the poultry industry. Therefore, the aim of this chapter is to explore the medicinal and nutritional importance of quinoa as a feed additive to boost both productivity and health performance in poultry farming. Another objective of this reappraisal is to highlight the most recent advances in the phytochemical compounds of quinoa and their contribution to the pharmacological aspects and potential health benefits of poultry.

NUTRITIONAL AND PHYTOCHEMICAL COMPOSITION OF THE QUINOA PLANT

The biological value and nutritional composition of quinoa and its grains have been estimated in many studies (Tables **1**, **2**, **3** and **4**). This plant has been characterized as a notable source of both α and γ-tocopherol, folic acid, riboflavin and thiamine. In comparison with other grains, it includes high concentrations of copper, magnesium, iron, calcium, potassium, zinc and phosphorus [7, 8]. It has also been reported as an important source of micronutrients such as protein, lipids, essential amino acids such as (cysteine, lysine and methionine), minerals (copper, calcium, manganese, iron and zinc) and vitamins (thiamine, riboflavin, niacin, folic acid and retinol) in addition to significant amounts of other bioactive components with health-promoting impacts, like phytosterols, flavonoids and polyphenols [9 - 11].

Table 1. Nutrient content of Quinoa.

Nutrient	Unit	Value Per 100 G
Proximal		
Water	g	13.28
Energy	kcal	368
Energy	kJ	1539
Protein	g	14.12
Total lipids (fat)	g	6.07
Ashes	g	2.38
Carbohydrates, by difference	g	64.16
Fibre, total dietary	g	7
Starch	g	52.22
Minerals		
Calcium, Ca	mg	47
Iron, Fe	mg	4.57
Magnesium,	Mg	197
Phosphorus,	P mg	457
Potassium, K	mg	563

(Table 1) cont.....

Nutrient	Unit	Value Per 100 G
Sodium, Na	mg	5
Zinc, Zn	mg	3.1
Copper, Cu	mg	0.59
Manganese, Mn	mg	2033
Selenium, Se	μg	8.5
Vitamins		
Thiamine	mg	0.36
Riboflavin	mg	0.318
Niacin	mg	1520
Pantothenic acid	mg	0.772
Vitamin B6	mg	0.487
Vitamin C., total ascorbic acid*	mg	22.39
Pholate, total	mg	184
Betaine	mg	630.4
Luteine + Zeaxantine	mg	163
Vitamin E (alpha-tocopherol)	mg	2.44
Tocopherol, beta	mg	0.08
Tocopherol, gamma	mg	4.55
Tocopherol, delta	mg	0.35
Lipids		
Fatty acids, total saturated	g	0.706
Fatty acids, total monounsaturated	g	1613
Fatty acids, total polyunsaturated	g	3292

*Source: reference [12].

Table 2. Approximate composition in genotypes of quinoa grain (g 100 g^{-1} dm).

Composition (%)	Kozioł [13]	Dini *et al.* [14]	Wright *et al.* [15]	Ogungbenle [16]	USDA [17]
Crude protein	16.5	13.7	16.7	15.2	16.3
Lipids	6.3	14.5	5.5	7.1	7
Fibre	3.8	2.6	10.5	10.7	7
Carbohydrates	69	65.7	74.7	65.6	74
Ash	3.8	3.5	3.2	1.4	2.7

Table 3. Composition of essential amino acid profile in quinoa, in relation to FAO standard (g amino acid 100 g^{-1} protein).

Amino Acid	References					
	Kozioł [13]	Dini *et al.* [14]	Repo-Carrasco *et al.* [18]	Wright *et al.* [15]	Gonz´alez *et al.* [19]	FAO [20]
Histidine	3.2	2	2.7	3.1	ND	1.7
Isoleucine	4.4	7.4	3.4	3.3	ND	4
Leucine	6.6	7.5	6.1	5.8	ND	7
Methionine + Cystine	4.8	4.5	4.8	2.0[a]	2.4[a]	3.5
Phenylalanine + Tyrosine	7.3	7.5	6.2	6.2	ND	6
Threonine	3.8	3.5	3.4	2.5	ND	4
Valine	4.5	6	4.2	4	ND	5
Lysine	6.1	4.6	5.6	6.1	6.6	5.5
Tryptophan	1.2	ND	1.1	ND	1.1	1

ND: not determine, a: only methionine reported.

Table 4. Vitamin concentration (mg 100 g^{-1} dry weight).

Vitamin	References	
	Kozioł [13]	Ruales and Nair [21]
Ascorbic acid (C)	4	16.4
α-Tocopherol (E)	5.37	2.6
Thiamin (B1)	0.38	0.4
Riboflavin (B2)	0.39	ND
Niacin (B3)	1.06	ND

ND, not detected.

Global Various Regions for Quinoa Cultivation

Currently, the quinoa crop is examined in several countries across the world [22, 23]. This global expansion of quinoa has been established through the global and multilateral system to permit the scientists, plant breeders and farmers to exchange plant genetic materials [24]. The quinoa seed exchange among different countries participated in quinoa investigations is shown in Fig (**1**). Collections of quinoa were reported during the 1980s by Wilson (1988, 1990) and were taken back to the United States. In Italy, The Cereal Research Centre (CER-CRA) had considered and investigated 100 accessions for cultivation and development of many varieties adapted to conditions of Mediterranean countries. After characterization and evaluation of germplasm, low-performing accessions were excluded and some of the chosen accessions were then distributed to some countries associated to a FAO regional project like Egypt and Iran [23, 24].

Traditional Use of Quinoa Grains

Besides, the whole plant has also been used as a substantial nutritional source in animal feeds, primarily poultry species [25]. A lot of published investigations have shown a wide range of health uses for quinoa, such as the treatment of fractures and wounds as well as promote gut health [25, 26].

BIOLOGICAL PROPERTIES AND FUNCTIONAL APPLICATIONS OF QUINOA

Anti-Oxidants and Immunomodulatory Effects

Currently, the seeds of quinoa are characterized as an excellent source of antioxidants [27]. Similarly, lipophilic antioxidants in quinoa and amaranth plants such as carotenoids, tocopherols, and fatty acids also contribute to the antioxidant activity of these grains. Most of the phenolic compounds and other extracts of the quinoa plant are capable of exhibiting anti-oxidant activity [28 - 30]. The anti-oxidant effect of iso-flavones has been stated clearly by Jiang *et al.* [31]. Supplementation of 40 or 80 mg/kg of iso-flavones significantly increased total antioxidant capacity and slightly improved total superoxide dismutase (SOD) and catalase (CAT) activity in the blood of chickens [32]. Considered as a whole, these evidence support the fact that quinoa could be used as a potential food supplement that is capable of improving an ordinary diet by providing sources of natural phenolic compounds. The aqueous and methanol extracts of quinoa have been determined to increase the activities of glutathione peroxidase (GPx) and SOD in hepatic tissue, and augment the production of 12-hydroxy-eicosate traenoic acid [33]. Nitric oxide is another signaling molecule that diminishes oxidative stress, thus being important in repairing the oxidative damages caused by the imbalance between the production of reactive oxygen species (ROS) and antioxidant defense [34].

In another study, quinoa has shown to significantly inhibit the overproduction of inflammatory mediators such as IL-6 and TNF-α from macrophages [35]. Quinoa polysaccharides were found to be very outstanding nutraceutical ingredients or functional foods for improving the immune system [36]. When the cereal grain was ingested by coeliac-disease patients, various immunogenic gluten peptides were produced and this would stimulate the immune system through multiple cellular channels and cause the premature aging of the mucus enterocytes which cover the lumen of the alimentary tract [37].

Anti-Inflammatory Effects

Polyphenols extracted from quinoa have been reported to reduce IL-1β, IL-8, and TNF cytokines in cultured colonic epithelial Caco-2 cells, prevent obesity-induced inflammation and promote gastrointestinal health in mice [38]. Quinoa saponins are important functional foods that could inhibit the overproduction of inflammatory mediators such as IL-6 and TNF-α thereby helping in the prevention and treatment of inflammatory problems [35]. It is demonstrated that the quinoa leaves and seeds have notable values of oleanolic acid due to the presence of aglycon in the seeds and hederagenin in the leaves [39], which have a role in several anti-inflammatory molecular mechanisms [40]. For considering the pharmaceutical potential of triterpene saponins, further investigations should concentrate on the application and characterization of quinoa saponins as anti-inflammatory and co-adjuvants agents in the absorption of certain drugs due to their capacity to induce alterations in intestinal resistance [18]. The current published literature has suggested that quinoa saponins play a major role in anti-inflammatory activity [42]. Recent studies have shown that extractable phenolic and polyunsaturated fatty acids (PUFA) of cooked quinoa significantly inhibit the release of pro-inflammatory factor IL-8, and reduce the mRNA expression of TNF-α, IL-1β, IL-8, IL-6, and COX-2 [35, 36, 43].

Antihypertensive and Hypocholesterolemic Effects

Moreover, the use of quinoa protein had revealed the binding activity to bile acids *in vitro* and can modulate the expression of 3-hydroxy-3-methylgluta-yl-coenzyme A (HMG-CoA) in the liver. Feeding of mice on a diet containing quinoa protein isolates can reduce the cholesterol level in liver and plasma probably due to the control of cholesterol synthesis and its catabolism and the prevention of bile-acid re-absorption in the small intestine [44]. Cholesterol absorbed through the diet and produced in the liver is essential for normal metabolic processes. Nevertheless, high levels of total cholesterol and elevated levels of low-density lipoproteins have been related to the high risk of coronary diseases [45]. Similarly, numerous investigations have demonstrated that the existence of sterols in plants prevents the absorption of cholesterol in intestines [46]. The investigation of phytosterol content in quinoa revealed the presence of β-sitosterol (63.7 mg/100g), which is greater than the seeds of maize, squash and barley [47].

Prebiotic Effects

Quinoa belongs to the group of the so-called "superfoods" and has a nutritional composition that confers health benefits. The gut's bacterial composition can be modified by different factors, including age, diseases, genetics and diet [48]. Therefore, it is advisable to introduce well known functional food and their ingredients in daily diets that can help in modulating the microbiota and improve colon health according to Gullón *et al.* [49] who suggested that these pseudo-cereals (quinoa) have the prebiotic potential and their intake could increase symbiosis or maintain the gastrointestinal health through a balanced intestinal microbiota, although additional studies are necessary to fully understand the prebiotic effects of quinoa in the poultry industry. Lamothe *et al.* [50], showed that quinoa represents a good source of dietary fiber(10%), which is much higher than that of wheat (2.7%), corn (1.7%), and rice (0.4%). Quinoa dietary insoluble fiber (78%) is mainly made up of homogalacturonans and RG-I with arabinan side chains (55–60%) xyloglucans (30%) and cellulose. The quinoa soluble fiber was mainly composed of arabinans and homogalacturonans as the predominant constituents.

Beneficial Uses of Quinoa in Poultry

Quinoa is one of the oldest crops and it has been extensively used as food and feed due to its high nutritional value [51]. As a result, quinoa has been used as a substitute source of protein for the poultry industry. The quinoa proteins contain a balanced composition of essential amino acids, similar to the composition of milk protein [52]. Previous studies have shown that the quinoa plant has been used in animal diets [53, 54]. The quinoa seed comprises crude protein (120-180 g/kg), which contains a better-balanced amino acid composition than conventional crops such as oilseed rape, pulses and cereals [55]. So it can be used as a supplementary protein, to improve the balance of amino acids in animal diets [56]. Currently, many studies have shown that dietary supplementation of grain derived from quinoa, either whole or ground in varying concentrations; can fulfill the needs of monogastric animals, particularly poultry. Jacobsen *et al.* [50], reported that the hulls of quinoa seeds (approximately 10% of the seed) that contain bitter saponins might inhibit the ingestion of quinoa grain, but it must be removed by being washed before the inclusion in the feed. Ward [57], reported that the broilers supplemented with a quinoa-based diet (30%) had achieved a better performance without any adverse effects. However, high levels of quinoa (with bitter saponin) can cause vitamin A deficiency. Generally, low doses of saponin perhaps not be absorbed through the gastrointestinal tract but might facilitate the absorption of other nutrients in the gut and thereby improving the health and protecting aganist various diseases [58]. Previous evidence has shown that saponin induces positive effects on the performance of ruminants, fish and monogastric animals [59, 60]. The dietary inclusion of saponins derived from *quillaja* had been reported to trigger the immune system in a pig model [61]. Another study also confirmed that the addition of saponin to chicken feed increased villus height in the small intestine [62]. As describe by Onning *et al.* [58], supplementary saponin had increased mucosal permeability in the gut of rats.

It is suggested that quinoa seed has the potential to be used as a poultry feed, but it use should not exceed the inclusion level of 150 g/kg of the diet, while it is observed that dehulling quinoa had slightly improved broiler performance [57]. Horsted and Hermansen [63], speculated that nutrient-restriction and high producing organic layer are capable of utilizing a considerable amount of quinoa without having any adverse effects on welfare or health. The residue obtained from milling has high nutritional content making it suitable for animals and the low-quality broken grains are used for poultry feed [64]. Another study elucidated that washing or polishing of quinoa before being used in feeding, or diluting the quinoa with another available feed are viable options which should be considered to improve the performance of broilers when quinoa is a major component in the diet [65]. Cardozo and Tapia [66], reported that the higher weight gain was determined in birds that were supplemented with washed and cooked quinoa, compared to unwashed and cooked quinoa. Gandarillas [67], reported no significant difference in the performance of broiler chickens supplemented with a diet contained 400 g/kg of washed and cooked quinoa seeds in comparison with maize. Cardozo [68], reported that unprocessed quinoa declined the live weight gain in broiler chickens. Thus, cooking or washing of the quinoa before being supplemented can be more practical in removing the growth decreasing factors in broiler chicken. Jacobsen *et al.* [52] concluded that quinoa could be used as an efficient feed additive in the broiler production industry. The biological activities of quinoa have been examined both *in vitro* and *in vivo,* in different animal models, although the poultry trials on the effectiveness of this plant have been poorly understood.

CONCLUSIONS

Quinoa is a grain-like, food crop with a higher nutritional value compared to other traditional cereals. Quinoa contains a good balance of methionine and lysine contents, carbohydrates, high-quality protein, and is rich in dietary fiber. Quinoa seeds have become quite popular due to their many physiological functions, such as; hypocholesterolemic, anti-inflammatory, anti-oxidant, antimicrobial, immune-modulatory, and cholesterol-lowering activities that have been examined both *in vitro* and *in vivo* in different poultry species. Moreover, quinoa contains a high protein and essential amino acid content (120-180 g/kg). Its high fat and starch content making it a high-quality feed additive in the poultry production industry. It is reported that quinoa seed has the potential to be used as a poultry feed additive, but its use should not exceed the inclusion level of 150 g/kg of the diet. So, this chapter highlighted the medicinal and nutritional importance of quinoa that could allow it to be considered as a feed additive to boost productivity and health performance in poultry farming. However, poultry trials on possible methods of quinoa supplementation in the diet have been poorly understood, so further studies are imperative to reveal its nutritional and therapeutic impacts in the poultry.

CONSENT FOR PUBLICATION

Not Applicable.

CONFLICT OF INTEREST

The author confirms that this chapter contents have no conflict of interest.

ACKNOWLEDGEMENTS

Declared none.

REFERENCES

[1]   Ruiz KB, Biondi S, Oses R, *et al.* Quinoa biodiversity and sustainability for food security under climate change. A review. Agron Sustain Dev 2014; 34: 349-59.

[2]   Kuljanabhagavad T, Thongphasuk P, Chamulitrat W, Wink M. Triterpene saponins from *Chenopodium quinoa* willd. Phytochemistry 2008; 69: 1919-26.

[3]   Mota C, Santos M, Mauro R, *et al.* Protein content and amino acids profile of pseudoccreals. Food Chem 2016; 193: 55-61.

[4]   Lintschinger J, Fuchs N, Moser H, *et al.* Uptake of various trace elements during germination of wheat, buckwheat and quinoa. Plant Foods Hum Nutr 1997; 50: 223-37. [Formerly Qualitas Plantarum].

[5]   Brady K, Ho CT, Rosen RT, Sang S, Karwe MV. Effects of processing on the nutraceutical profile of quinoa. Food Chem 2007; 100: 1209-16.

[6]   Tang Y, Li X, Zhang B, Chen PX, Liu R, Tsao R. Characterisation of phenolics, betanins and antioxidant activities in seeds of three *Chenopodium quinoa* willd. Genotypes. Food Chem 2015; 166: 380-8.

[7]   Abugoch James LE. Quinoa (*Chenopodium quinoa* Willd.): composition, chemistry, nutritional, and functional properties. Adv Food Nutr Res 2009; 58: 1-31.

[8]   Jancurová M, Minarovicová L, Dandar A. Quinoa–a review. Czech J Food Sci 2009; 27: 71-9.

[9]   Nascimento AC, Mota C, Coelho I, *et al.* Characterisation of nutrient profile of quinoa (*Chenopodium quinoa*), amaranth (*Amaranthus caudatus*), and purple corn (Zea mays L.) consumed in the North of Argentina: proximates, minerals and trace elements. Food Chem 2014; 148: 420-6.

[10]   Taylor JRN, Belton PS, Beta T, Duodu KG. Increasing the utilisation of sorghum, millets and pseudocereals: Developments in the science of their phenolic phytochemicals, biofortification and protein functionality. J Cereal Sci 2014; 59: 257-75.

[11]   Filho AM, Pirozi MR, Borges JT, Pinheiro Sant'ana HM, Chaves JB, Coimbra JS. Quinoa: Nutritional, functional, and antinutritional aspects. Crit Rev Food Sci Nutr 2017; 57: 1618-30.

[12]   Usda, Department of Agriculture. Agricultural Research Service, USDA National Nutrient Database for Standard Reference, Release 26. Nutrient Data Laboratory Home. Page 2013. http://www.ars.usda.gov/ ba/bhnrc/nd

[13]   Kozioł M. Chemical composition and nutritional evaluation of Quinoa. (*Chenopodium quinoa* Willd). J Food Compos Anal 1992; 5: 35-68.

[14]   Dini A, Rastrelli L, Saturnino P, Schettino O. A compositional study of *Chenopodium quinoa* seeds. Nahrung 1992; 36: 400-4.

[15]   Wright KH, Pike OA, Fairbanks DJ, Huber SC. Composition of Atriplex hortensis, sweet and bitter *Chenopodium quinoa* seeds. Food Chem Toxicol 2002; 67: 1383-5.

[16]   Ogungbenle NH. Nutritional evaluation and functional properties of quinoa (*Chenopodium quinoa*) flour. Int J Food Sci Nutr 2003; 54: 153-8.

[17]   Usda, United States Department of Agriculture – Agricultural Research Service. National Nutrient Database for Standard Reference, Release 27. Nutrient Data Laboratory 2011. Available in: http://www.nal.usda.gov/fnic/foodcomp/search

[18]   Repo-Carrasco R, Espinoza C, Jacobsen SE. Nutritional value and use of the andean crops quinoa (*Chenopodium quinoa*) and kañiwa (*chenopodium pallidicaule*). Food Rev Int 2003; 19: 179-89.

[19]   Gonz'Alez JA, Rold'An A, Gallardo M, Escudero T, Prado FE. Quantitative determinations of chemical compounds with nutritional value from inca crops: *Chenopodium quinoa* ('quinoa'). Plant Foods Hum Nutr 1989; 39: 331-7.

[20]   Fao/Who/Unu. Food and Agriculture Organization of the United States/World Health Organization/United Nations University, Energy and protein requirements Report of a joint FAO/WHO/UNU meeting. Geneva: World Health Organization 1985.

[21]   Ruales J, Nair BM. Contents of fat, vitamins and minerals in quinoa (*Chenopodium quinoa* Willd.) seeds. Food Chem 1993; 48: 131-7.

[22]   FAO & CIRAD. State of the Art Report of Quinoa in the World in 2013. In: Bazile D, Bertero D, Nieto C, (Eds). Rome 2015.

[23]   Bazile D, Jacobsen SE, Verniau A. The global expansion of quinoa: Trends and limits. Front Plant Sci 2016; 7: 622.

[24]   Louafi S, Bazile D, Noyer JL. Conserving and cultivating agricultural genetic diversity: Transcending established divides. Cultivating Biodiversity to Transform Agriculture. Springer 2013; pp. 181-220.

[25]   Bhargava A, Shukla S, Ohri D. *Chenopodium quinoa*-an indian perspective. Ind Crops Prod 2006; 23: 73-87.

[26]   FAO. Quinoa: an ancient crop to contribute to world food security 2011. http://www.fao.org/docrep/017/aq287e/aq287e.pdf

[27]   Kraujalis P, Venskutonis PR, Kraujalienė V, Pukalskas A. Antioxidant properties and preliminary evaluation of phytochemical composition of different anatomical parts of amaranth. Plant Foods Hum Nutr 2013; 68: 322-8.

[28]   Pasko P, Barton H, Zagrodzki P, *et al.* Effect of diet supplemented with quinoa seeds on oxidative status in plasma and selected tissues of high fructose-fed rats. Plant Foods Hum Nutr 2010; 65: 146-51.

[29]   Tang Y, Tsao R. Phytochemicals in quinoa and amaranth grains and their antioxidant, anti-inflammatory and potential health beneficial effects: A review. Mol Nutr Food Res 2017; 61(7) [http://dx.doi.org/10.1002/mnfr.201600767]

[30]   Nsimba RY, Kikuzaki H, Konishi Y. Antioxidant activity of various extracts and fractions of *Chenopodium quinoa* and amaranthus spp. Seeds. Food Chem 2008; 106: 760-6.

[31]   Jiang Q, Payton-Stewart F, Elliott S, *et al.* Effects of 7-o substitutions on estrogenic and anti-estrogenic activities of daidzein analogues in mcf-7 breast cancer cells. J Med Chem 2010; 53: 6153-63.

[32]   Jiang Z. Effects of soybean isoflavone on growth performance, meat quality, and antioxidation in male broilers. Poult Sci 2007; 86: 1356-62.

[33]   Matsuo M. *In vivo* antioxidant activity of methanol extract from quinoa fermented with *rhizopus oligosporus*. J Nutr Sci Vitaminol (Tokyo) 2005; 51: 449-52.

[34]   Tang Y, Zhang B, Li X, *et al.* Bound phenolics of quinoa seeds released by acid, alkaline, and enzymatic treatments and their antioxidant and α-glucosidase and pancreatic lipase inhibitory effects. J Agric Food Chem 2016; 64: 1712-9.

[35]   Yao Y, Yang X, Shi Z, Ren G. Anti-inflammatory activity of saponins from quinoa (*Chenopodium quinoa* willd.) seeds in lipopolysaccharide-stimulated raw 264.7 macrophages cells. J Food Sci 2014; 79: H1018-23. b

[36]   Yao Y, Shi Z, Ren G. Antioxidant and immunoregulatory activity of polysaccharides from quinoa (*Chenopodium quinoa* willd.). Int J Mol Sci 2014; 15: 19307-18. a

[37]   Tjon AS, Nicolaas JS, Kwekkeboom J, *et al.* Increased incidence of early *de novo* cancer in liver graft recipients treated with cyclosporine: An association with C_2 monitoring and recipient age. Liver Transpl 2010; 16: 837-46.

[38]   Noratto G, Carrion-Rabanal R, Medina G, *et al.* Quinoa protective effects against obesity-induced intestinal inflammation. FASEB J 2015; 29: 602-9.

[39]   Mastebroek HD, Limburg H, Gilles T, Marvin HJP. Occurrence of sapogenins in leaves and seeds of quinoa (*Chenopodium quinoa* willd). J Sci Food Agric 2000; 80: 152-6.

[40]   Wang X, Liu R, Zhang W, *et al.* Oleanolic acid improves hepatic insulin resistance *via* antioxidant, hypolipidemic and anti-inflammatory effects. Mol Cell Endocrinol 2013; 376: 70-80.

[41]   Gee J, Price K, Ridout C, Johnson I, Fenwick G. Effects of some purified saponins on transmural potential difference in mammalian small intestine. Toxicol *In Vitro* 1989; 3: 85-90.

[42]   Mujica A. Andean grains and legumes. Neglected crops: 1492 from a different perspective In: Bermujo Hernando, Leon, J JE, Eds. 1994; 26: 131-48. http://www.hort.purdue.edu/newcrop/1492/grains.html

[43]   Marino R, Mariangela C, Giovanni A, *et al.* Effect of diet supplementation with quinoa seed and/or linseed on immune response, productivity and meat quality in merinos derived lambs. Animals (Basel) 2018; 8: 204. [http://dx.doi.org/10.3390/ani8110204]

[44]   Ogawa H, Watanabe K, Mitsunaga T, Meguro T. Effect of quinoa on blood pressure and lipid metabolism in diet-induced hyperlipidemic spontaneously hypertensive rats (shr). J Jpn Soc Nutr Food Sci 2001; 54(4): 221-7.

[45]   Quilez J, Garcia-Lorda P, Salas-Salvado J. Potential uses and benefits of phytosterols in diet: Present situation and future directions. Clin Nutr 2003; 22: 343-51.

[46]   Moreau RA, Whitaker BD, Hicks KB. Phytosterols, phytostanols, and their conjugates in foods: Structural diversity, quantitative analysis, and health-promoting uses. Prog Lipid Res 2002; 41: 457-500.

[47] Ryan E, Galvin K, O'connor T, Maguire A, O'brien N. Phytosterol, squalene, tocopherol content and fatty acid profile of selected seeds, grains, and legumes. Plant Foods Hum Nutr 2007; 62: 85-91.

[48] Benson AK, Kelly SA, Legge R, *et al*. Individuality in gut microbiota composition is a complex polygenic trait shaped by multiple environmental and host genetic factors. Proc Natl Acad Sci USA 2010; 107: 18933-8.

[49] Gullón B, Gullón P, Tavaria FK, Yáñez R. Assessment of the prebiotic effect of quinoa and amaranth in the human intestinal ecosystem. Food Funct 2016; 7: 3782-8.

[50] Lamothe LM, Srichuwong S, Reuhs BL, Hamaker BR. Quinoa (*Chenopodium quinoa* W.) and Amaranth (*Amaranthus caudatus* L.) Provide dietary fibres high in pectic substances and xyloglucans. Food Chem 2015; 167: 490-6.

[51] Repo-Carrasco-Valencia R, Cruz AADL, Alvarez JCI, Kallio H. Chemical and functional characterization of kañiwa (c henopodium pallidicaule) grain, extrudate and bran. Plant Foods Hum Nutr 2009; 64: 94-101.

[52] Jacobsen SE, Hill J, Stolen O. Stability of quantitative traits in quinoa (*Chenopodium quinoa*). Theor Appl Genet 1996; 93: 110-6.

[53] Bonifacio A. Chenopodium Sp.: Genetic resources, ethnobotany, and geographic distribution. Food Rev Int 2003; 19: 1-7.

[54] Galwey N, Leakey CLA, Price KR, Fenwick GR. Chemical composition and nutritional characteristics of quinoa (*Chenopodium quinoa* willd). Food Sci Nutr 1990; 245-61.

[55] Jacobsen SE. The worldwide potential for quinoa (*Chenopodium quinoa* willd.). Food Rev Int 2003; 19: 167-77.

[56] Jacobsen EE, Skadhauge B, Jacobsen SE. Effect of dietary inclusion of quinoa on broiler growth performance. Anim Feed Sci Technol 1997; 65: 5-14.

[57] Ward SM. Response to selection for reduced grain saponin content in quinoa (*Chenopodium quinoa* willd.). Field Crops Res 2000; 68: 157-63.

[58] Onning G, Wang Q, Weström BR, Asp NG, Karlsson BW. Influnce of oat saponins on intestinal permeability *in vitro* and *in vivo* in the rat. Br J Nutr 1996; 76: 141-51.

[59] Francis G, Kerem Z, Makkar HP, Becker K. The biological action of saponins in animal systems: A review. Br J Nutr 2002; 88: 587-605.

[60] Cheeke PR, Otero R. Yucca, quillaja may have role in animal nutrition. Feedstuffs 2005; 77: 11-4.

[61] Ilsley SE, Miller HM, Kamel C. Effects of dietary quillaja saponin and curcumin on the performance and immune status of weaned piglets. J Anim Sci 2005; 83: 82-8.

[62] Alfaro DM, Silva AVF, Borges SA, Maiorka FA, Vargas S, Santin E. Use of yucca schidigera extract in broiler diets and its effects on performance results obtained with different coccidiosis control methods. J Appl Poult Res 2007; 16: 248-54.

[63] Horsted K, Hermansen JE. Whole wheat *versus* mixed layer diet as supplementary feed to layers foraging a sequence of different forage crops. Animal 2007; 1(4): 575-85.

[64] León H. Cultivo de la quinua en puno–perú. Descripción, manejo y producción. Universidad Nacional del Altillano-Facultad de Ciencias Agrarias 2003.

[65] Improta F, Kellems RO. Comparison of raw, washed and polished quinoa (*Chenopodium quinoa* Willd.) to wheat, sorghum or maize based diets on growth and survival of broiler chicks. Livest Res Rural Dev 2001; 13: 1. Retrieved December 7, 2020, from http://www.lrrd.org/lrrd13/1/impr131.htm

[66] Cardozo A, Tapia M. Valor nutritivo Quinoa y Kañiwa Cultivos andinos Editorial IICA Centro Internacional de Investigaciones para el Desarrollo (CIID) Instituto Interamericano de Ciencias Agrícolas. Bogotá, Colombia: IICA 1979; pp. 149-92.

[67]   Gandarillas H. Efecto fisiol6gico de la saponina de la quinua en 10s animales. Rev Agric (Piracicaba) 1948; 4: 52-6.

[68]   Cardozo E. El Paraguay colonial: las raíces de la nacionalidad. Ediciones Nizza 1959.

CHAPTER 8

Turmeric (*Curcuma longa*) as a Useful Feed Supplement in Poultry

Mohamed E. Abd El-Hack[1,*], Mohammed A. E. Naiel[2], Samar S. Negm[3], Asmaa F. Khafaga[4], Sabry A.A. El-Sayed[5], Sarah Y.A. Ahmed[6], Mayada R. Farag[7] and Mahmoud Alagawany[1,*]

[1] *Department of Poultry, Faculty of Agriculture, Zagazig University, Zagazig 44511, Egypt*

[2] *Department of Animal Production, Faculty of Agriculture, Zagazig University, Zagazig 44511, Egypt*

[3] *Fish Biology and Ecology Department, Central Lab for Aquaculture Research Abassa, Agriculture Research Centre, Giza, Egypt*

[4] *Department of Pathology, Faculty of Veterinary Medicine, Alexandria University, Edfina 22758, Egypt*

[5] *Department of Nutrition and Clinical Nutrition, Faculty of Veterinary Medicine, Zagazig University, Zagazig, Egypt*

[6] *Department of Microbiology, Faculty of Veterinary Medicine, Zagazig University, Zagazig, Egypt*

[7] *Forensic Medicine and Toxicology Department, Veterinary Medicine Faculty, Zagazig University, Zagazig 44519, Egypt*

Abstract: In the last decade, poultry nutritionists were particularly interested in inspecting relevant natural antibiotic alternatives to be used in poultry feeding to reduce the competitive efficacy of bacterial resistance and its residuals in poultry products. Using antibiotics and hormones in feed not only raises production costs but they also get incorporated into the processing of meat and eggs and increase microbial resistance. Several synthetic medicine and growth promoters are fortified into broilers diets for fast growth. However, their use still shows some drawbacks, such as high costs, adverse side effects on bird health, and extended residual properties. Thus, the primary aim of poultry production is to obtain higher performance through increasing the feed efficiency besides getting safety products for consumption. Due to their nutritional and immunological effects, such as improved feed efficiency, regulation of endogenous digestive enzymes, immune response stimulation, antiviral, antibacterial, and antioxidant properties, medicinal plants seem to be of great importance. Turmeric (*Curcuma longa*) is a useful medicinal herb belonging to the ginger family, Zingiberaceae which is inherent to the Asian subcontinent.

* **Corresponding authors Mahmoud Alagawany and Mohamed E. Abd El-Hack:** Poultry Department, Faculty of Agriculture, Zagazig University, Zagazig, Egypt; E-mails: mmalagwany@zu.edu.eg and m.ezzat@zu.edu.eg

It has numerous medicinal properties, such as antimicrobial, anti-inflammatory, antimutagenic activities, and other beneficial health applications. Furthermore, turmeric contains several biologically active compounds such as curcumin, bisdemethoxy curcumin, demethoxy-curcumin, and tetrahydrocurcuminoids, which may be responsible for these beneficial effects. Besides, turmeric is safe due to its low toxicity index and could be effective against aflatoxin-induced mutagenicity and hepatocarcinogenicity. In this chapter, we will discuss the valuable effects of turmeric in terms of the production, carcass traits, and ameliorative role in bird .

Keywords: Growth promoter, Immunomodulation, Poultry, Turmeric.

INTRODUCTION

Feed additives are often used in the production of poultry to enhance the quality of production, performance and bird health [1]. Using low prophylactic levels of antibiotics to improve growth, as well as gastrointestinal health, has become a common procedure in modern poultry production industries [2]. Furthermore, inappropriate and unnecessary use of antibiotics may lead to the development of antibiotic-resistant bacterial strains, which adversely affect both bird and consumers' health [3]. Thus, using safe, natural herbs as feed additives to substitute the antibiotics as growth promoters and efficiency enhancers has a tremendous and critical demand for the poultry industry [4]. Several medicinal plants show potential as growth promoters, antibacterials, immunostimulants, antioxidants, and anti-stress agents [5 - 8]. They could also be valuable for the prevention and cure of various types of diseases, disorders, and illnesses [9].

Turmeric (*Curcuma longa*) is a seasonal flowering plant of the family Zingiberaceae, and grows predominantly in tropical regions of India and Southern East Asia [10]. It is a three to five feet high stemless plant with yellowish leaves, yellow rhizome/root, and white clustered flowers [11]. Generally, turmeric is a medicinal plant used as an ingredient in the diet to enhance the appearance, flavor, palatability, and preservation of feed [12]. Also, it has antioxidant, antibacterial, antifungal, antiprotozoal, antiviral, anti-inflammation, anticarcinogenic, antihypertensive, and hypo-cholesteric activities [13]. Curcuminoid and a polyphenol present in the form of curcumin are the active principles of the turmeric mode of action [14]. Curcumin is an orange-yellow turmeric pigment derived by extracting 40% of the oleoresin turmeric oil content [15]. The turmeric oil contains mainly turmerone and curlone compounds, which have also been tested against several bacterial strains (*Staphylococcus aureus, Bacillus cereus, Bacillus coagulans, Bacillus subtilis, Escherichia coli,* and *Pseudomonas aeruginosa*) [16]. Besides, numerous medicinal properties of turmeric are well documented in several poultry studies [17 - 20]. The use of herbal products is gaining increasing attention in both the industry and scientific circles. Thus, the present chapter will discuss the beneficial applications and mode of actions of *Curcuma longa*, including its health impact and preventive action on diseases. Also, we will present the nutritional role of turmeric and its effect on production and carcass traits in broilers and hens. The chapter will be useful for veterinary professionals, people involved in pharmaceutical industries, researchers, scientists, and the poultry industry.

TURMERIC ACTIVE CONSTITUENTS

Turmeric is commonly used as the primary provenance of curcumin in several medications (Fig. **1**) [21].

The chemical analysis of turmeric powder shows that it consists of nearly 60–70% carbohydrates, 6–13% moisture, 6–8% crude protein, 5–10% crude fat, 3–7% minerals, 3–7% essential oils, 2–7% fiber, and 1–6% of curcumin-related compounds [22]. Several active ingredients in turmeric rhizomes are volatile and non-volatile components [23]. Within turmeric, there are 34 essential oils, including, for example, turmerone, germacrone, atlantone and zingiberene [24]. Coloring agents, which are the primary sources of several phenolic compounds such as demethoxycurcumin, curcumin, tetrahydrocurcumin, and bisdemethoxycurcumin, in addition to the colorless metabolites, are the main active substances in non-volatile compounds [25]. While curcuminoids are the principal active substances in volatile oil [26]. Turmeric powder contains approximately 3.14% curcumin, the content of which differs among *Curcuma longa* species [27]. Curcumin "diferuloylmethane" with the chemical formula of (1,7-bis(4-hydroxy-3-methoxyphenyl)-1,6-heptadiene-3,5-dione) and with 368,379 molecular weight and other curcuminoids are the major phytochemicals of *Curcuma longa* L. belonging to the family of Zingiberaceae, rhizome [28]. Curcumin can be metabolized with catabolic products, including vanillic acid and ferulic acid, into curcumin-sulfate, curcumin-glucuronide [29]. Thus, curcumin has a surprisingly wide range of pleiotropic beneficial properties and activities, including survival pathways regulated by NF-κBand Akt, the growth factors; Nrf2 mediated cytoprotective pathways, metastatic and angiogenic pathways and acts as a free radical scavenger and hydrogen donor with pro- and antioxidant activity due to demethoxycurcumin and bisdemethoxycurcumin, in addition to the anti-inflammatory, hypolipidemic, antioxidant, antiviral, antibacterial, antifungal, anticancer and chemotherapeutic activities [30 - 32].

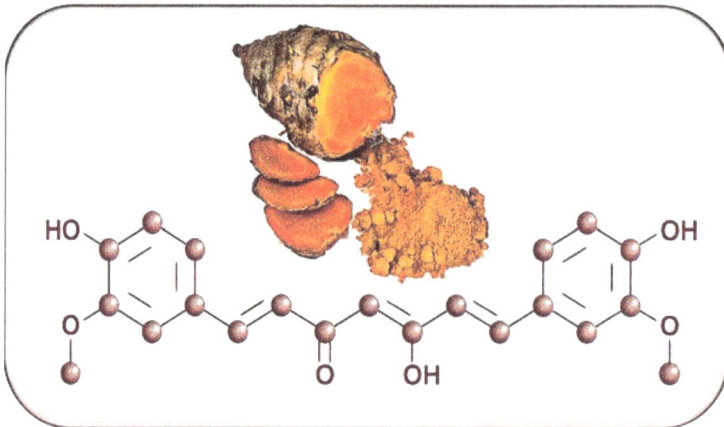

Fig. (1). Chemical structure of enol turmeric.

THE BENEFICIAL APPLICATIONS OF TURMERIC IN POULTRY PRODUCTION

Previous studies have shown that turmeric has diverse biological, clinical and pharmacological applications [33]. Curcumin's beneficial biological properties include cellular and molecular mechanisms that support its use as an anti-inflammatory and healing enhancer [34]. In poultry studies, turmeric has beneficial effects on blood parameters in broilers and laying hens [35]. Fat metabolism studies using male Wanjiang Yellow [36] and Arbor Acres [37] broiler chickens exhibited that dietary supplementation of 0.35 g kg^{-1} turmeric reliably stimulated hormone-sensitive lipase (HSL) and tended to increase the high-density lipoprotein (HDL) content in the serum. Moreover, broiler diets supplemented with turmeric reduced the total cholesterol concentration, total triglycerides and very-low-density lipoprotein (VLDL) content in the serum [38]. Additionally, the dietary supplementation of Hy-Line W-38 laying hen's diets with 0.5 g kg^{-1} turmeric increased the HDL-cholesterol and reduced the triglyceride and total LDL-cholesterol levels in the serum [39].

The curcumin's antioxidant function is primarily due to the presence of phenolic hydroxyl (OH) group, and the substitution or elimination of this group resulted in the loss of antioxidant properties and the scavenging of free radicals in the cells [40]. Also, curcumin can improve the production of inducible nitric oxide synthase (iNOS), which plays a vital role in the synthesis of nitric oxide in large amounts by macrophages to eliminate pathogens. Consequently, curcumin could minimize the activity of iNOS, thereby reducing the development of harmful nitric oxide leading to a reduction of reactive oxygen species in cells [41]. The antioxidant properties of curcumin have been shown to prevent liver damage caused by oxidative stress during liver diseases [42]. The valuable applications and mode of actions of *Curcuma longa,* including its health impact and role in preventing infections in poultry, will be presented later in detail.

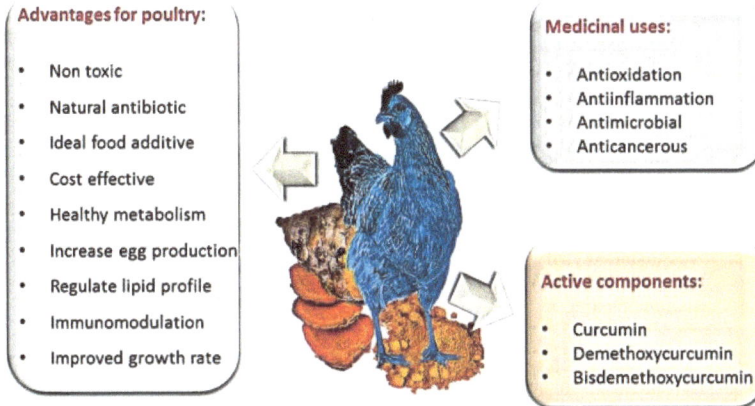

Fig. (2). Active component, medicinal use, and advantages of turmeric in poultry.

Immunostimulatory Role of Turmeric

Turmeric powder has been verified as an effective immunostimulating agent that can regulate the stimulation of T cells, B cells, K cells, neutrophils, macrophages and dendritic cells [43]. The immune response of poultry fed on turmeric supplemented diets was evaluated where the dietary supplementation of turmeric at the level of 0.5 g kg^{-1} decreased the harmful effect of aflatoxin B1 on the immune system by stimulating the humoral immune system in poultry [44]. Some studies revealed that supplementation of either 0.5% or 1.0% turmeric powder improved the immune response and antioxidant enzymes concentration in broiler chickens [45].

Turmeric ameliorated the deleterious effects of ochratoxin A on the haemato-biochemical and the immune system of laying hens [46]. Besides, it has an immunomodulatory impact against parasitic infection in broiler chickens [47]. When curcumin-enriched food was used for five weeks, it reduced digestive problems, pancreatitis and liver damage and prevented protozoan diseases such as amoebic dysentery [48]. Also, Mitogenic responses of splenic lymphocytes were increased by using turmeric in the poultry diet [49]. In addition, turmeric supplementation (5.0 g kg^{-1}) in broiler diet stimulated the antioxidant and immune-related genes expression in broiler chickens defense system (such as interleukins 6 and 2; IL-6 and IL-2) [50]. Also, broilers fed on turmeric supplemented diets had a significantly high expression level of pro-inflammatory cytokine (IL-1K) in the duodenum [51], and increased IL-6, IL-15 and IFN-L expression levels.

The turmeric treatment increased the number of mucosal CD4 (+) T and B cells, and regulated the lymphocyte immune functions [52]. These improvements could be attributed to the activity of turmeric as an immunostimulant agent [53]. Studies on broilers with *Piper nigrum* and *Curcuma longa* showed that the combination of these two herbs as feed additives increased antibody and total protein levels while reduced glucose level in serum, which reflects the beneficial role of curcumin in augmenting growth performance and inducing humoral immune responses of broiler chickens [54]. Curcumin increased the antibody level and reduced cholesterol and LDL in hens [55]. Curcumin also reduced lymphocyte proliferation, cell-mediated cytotoxicity and cytokine production by inhibiting NF-kappaB genes [53].

Anti-Inflammatory Effect

Turmeric has been known to possess anti-inflammatory activity by suppressing the production of inflammatory mediators [56]. The curcumin mechanism, which provokes its anti-inflammatory properties, still has to be explained. Very few studies revealed that peroxisome proliferator-activated receptor gamma (PPAR-γ) might be correlated with anti-inflammatory efficiency. In some studies it is mentioned that during ligand binding, the heterodimer forms of PPAR-ÿ with the retinoid X receptor bind to a peroxisome proliferation response element (PPRE) in a gene promoter, which leads to regulation of gene transcription. Thus, it was found that curcumin pretreatment for three days at 0.24 μmol kg^{-1} body weight increased the production of PPAR-γ mRNA and protein levels up to 45% and 65%, respectively [57]. In the ligand binding phase, curcumin could activate the PPAR-π receptor, heterodimerize with the receptor of retinoic acid and bind directly to the TNF-α gene PPRE itself or its encoding genes, thence inactivating its endogenous intermediaries. Additionally, curcumin binds to its receptor and the interaction between the ligand-binding phase and receptor triggers signaling pathways leading to the up-regulation and subsequent suppression of the inflammatory cytokines' activation. The exact mechanism of the anti-inflammatory effects caused by curcumin has been studied *in vitro* using macrophage cells [58]. Possible anti-inflammatory mechanisms of curcumin include inhibition of the Cox-2 pathway by inhibiting the phorbol ester-induced expression of cyclooxygenase-2 and prostaglandin E2 development throughout suppressing kinase activity and activation of NF-kappa B and by inducing detoxifying enzymes such as glutathione S-transferase [59]. Also, curcumin was found to prevent the immunostimulatory role of dendritic cells, reduce the proliferation of stimulated mitogenic lymphocytes, inhibit the release of lysosomal enzymes, eicosanoids, IL-2 signals and inflammatory cytokines from peripheral blood monocytes and alveolar macrophages, and induce nitric oxide synthesis in activated macrophages [60]. The anti-inflammatory effect is mediated by the inflammatory mediator enzyme, iNOS, and the excessive upregulation of this enzyme causes health problems linked to the inflammatory disorders. Additionally, volatile oil obtained from *Curcuma longa* showed anti-inflammatory effects against osteoarthritis and rheumatoid arthritis [61].

PREVENTING INFECTIOUS DISEASES

The *Curcuma longa* has usually been used as an antibacterial agent and antipathetic agent for insects [62]. *Curcuma longa* has been reported to be beneficial for preventing and treating intestinal disorders like diarrhea [32]. Also, turmeric oil extracted from *Curcuma longa* has antiviral, antimicrobial and anti-fungal efficacy. Besides, *Curcuma longa* inhibits the intestinal population of *E. coli* and enhances the growth of *lactobacillus* [63].

Antibacterial Activity

The *Curcuma longa* aqueous extract demonstrated antibacterial properties against *S. epidermis* ATCC 12228, *Staphylococcus aureus* ATCC 25923, *Klebsiella pneumoniae* ATCC 10031, and *E. coli* ATCC 25922 with the minimum inhibitory concentration (MIC) values of 4 to 16 g L^{-1} and minimum bactericidal concentration (MBC) values of 16 to 32 g L^{-1} [64]. Also, curcumin has been found useful in providing protecting from *Klebsiella pneumonia* induced lung inflammation in Balb-C mice and it blocks the mitogenic response in *Helicobacter pylori*-infected epithelial cells. Extracted curcuminoid compounds from *Curcuma longa* using hexane or ethanol (containing 86.5% curcumin) showed the highest antimicrobial activity against 24 pathogenic isolated bacteria from the chicken with the MIC value of 3.91 to 125 ppt. Additionally, extracts of *Curcuma longa* active compounds in hexane and methanol solutions demonstrated an antibacterial efficiency against thirteen bacterial strains, such as *S. aureus, Vibrio harveyi, V. alginolyticus, Bacillus subtilis, V. vulnificus, V. parahae molyticus, V. cholerae, B. cereus, Aeromonas hydrophila*, and *Streptococcus agalactiae* [65]. However, using curcumin extract solution with 125–250 μg mL^{-1} showed the highest MIC levels against methicillin-resistant *Staph. aureus* strains (MRSA) [66]. Also, curcumin displayed significant antibacterial efficiency with MIC values between 5 and 50 μg mL^{-1} against 65 clinical isolates of *H. pylori*. Besides, it is a potent growth inhibitor of *H. pylori* strains by causing non-competitive inhibition of shikimate dehydrogenase (SDH) enzyme activity, which is required by the *H. pylori* for the synthesis of various important amino acids and bacterial metabolites to counteract antimicrobial action of drugs. Curcumin therapy completely abolishes *H. pylori* bacterial infection and other *H. pylori*-associated gastroduodenal diseases and restores the glandular atrophy and damage of mucosa and submucosa of gastric tissue [67].

The antibacterial activity of curcumin could be due to inhibition of the bacterial cell proliferation by hampering bacterial cell division by disrupting the bacterial protofilament FtsZ, which coordinates Z ring formation in bacteria [68]. A combination of curcumin, along with ampicillin, has yielded excellent results against *Staphylococcus aureus* [69, 70]. Similarly, curcumin along with subtilisin inhibited *L. monocytogenes*. Also, there was a synergistic effect of curcumin and various antibiotic drugs such as norfloxacin, ampicillin, *etc.*, against methicillin resistance *S. aureus* bacterial strain [71, 72]. Curcumin synergism is not only restricted to antibiotics, but it is also seen with various metals like cobalt, which have a good effect on *E. coli* [73]. In addition, the encapsulated curcumin combined with *Bacteriocin subtilisin* isolated from *B. amyloliquefaciensin* showed partial synergism against nisin sensitive *L. monocytogenes* Scott A strains [71].

Curcumin was also reported to have an anti-biofilm forming capacity [74]. It exhibited the potential for the reduction of biofilm initiation genes and the reserve of 31 quorum sensing (QS) genes. It could also downregule some virulence factors, as well as acyl-homoserine lactone (HSL) production, elastase or protease activity, and biosynthesis of pyocyanin. Moreover, the antibacterial properties reduce the *Arabidopsis thaliana* and *Caenorhabditis elegans* pathogenicity in animal models infected with *P. aeruginosa* [62].

Antifungal Activity

The dietary addition of curcumin and turmerones may function as a natural antibiotic in poultry feed. It may contribute to the promotion of meat growth and carcass traits besides the prevention of fungal infections. The use of 0.8 and 1.0 g L^{-1} of turmeric powder displayed antifungal properties in contaminated diets [75]. Specifically, curcumin can inhibit *Plasmopara viticol* and *Phomopsis obscurans,* which are common fungal pathogens derived from plants [76]. Besides, turmeric methanol extract showed antifungal efficiency against *Cryptococcus neoformans* and *Candida albicans* with MIC levels of 128 and 256 μg mL^{-1}, respectively [77]. While turmeric extract with hexane showed antifungal properties against *Rhizoctonia solani*, *Phytophthora infestans* and *Erysiphe graminis*. Additionally, extracting *Curcuma longa* by ethyl acetate exhibited inhibitory efficiency against *R. solani*, *P. infestans*, *Puccinia recondita*, and *Botrytis cinereal* strains. Likewise, the aqueous solution of curcumin at a concentration of 500 mg L^{-1} revealed antifungal activity against *R. solani*, *Pu.*

recondita, and *P. infestans* [78]. Similarly, turmeric oil exerted an antifungal effect against *Fusarium solani, Helminthosporium oryzae, F. solani* and *H. oryzae* [79]. The crude methanol extract of *Curcuma longa* showed an inhibitory effect against some clinical isolates of dermatophytes [80].

The curcuminby-product compounds exhibited more antifungal effects against *Paracoccidioides brasiliensis* than *fluconazole*, although it did not show any effect against the development of *Aspergillus* species [81]. In contrast, the hyphae development was impeded by curcumin through obstructing the global suppressor thymidine uptake 1 (TUP1) [82]. Also, curcumin has an inhibitory influence against *cryptococcus neoformans* and *candida dubliniensis* strains [81]. It has been used for candidosis treatment in murine model of asthma where it reduced the *candida albicans, candida glabrata*, and *candida tropicalis* biofilm biomass [83]. The synergistic effects of curcumin and ascorbic acid mixture revealed antifungal activity against different strains of candida. Besides, the combination of curcumin and different fungicide materials significantly elicited synergistic properties against fungal infections [84].

Antiviral and Parasitic Infections

Curcumin, as a plant derivative, has an extensive range of antiviral efficiency against different viruses. It has a non-competitive or competitive effect against inosine monophosphate dehydrogenase as a potent antiviral compound revealing notable antiviral activity against vesicular stomatitis virus (VSV), feline infectious peritonitis virus (FIPV) and feline herpes virus (FHV) [85]. Also, curcumin by-products such as allyl-curcumin, and tocopheryl-curcumin, presented 70% to 85% inhibition in Tat protein transactivation of HIV-1 LTR (human immune deficiency) [86]. However, curcumin can be an effective compound for combinatorial HIV therapy by affecting the acetyltransferase proteins of p300/CREB binding protein and inhibiting HIV-1 and HIV-2 protease [87]. The antiviral effect of curcumin aqueous extract in HepG2 Cells containing hepatitis B virus (HBV) genomes exhibited suppression of the HBsAg release from hepatocytes without inducing any cytotoxic effect. Similarly, the extract of *Curcuma longa* restricted HBV virus replication by increasing the p53 protein levels, improving the protein stability as well as promoting the p53 gene transcription. Curcumin's inclusive antiviral effects on various viruses show its ability to be utilized as a natural resource for the production of antiviral drugs [88].

Several combinations and concentrations of curcumin and curcumin liposomal formulations can act as antileishmanial agents. Curcumin showed potential activity against *Eimeria maxima,* which is the cause of coccidiosis in broiler chicken, but the exact mechanism needs further studies [89]. Additionally, hexane fraction derived from *Curcuma longa* cortex, incorporated in the liposomal formulation (LipoRHIC) could be used in the production of new antileishmanial agents [90].

ASPECTS OF USING TURMERIC IN POULTRY PRODUCTION

Broiler Performance

Several studies have demonstrated the effect of dietary turmeric supplementation in broiler production traits. For instance, Kumari *et al.* [91], found that feeding of 42-d old broiler chickens with 1.0 g kg^{-1} turmeric meal enhanced all growth performance parameters. Also, The diets supplemented with turmeric up to 5.0 g kg^{-1} increased the final body weight and improved the feed conversion ratio (FCR) of broiler chickens [92]. At the same trend, turmeric induced a significant enhancement in body weight gain and feed efficiency parameters in broilers without any adverse effects on the mortality rate at a high level [93]. Whereas, turmeric supplementation improved the retarded growth induced under *Eimeria* infection [94]. In addition, supplementation of broiler chickens diet with 0.2 g kg^{-1} pure curcumin improved the body weight gain and reduced the FCR values *via* increasing the villus length and weight in the duodenum, jejunum and ceca [95].

Supporting the previous studies, Al-Kassie *et al.* [96], revealed improvements in body weight gain, feed intake and feed conversion ratio of broilers fed with 0.75% and 1% turmeric. Similarly, Ahmadi [97] found that the FCR level was reduced by increasing turmeric powder concentration (0.9%) in broiler chickens diet. While feeding aflatoxin-exposed chicks with diets supplemented by with 0.5% turmeric enhanced weight gain [50]. Improvement in the performance of broilers may be due to the role of curcumin and essential oils in enhancing the feeding digestibility throughout increasing the secretion of digestive enzymes such as pancreatic lipase, amylase, trypsin and chymotrypsin [96]. According to Radwan *et al.* [98], this enhancement may be due to the quality of essential oils with active ingredients having antibacterial and antioxidant activity, that could increase the utilization of dietary nutrients by birds. Some other scientists have also attributed weight gain improvements to this plant's antioxidant properties and enhanced synthesis of protein through the activation of co-enzymes [92, 99, 100].

Conversely, some authors showed no significant effect of turmeric supplemented diets on broiler performance. For example, Emadi and Kermanshahi [39] reported that turmeric supplemented diets did not affect broiler chicks' growth and feed efficiency. Also, Nouzarian *et al.* [101], found that supplemented broiler chickens diets with 3.3, 6.6 and 10 g kg^{-1} turmeric powder exhibited no significant effect on the carcass yield. Both of these negligible outcomes can be a dose-dependent concern.

Laying Hen Performance

Few studies have demonstrated the efficiency of turmeric as feed additives on laying hen performance. In a study using a commercial substance, the addition of a herbo-mineral toxin binder product containing turmeric alleviated the adverse effect of Ochratoxin A on egg production [46]. Additionally, dietary turmeric supplementation of 5.0 up to 10.0 g kg^{-1} increased egg production (weight and mass) and the yolk weight and index of laying hens [98]. While supplementing layer diets with turmeric improved the uterine environment and increased shell weight and thickness [102]. Conversely, Nouzarian *et al.* [103], reported that supplementing laying hens with several turmeric levels (0.0, 0.5, 1.0, 1.5 and 2.0 g kg^{-1}) revealed no significant influence on the egg specific gravity, eggs shell weight to egg weight ratio, and eggshell thickness and weight.

Carcass Traits

Turmeric has beneficial effects on broiler carcass characteristics as it contains beneficial phytochemicals such as curcumin, ar-turmerone, methyl-curcumin and other substances. The curcumin supplemented diet (0.35 g kg^{-1}) decreased the abdominal, intermuscular and visceral fat content and thickness as well as liver fatness of male chickens [36]. Besides, the higher level of dietary turmeric supplementation (5.0 g kg^{-1}) reduced fat content, increased carcass quality, dressing percentage, and the giblet and breast weight in broiler chickens [93]. Although, some studies investigated no significant influence of turmeric supplementation at 1.0 g kg^{-1} [104] or 2.0 g kg^{-1} levels [100] on carcass characterization, at low levels, turmeric supplemented diets reduced the cost per click ratio and enhanced economic efficiency ratio. Moreover, curcumin improved bile development and promoted fat digestion as well as increased the percentage of crude protein in breast meat and its weight owing to its role in activating the digestive enzymes in poultry [105].

CONCLUDING REMARKS

The use of turmeric as a medication for a variety of ailments provides hopes that it can be a novel drug soon. *Curcuma longa* is a valuable alternative to antibiotics in poultry production owing to its widespread safety margin and its applications in promoting the growth performance. The enhancement in growth performance is attributed to the improved enteric health status, immunomodulatory system, digestive system, and energy utilization. Extensive studies on curcumin are required to explore the full use of this useful herb so that it could be used as a phytogenic feed additive in poultry diets without any harmful effects. Hence, for optimizing the turmeric meal supplementation efficacy in poultry diets, future research should focus more on the mechanism of action, optimum dose of supplementation, as well as the duration of application.

CONSENT FOR PUBLICATION

Not applicable.

CONFLICT OF INTEREST

The author declares no conflict of interest, financial or otherwise.

ACKNOWLEDGEMENTS

Declared none.

REFERENCES

[1]   Abd El-Hack ME, Abdelnour SA, Taha AE, *et al.* Herbs as thermoregulatory agents in poultry: An overview. Sci Total Environ 2020; 703: 134399.
[http://dx.doi.org/10.1016/j.scitotenv.2019.134399] [PMID: 31757531]

[2]   Ogbuewu I, Mbajiorgu C, Okoli I. Antioxidant activity of ginger and its effect on blood chemistry and production physiology of poultry. Comp Clin Pathol 2019; 28(3): 655-60.
[http://dx.doi.org/10.1007/s00580-017-2536-x]

[3]   Chung A, Perera R, Brueggemann AB, *et al.* Effect of antibiotic prescribing on antibiotic resistance in individual children in primary care: prospective cohort study. BMJ 2007; 335(7617): 429.
[http://dx.doi.org/10.1136/bmj.39274.647465.BE] [PMID: 17656505]

[4]   Suresh G, Das RK, Kaur Brar S, *et al.* Alternatives to antibiotics in poultry feed: molecular perspectives. Crit Rev Microbiol 2018; 44(3): 318-35.
[http://dx.doi.org/10.1080/1040841X.2017.1373062] [PMID: 28891362]

[5]   Jyotsana P K, Berwal R. Evaluation of the effect of supplementation of Ashwagandha (Withania somnifera) root powder in the broiler's ration on gut morphology and bacteriology. A Wartazoa 2013; 23(1): 41-9.

[6]   Saeed M, Abd El-Hack ME, Alagawany M, *et al.* Determination of the antimicrobial capacity of green tea (*Camellia sinensis*) against the potentially pathogenic microorganisms *Escherichia coli*, *Salmonella enterica*, *Staphylococcus aureus*, *Listeria monocytogenes*, Candida albicans and Aspergillus niger. Int J Pharmacol 2005; 13: 807-12.

[7]   Qureshi S, Adil S, Abd El-Hack M, Alagawany M, Farag M. Beneficial uses of dandelion herb (Taraxacum officinale) in poultry nutrition. Worlds Poult Sci J 2017; 73(3): 591-602.
[http://dx.doi.org/10.1017/S0043933917000459]

[8]   Saeed M, Abd El-Hack M, Alagawany M, *et al.* Phytochemistry, modes of action and beneficial health applications of green tea (Camellia sinensis) in humans and animals. Int J Pharmacol 2017; 13(7): 698-708.
[http://dx.doi.org/10.3923/ijp.2017.698.708]

[9]   Tiwari R, Chakraborty S, Dhama K, Wani MY, Kumar A, Kapoor S. Wonder world of phages: potential biocontrol agents safeguarding biosphere and health of animals and humans- current scenario and perspectives. Pak J Biol Sci 2014; 17(3): 316-28.
[http://dx.doi.org/10.3923/pjbs.2014.316.328] [PMID: 24897785]

[10]   Devi NB, Singh P, Das AK. Ethnomedicinal utilization of Zingiberaceae in the valley districts of Manipur. J Environ Sci Toxicol Food Technol 2014; 8: 21-30.

[11]   Krup V, Prakash L, Harini A. Pharmacological activities of turmeric (*Curcuma longa* Linn): A review. J Homeop Ayurv Med 2013; 2: 133.
[http://dx.doi.org/10.4172/2167-1206.1000133]

[12]   Sethy K, Swain P, Behera K, *et al.* Effect of turmeric (*Curcuma longa*) supplementation on growth and blood chemistry of broilers. Explor Anim Med Res 2016; 6: 75-9.

[13]   Chen HW, Huang HC. Effect of curcumin on cell cycle progression and apoptosis in vascular smooth muscle cells. Br J Pharmacol 1998; 124(6): 1029-40.
[http://dx.doi.org/10.1038/sj.bjp.0701914] [PMID: 9720770]

[14]   Ramsewak RS, DeWitt DL, Nair MG. Cytotoxicity, antioxidant and anti-inflammatory activities of curcumins I-III from *Curcuma longa*. Phytomedicine 2000; 7(4): 303-8.
[http://dx.doi.org/10.1016/S0944-7113(00)80048-3] [PMID: 10969724]

[15]   Sanagi MM, Ahmad UK, Smith RM. Application of supercritical fluid extraction and chromatography to the analysis of turmeric. J Chromatogr Sci 1993; 31(1): 20-5.
[http://dx.doi.org/10.1093/chromsci/31.1.20]

[16]   Naz S, Ilyas S, Jabeen S, Parveen Z. Composition and antibacterial activity of the essential oil from the rhizome of turmeric (*Curcuma longa* L.). Asian J Chem 2011; 23: 1639.

[17]   Samarasinghe K, Wenk C, Silva K, Gunasekera J. Turmeric (*Curcuma longa*) root powder and mannanoligosaccharides as alternatives to antibiotics in broiler chicken diets. Asian-Australas J Anim Sci 2003; 16(10): 1495-500.
[http://dx.doi.org/10.5713/ajas.2003.1495]

[18]   Abbas R, Colwell D, Gilleard J. Botanicals: an alternative approach for the control of avian coccidiosis. Worlds Poult Sci J 2012; 68(2): 203-15.
[http://dx.doi.org/10.1017/S0043933912000268]

[19]   Kim DK, Lillehoj HS, Lee SH, Jang SI, Lillehoj EP, Bravo D. Dietary *Curcuma longa* enhances resistance against *Eimeria* maxima and *Eimeria* tenella infections in chickens. Poult Sci 2013; 92(10): 2635-43.
[http://dx.doi.org/10.3382/ps.2013-03095] [PMID: 24046410]

[20]   Dono ND. Turmeric (*Curcuma longa* Linn.) supplementation as an alternative to antibiotics in poultry diets. WARTAZOA 2013; 23: 41-9.
[http://dx.doi.org/10.14334/wartazoa.v23i1.958.]

[21]   Araújo CC, Leon LL. Biological activities of *Curcuma longa* L. Mem Inst Oswaldo Cruz 2001; 96(5): 723-8.
[http://dx.doi.org/10.1590/S0074-02762001000500026] [PMID: 11500779]

[22]   Ikpeama A, Onwuka G, Nwankwo C. Nutritional composition of Tumeric (*Curcuma longa*) and its antimicrobial properties. Int J Sci Eng Res 2014; 5: 1085-9.

[23]   Jayaprakasha G, Rao LJ, Sakariah K. Chemistry and biological activities of *C. longa*. Trends Food Sci Technol 2005; 16(12): 533-48.
[http://dx.doi.org/10.1016/j.tifs.2005.08.006]

[24]   Chane-Ming J, Vera R, Chalchat JC, Cabassu P. Chemical composition of essential oils from rhizomes, leaves and flowers of *Curcuma longa* L. from Reunion Island. J Essent Oil Res 2002; 14(4): 249-51.

[http://dx.doi.org/10.1080/10412905.2002.9699843]

[25]   Huang MT, Ma W, Lu YP, *et al.* Effects of curcumin, demethoxycurcumin, bisdemethoxycurcumin and tetrahydrocurcumin on 12-O-tetradecanoylphorbol-13-acetate-induced tumor promotion. Carcinogenesis 1995; 16(10): 2493-7.
[http://dx.doi.org/10.1093/carcin/16.10.2493] [PMID: 7586157]

[26]   He XG, Lin LZ, Lian LZ, Lindenmaier M. Liquid chromatography–electrospray mass spectrometric analysis of curcuminoids and sesquiterpenoids in turmeric (*Curcuma longa*). J Chromatogr A 1998; 818(1): 127-32.
[http://dx.doi.org/10.1016/S0021-9673(98)00540-8]

[27]   Tayyem RF, Heath DD, Al-Delaimy WK, Rock CL. Curcumin content of turmeric and curry powders. Nutr Cancer 2006; 55(2): 126-31.
[http://dx.doi.org/10.1207/s15327914nc5502_2] [PMID: 17044766]

[28]   Ammon HP, Wahl MA. Pharmacology of *Curcuma longa*. Planta Med 1991; 57(1): 1-7.
[http://dx.doi.org/10.1055/s-2006-960004] [PMID: 2062949]

[29]   Mahran RI, Hagras MM, Sun D, Brenner DE. Bringing curcumin to the clinic in cancer prevention: a review of strategies to enhance bioavailability and efficacy. AAPS J 2017; 19(1): 54-81.
[http://dx.doi.org/10.1208/s12248-016-0003-2] [PMID: 27783266]

[30]   Chiablaem K, Lirdprapamongkol K, Keeratichamroen S, Surarit R, Svasti J. Curcumin suppresses vasculogenic mimicry capacity of hepatocellular carcinoma cells through STAT3 and PI3K/AKT inhibition. Anticancer Res 2014; 34(4): 1857-64.
[PMID: 24692720]

[31]   Lai PK, Roy J. Antimicrobial and chemopreventive properties of herbs and spices. Curr Med Chem 2004; 11(11): 1451-60.
[http://dx.doi.org/10.2174/0929867043365107] [PMID: 15180577]

[32]   Anand P, Kunnumakkara AB, Newman RA, Aggarwal BB. Bioavailability of curcumin: problems and promises. Mol Pharm 2007; 4(6): 807-18.
[http://dx.doi.org/10.1021/mp700113r] [PMID: 17999464]

[33]   Duvoix A, Blasius R, Delhalle S, *et al.* Chemopreventive and therapeutic effects of curcumin. Cancer Lett 2005; 223(2): 181-90.
[http://dx.doi.org/10.1016/j.canlet.2004.09.041] [PMID: 15896452]

[34]   Joe B, Vijaykumar M, Lokesh BR. Biological properties of curcumin-cellular and molecular mechanisms of action. Crit Rev Food Sci Nutr 2004; 44(2): 97-111.
[http://dx.doi.org/10.1080/10408690490424702] [PMID: 15116757]

[35]   Riasi A, Kermanshahi H, Mahdavi A. Production performance, egg quality and some serum metabolites of older commercial laying hens fed different levels of turmeric rhizome (*Curcuma longa*) powder. J Med Plants Res 2012; 6: 2141-5.
[http://dx.doi.org/10.5897/JMPR11.1316]

[36]   Zhongze H, Like W, Aiyou W. Effect of curcumin on fat metabolism in Wanjiang Yellow chickens. Cereal Feed Ind 2008; 4: 12.

[37]   Hu Z, Hu Yq, Wang Lk, Wem Ay. Effect of Curcumin on Metabolism of Fat for Broilers. J of Anhui Sci and Techno Univer 2007; 6.

[38]   Zhongze H. Effect of curcumin on fat deposition and its mechanism in different breeds chickens. Anhui Agric Sci Bull 2009; 15: 107.

[39]   Emadi M, Kermanshahi H. Effect of turmeric rhizome powder on immunity responses of broiler chickens. J Anim Vet Adv 2007; 6: 833-6.

[40]   Park J, Conteas CN. Anti-carcinogenic properties of curcumin on colorectal cancer. World J Gastrointest Oncol 2010; 2(4): 169-76.

[http://dx.doi.org/10.4251/wjgo.v2.i4.169] [PMID: 21160593]

[41]   Jung KK, Lee HS, Cho JY, *et al.* Inhibitory effect of curcumin on nitric oxide production from lipopolysaccharide-activated primary microglia. Life Sci 2006; 79(21): 2022-31.
[http://dx.doi.org/10.1016/j.lfs.2006.06.048] [PMID: 16934299]

[42]   Thent ZC, Das S. Involvement of liver in diabetes mellitus: herbal remedies. Clin Ter 2014; 165(4): 223-30.
[PMID: 25203338]

[43]   Jagetia GC, Aggarwal BB. "Spicing up" of the immune system by curcumin. J Clin Immunol 2007; 27(1): 19-35.
[http://dx.doi.org/10.1007/s10875-006-9066-7] [PMID: 17211725]

[44]   Arslan M, Haq A. effect of turmeric (*Curcuma longa*) supplementation on growth performance, immune response, carcass characteristics and cholesterol profile in broilers. Veterinaria 2017; 66(1): 16-20.

[45]   Sethy K, Swain P, Behera K, *et al.* Effect of turmeric (*Curcuma longa*) supplementation on antioxidants and immunity of broiler birds. J Livestock Sci 2017; 103-6.

[46]   Sawale G, Gosh R, Ravikanth K, Maini S, Rekhe D. Experimental mycotoxicosis in layer induced by ochratoxin A and its amelioration with herbomineral toxin binder 'Toxiroak'. Int J Poult Sci 2009; 8(8): 798-803.
[http://dx.doi.org/10.3923/ijps.2009.798.803]

[47]   Lee SH, Jang SI, Kim DK, Ionescu C, Bravo D, Lillehoj HS. Effect of dietary Curcuma, Capsicum, and Lentinus on enhancing local immunity against *Eimeria acervulina* infection. J Poult Sci 2009; 0912030019-.

[48]   Tiwari R, Latheef SK, Ahmed I, *et al.* Herbal immunomodulators-a remedial panacea for designing and developing effective drugs and medicines: current scenario and future prospects. Curr Drug Metab 2018; 19(3): 264-301.
[http://dx.doi.org/10.2174/1389200219666180129125436] [PMID: 29380694]

[49]   Yasni S, Yoshiie K, Oda H, Sugano M, Imaizumi K. Dietary Curcuma xanthorrhiza Roxb. increases mitogenic responses of splenic lymphocytes in rats, and alters populations of the lymphocytes in mice. J Nutr Sci Vitaminol (Tokyo) 1993; 39(4): 345-54.
[http://dx.doi.org/10.3177/jnsv.39.345] [PMID: 8283313]

[50]   Yarru LP, Settivari RS, Gowda NK, Antoniou E, Ledoux DR, Rottinghaus GE. Effects of turmeric (*Curcuma longa*) on the expression of hepatic genes associated with biotransformation, antioxidant, and immune systems in broiler chicks fed aflatoxin. Poult Sci 2009; 88(12): 2620-7.
[http://dx.doi.org/10.3382/ps.2009-00204] [PMID: 19903961]

[51]   Lee KS, Lee BS, Semnani S, *et al.* Curcumin extends life span, improves health span, and modulates the expression of age-associated aging genes in Drosophila melanogaster. Rejuvenation Res 2010; 13(5): 561-70.
[http://dx.doi.org/10.1089/rej.2010.1031] [PMID: 20645870]

[52]   Mollazadeh H, Cicero AFG, Blesso CN, Pirro M, Majeed M, Sahebkar A. Immune modulation by curcumin: The role of interleukin-10. Crit Rev Food Sci Nutr 2019; 59(1): 89-101.
[http://dx.doi.org/10.1080/10408398.2017.1358139] [PMID: 28799796]

[53]   Gao X, Kuo J, Jiang H, *et al.* Immunomodulatory activity of curcumin: suppression of lymphocyte proliferation, development of cell-mediated cytotoxicity, and cytokine production *in vitro*. Biochem Pharmacol 2004; 68(1): 51-61.
[http://dx.doi.org/10.1016/j.bcp.2004.03.015] [PMID: 15183117]

[54]   Abou-Elkhair R, Ahmed HA, Selim S. Effects of black pepper (piper nigrum), turmeric powder (*Curcuma longa*) and coriander seeds (coriandrum sativum) and their combinations as feed additives on growth performance, carcass traits, some blood parameters and humoral immune response of

broiler chickens. Asian-Australas J Anim Sci 2014; 27(6): 847-54.
[http://dx.doi.org/10.5713/ajas.2013.13644] [PMID: 25050023]

[55]   Arshami J, Pilevar M, Aami Azghadi M, Raji AR. Hypolipidemic and antioxidative effects of curcumin on blood parameters, humoral immunity, and jejunum histology in Hy-line hens. Avicenna J Phytomed 2013; 3(2): 178-85.
[PMID: 25050272]

[56]   Lantz RC, Chen GJ, Solyom AM, Jolad SD, Timmermann BN. The effect of turmeric extracts on inflammatory mediator production. Phytomedicine 2005; 12(6-7): 445-52.
[http://dx.doi.org/10.1016/j.phymed.2003.12.011] [PMID: 16008121]

[57]   Siddiqui AM, Cui X, Wu R, *et al.* The anti-inflammatory effect of curcumin in an experimental model of sepsis is mediated by up-regulation of peroxisome proliferator-activated receptor-γ. Crit Care Med 2006; 34(7): 1874-82.
[http://dx.doi.org/10.1097/01.CCM.0000221921.71300.BF] [PMID: 16715036]

[58]   Jacob A, Wu R, Zhou M, Wang P. Mechanism of the anti-inflammatory effect of curcumin: PPAR-γ activation. PPAR Res 2007; 2007: 89369.
[http://dx.doi.org/10.1155/2007/89369] [PMID: 18274631]

[59]   Leclercq IA, Farrell GC, Sempoux C, dela Peña A, Horsmans Y. Curcumin inhibits NF-kappaB activation and reduces the severity of experimental steatohepatitis in mice. J Hepatol 2004; 41(6): 926-34.
[http://dx.doi.org/10.1016/j.jhep.2004.08.010] [PMID: 15582125]

[60]   Kim DC, Kim SH, Choi BH, *et al. Curcuma longa* extract protects against gastric ulcers by blocking H2 histamine receptors. Biol Pharm Bull 2005; 28(12): 2220-4.
[http://dx.doi.org/10.1248/bpb.28.2220] [PMID: 16327153]

[61]   Narang H, Krishna M. Inhibition of radiation induced nitration by curcumin and nicotinamide in mouse macrophages. Mol Cell Biochem 2005; 276(1-2): 7-13.
[http://dx.doi.org/10.1007/s11010-005-2241-y] [PMID: 16132679]

[62]   Rudrappa T, Bais HP. Curcumin, a known phenolic from *Curcuma longa*, attenuates the virulence of Pseudomonas aeruginosa PAO1 in whole plant and animal pathogenicity models. J Agric Food Chem 2008; 56(6): 1955-62.
[http://dx.doi.org/10.1021/jf072591j] [PMID: 18284200]

[63]   Faghani M, Rafiee A, Namjoo AR, Rahimian Y. Performance, cholesterol profile and intestinal microbial population in broilers fed turmeric extract. Res Opin Anim Vet Sci 2014; 4: 500-3.

[64]   Niamsa N, Sittiwet C. Antimicrobial activity of *Curcuma longa* aqueous extract. J Pharmacol Toxicol 2009; 4(4): 173-7.
[http://dx.doi.org/10.3923/jpt.2009.173.177]

[65]   Lawhavinit Oa, Kongkathip N, Kongkathip B. Antimicrobial activity of curcuminoids from *Curcuma longa* L. on pathogenic bacteria of shrimp and chicken. Witthayasan Kasetsat Witthayasat 2010; 44: 364-71.

[66]   Tajbakhsh S, Mohammadi K, Deilami I, *et al.* Antibacterial activity of indium curcumin and indium diacetylcurcumin. Afr J Biotechnol 2008; 7-12.

[67]   De R, Kundu P, Swarnakar S, *et al.* Antimicrobial activity of curcumin against *Helicobacter pylori* isolates from India and during infections in mice. Antimicrob Agents Chemother 2009; 53(4): 1592-7.
[http://dx.doi.org/10.1128/AAC.01242-08] [PMID: 19204190]

[68]   Bansal S, Chhibber S. Curcumin alone and in combination with augmentin protects against pulmonary inflammation and acute lung injury generated during Klebsiella pneumoniae B5055-induced lung infection in BALB/c mice. J Med Microbiol 2010; 59(Pt 4): 429-37.
[http://dx.doi.org/10.1099/jmm.0.016873-0] [PMID: 20056776]

[69]   Karthik K, Muneeswaran NS, Manjunathachar HV, Gopi M, Elamurugan A, Kalaiyarasu S.

Bacteriophages: effective alternative to antibiotics. Adv Anim Vet Sci 2014; 2(3S): 1-7.
[http://dx.doi.org/10.14737/journal.aavs/2014/2.3s.1.7]

[70] Moghaddam KM, Iranshahi M, Yazdi MC, Shahverdi AR. The combination effect of curcumin with different antibiotics against *Staphylococcus aureus*. Intern Jour of Green Pharm. 2009; 3.(9)
[http://dx.doi.org/10.4103/0973-8258.54906]

[71] Amrouche T, Sutyak Noll K, Wang Y, Huang Q, Chikindas ML. Antibacterial activity of subtilosin alone and combined with curcumin, poly-lysine and zinc lactate against *Listeria monocytogenes* strains. Probiotics Antimicrob Proteins 2010; 2(4): 250-7.
[http://dx.doi.org/10.1007/s12602-010-9042-7] [PMID: 26781320]

[72] Mun SH, Joung DK, Kim YS, *et al.* Synergistic antibacterial effect of curcumin against methicillin-resistant *Staphylococcus aureus*. Phytomedicine 2013; 20(8-9): 714-8.
[http://dx.doi.org/10.1016/j.phymed.2013.02.006] [PMID: 23537748]

[73] Hatamie S, Nouri M, Karandikar S, *et al.* Complexes of cobalt nanoparticles and polyfunctional curcumin as antimicrobial agents. Mater Sci Eng C 2012; 32(2): 92-7.
[http://dx.doi.org/10.1016/j.msec.2011.10.002]

[74] Karaman M, Fırıncı F, Arıkan Ayyıldız Z, Bahar IH. Effects of Imipenem, Tobramycin and Curcumin on biofilm formation of Pseudomonas aeruginosa strains. Mikrobiyol Bul 2013; 47(1): 192-4.
[http://dx.doi.org/10.5578/mb.3902] [PMID: 23390919]

[75] Upendra R, Khandelwal P, Reddy A. Turmeric powder (*Curcuma longa* Linn.) as an antifungal agent in plant tissue culture studies. Int J Eng Sci 2011; 3: 7899-904.

[76] Radwan MM, Tabanca N, Wedge DE, Tarawneh AH, Cutler SJ. Antifungal compounds from turmeric and nutmeg with activity against plant pathogens. Fitoterapia 2014; 99: 341-6.
[http://dx.doi.org/10.1016/j.fitote.2014.08.021] [PMID: 25173461]

[77] Ungphaiboon S, Supavita T, Singchangchai P, Sungkarak S, Rattanasuwan P, Itharat A. Study on antioxidant and antimicrobial activities of turmeric clear liquid soap for wound treatment of HIV patients. Songklanakarin J Sci Technol 2005; 27: 269-578.

[78] Kim MK, Choi GJ, Lee HS. Fungicidal property of *Curcuma longa* L. rhizome-derived curcumin against phytopathogenic fungi in a greenhouse. J Agric Food Chem 2003; 51(6): 1578-81.
[http://dx.doi.org/10.1021/jf0210369] [PMID: 12617587]

[79] Islam MK, Chowdhury MM, Moinuddin SM. Effects of turmeric and garlic on blood cholesterol level in guinea pig. Bangladesh J Pharmacol 2008; 3(1): 17-20.
[http://dx.doi.org/10.3329/bjp.v3i1.824]

[80] Wuthi-udomlert M, Grisanapan W, Luanratana O, Caichompoo W. Antifungal activity of *Curcuma longa* grown in Thailand. Southeast Asian J Trop Med Public Health 2000; 31 (Suppl. 1): 178-82.
[PMID: 11414453]

[81] Martins CV, da Silva DL, Neres AT, *et al.* Curcumin as a promising antifungal of clinical interest. J Antimicrob Chemother 2009; 63(2): 337-9.
[http://dx.doi.org/10.1093/jac/dkn488] [PMID: 19038979]

[82] Sharma M, Manoharlal R, Puri N, Prasad R. Antifungal curcumin induces reactive oxygen species and triggers an early apoptosis but prevents hyphae development by targeting the global repressor TUP1 in Candida albicans. Biosci Rep 2010; 30(6): 391-404.
[http://dx.doi.org/10.1042/BSR20090151] [PMID: 20017731]

[83] Dovigo LN, Pavarina AC, Carmello JC, Machado AL, Brunetti IL, Bagnato VS. Susceptibility of clinical isolates of Candida to photodynamic effects of curcumin. Lasers Surg Med 2011; 43(9): 927-34.
[http://dx.doi.org/10.1002/lsm.21110] [PMID: 22006736]

[84] Khalil OA, De Faria Oliveira OM, Vellosa JC, *et al.* Curcumin antifungal and antioxidant activities are increased in the presence of ascorbic acid. Food Chem 2012; 133(3): 1001-5.

[http://dx.doi.org/10.1016/j.foodchem.2012.02.009]

[85]　Dairaku I, Han Y, Yanaka N, Kato N. Inhibitory effect of curcumin on IMP dehydrogenase, the target for anticancer and antiviral chemotherapy agents. Biosci Biotechnol Biochem 2010; 74(1): 185-7.
[http://dx.doi.org/10.1271/bbb.90568] [PMID: 20057137]

[86]　Barthelemy S, Vergnes L, Moynier M, Guyot D, Labidalle S, Bahraoui E. Curcumin and curcumin derivatives inhibit Tat-mediated transactivation of type 1 human immunodeficiency virus long terminal repeat. Res Virol 1998; 149(1): 43-52.
[http://dx.doi.org/10.1016/S0923-2516(97)86899-9] [PMID: 9561563]

[87]　Balasubramanyam K, Varier RA, Altaf M, *et al.* Curcumin, a novel p300/CREB-binding protein-specific inhibitor of acetyltransferase, represses the acetylation of histone/nonhistone proteins and histone acetyltransferase-dependent chromatin transcription. J Biol Chem 2004; 279(49): 51163-71.
[http://dx.doi.org/10.1074/jbc.M409024200] [PMID: 15383533]

[88]　Moghadamtousi SZ, Kadir HA, Hassandarvish P, Tajik H, Abubakar S, Zandi K. A review on antibacterial, antiviral, and antifungal activity of curcumin. BioMed Res Int 2014; 2014: 186864.
[PMID: 24877064]

[89]　Almeida GF, Thamsborg SM, Madeira AM, *et al.* The effects of combining *Artemisia annua* and *Curcuma longa* ethanolic extracts in broilers challenged with infective oocysts of *Eimeria acervulina* and *E. maxima*. Parasitology 2014; 141(3): 347-55.
[http://dx.doi.org/10.1017/S0031182013001443] [PMID: 24553078]

[90]　Amaral AC, Gomes LA, Silva JR, *et al.* Liposomal formulation of turmerone-rich hexane fractions from *Curcuma longa* enhances their antileishmanial activity. BioMed Res Int 2014; 694934.
[http://dx.doi.org/10.1155/2014/694934] [PMID: 25045693]

[91]　Kumari P, Gupta MK, Ranjan R, Singh KK, Yadava R. *Curcuma longa* as feed additive in broiler birds and its patho-physiological effects. Indian J Exp Biol 2007; 45(3): 272-7.
[PMID: 17373373]

[92]　Al-Sultan S. S. I. AL-Sultan. The effect of *Curcuma longa* (turmeric) on overall performance of broiler chickens. Int J Poult Sci 2003; 2(5): 351-3.
[http://dx.doi.org/10.3923/ijps.2003.351.353]

[93]　Durrani F, Ismail M, Sultan A, Suhail S, Chand N, Durrani Z. Effect of different levels of feed added turmeric (*Curcuma longa*) on the performance of broiler chicks. J Agric Biol Sci 2006; 1: 9-11.

[94]　Abbas RZ, Iqbal Z, Khan MN, Zafar MA, Zia MA. Anticoccidial activity of *Curcuma longa* L. in broilers. Braz Arch Biol Technol 2010; 53(1): 63-7.
[http://dx.doi.org/10.1590/S1516-89132010000100008]

[95]　Rajput N, Muhammah N, Yan R, Zhong X, Wang T. Effect of dietary supplementation of curcumin on growth performance, intestinal morphology and nutrients utilization of broiler chicks. J Poult Sci 2012; 50(1): 44-52.
[http://dx.doi.org/https://doi.org/10.2141/jpsa.0120065]

[96]　Al-Kassie GA, Mohseen AM, Abd-Al-Jaleel RA. Modification of productive performance and physiological aspects of broilers on the addition of a mixture of cumin and turmeric to the diet. Res Opin Anim Vet Sci 2011; 1(1): 31-4.

[97]　Ahmadi F. Effect of turmeric (*Curcumin longa*) powder on performance, oxidative stress state and some of blood parameters in broiler fed on diets containing aflatoxin B1. Glob Vet 2010; 5: 312-7.

[98]　Radwan NL, Hassan R, Qota E, Fayek H. Effect of natural antioxidant on oxidative stability of eggs and productive and reproductive performance of laying hens. Int J Poult Sci 2008; 7: 134-50.
[http://dx.doi.org/10.3923/ijps.2008.134.150]

[99]　Alagawany MM, Farag MR, Dhama K. Nutritional and biological effects of turmeric (*Curcuma longa*) supplementation on performance, serum biochemical parameters and oxidative status of broiler chicks exposed to endosulfan in the diets. Asian J Anim Vet Adv 2015; 10(2): 86-96.

[http://dx.doi.org/10.3923/ajava.2015.86.96]

[100] El-Hakim AA, Cherian G, Ali M. Use of organic acid, herbs and their combination to improve the utilization of commercial low protein broiler diets. Int J Poult Sci 2009; 8(1): 14-20.
[http://dx.doi.org/10.3923/ijps.2009.14.20]

[101] Nouzarian R, Tabeidian S, Toghyani M, Ghalamkari G, Toghyani M. Effect of turmeric powder on performance, carcass traits, humoral immune responses, and serum metabolites in broiler chickens. J Anim Feed Sci 2011; 20(3): 20.
[http://dx.doi.org/10.22358/jafs/66194/2011]

[102] Park SS, Kim JM, Kim EJ, Kim HS, An BK, Kang CW. Effects of dietary turmeric powder on laying performance and egg qualities in laying hens. Kor J Poult Sci 2012; 39(1): 27-32.
[http://dx.doi.org/10.5536/KJPS.2012.39.1.027]

[103] Riasi A, Kermanshahi H, Fathi M. Effect of Turmeric rhizome powder (*Curcuma longa*) on performance, egg quality and some blood serum parameters of laying hens. Greece: Proceeding 1st Mediterranean Summit of World Poultry Science Association 2008.

[104] Rahmatnejad E, Roshanfekr H, Ashayerizadeh O, Mamooee M, Ashayerizadeh A. Evaluation the effect of several non-antibiotic additives on growth performance of broiler chickens. J Anim Vet Adv 2009; 8: 1757-60.

[105] Hernández F, Madrid J, García V, Orengo J, Megías MD. Influence of two plant extracts on broilers performance, digestibility, and digestive organ size. Poult Sci 2004; 83(2): 169-74.
[http://dx.doi.org/10.1093/ps/83.2.169] [PMID: 14979566]

CHAPTER 9

Nutritional and Promising Therapeutic Potential of Chia Seed as a Feed Additive in Poultry

Muhammad Saeed[1], Muhammad Sajjad Khan[1], Muhammad Asif Arain[2], Mohamed E. Abd El-Hack[3], Mayada R. Farag[4] and Mahmoud Alagawany[3,*]

[1] *Cholistan University of Veterinary and Animal Sciences Bahawalpur - 63100, Pakistan*

[2] *Faculty of Veterinary and Animal Sciences, Lasbela University of Agriculture, Water and Marine Sciences, Uthal, Balochistan - 3800, Pakistan*

[3] *Department of Poultry, Faculty of Agriculture, Zagazig University, Zagazig 44511 , Egypt*

[4] *Forensic Medicine and Toxicology Department, Veterinary Medicine Faculty, Zagazig University, Zagazig 44511 , Egypt*

Abstract: Chia (*Salvia hispanica* L.) is an annual summer crop that belongs to the Labiate family. Chia seeds are a rich source of nutrients like polyunsaturated omega-3 fatty acids (PUFA), which safeguard against inflammation, improve performance and could be used for the enrichment of eggs and meat with omega-3 contents in poultry. These seeds are also rich in polyphenols, which can protect the body against cancer, aging and free radicals. Quercetin, chlorogenic acid, kaempferol, caffeic acid, and myricetin are reported as valuable sources of antioxidants in chia seed. It is believed that these seeds have antidepressant, anti-blood clotting, and hepato-protective features, along with anti-inflammatory and anti-carcinogenic effects. They have a positive role in diabetes, dyslipidemia, antianxiety, hypertension and constipation in humans. Furthermore, it is a potential source of dietary fiber, which helps to support the gastrointestinal function. Chia seeds also have a high concentration of beneficial unsaturated fatty acids, phenolic compounds, vitamins and minerals. Chia seeds contain a good balance of non-essential and essential amino acids. The addition of chia seed in poultry feed resulted in an increase of omega-3 fatty acids content in both eggs and meat. Moreover, it also offers advantages over other sources of PUFA for poultry feeding due to the absence of adverse effects on bird's health. Chia seeds do not have any toxic compounds or anti-nutritional factors and have been added to poultry feed up to 30%, which proved it as a safe feed ingredient for poultry diets. However, further studies are required to explore its potential application as a promising feed additive, growth promoter and antioxidant for commercial poultry diets.

Keywords: Antioxidant, Feed additive, Nutritional value, Poultry, *Salvia hispanica* seed.

---

* **Corresponding author Mahmoud Alagawany:** Department of Poultry, Faculty of Agriculture, Zagazig University, Zagazig - 44511, Egypt; E-mail: mmalagwany@zu.edu.eg

Mahmoud Alagawany & Mohamed E. Abd El-Hack (Eds.)

INTRODUCTION

In many countries particularly the European Union, due to the ban on the use of chemical growth promoters (antibiotics) as a growth factor, the researchers have tried to find and replace them with natural feed additives such as herbal plants, prebiotics, and probiotics in animal nutrition [1, 2]. These alternatives should be efficient against the pathogenic gastrointestinal microorganisms by improving immunity and feed efficiency. Thus, one of the best options for replacing synthetic antibiotics as growth enhancers is the incorporation of medicinal plants and their extracts [3, 4]. As a result, many experiments have been conducted to evaluate the effects of medicinal/herbal plant materials and their extracts as an alternative for antimicrobial growth promoter (AGP) sources and they have reported some significant effects on chicken growth performance [5 - 12]. *Salvia hispanica* L. is known as chia that is native to Southern Mexico and Northern Guatemala and is well-known as a medicinal herbaceous plant [13]. The genus *Salvia* consists of about 900 species and its name is derived from the Latin word "salvere", referring to the therapeutic activities of *Salvia officinalis* that is also known as a medicinal herb [14]. Chia contains high levels of α-linolenic acid, which does not contain any of the vitamin B6 antagonists or anti-nutritional factors [15, 16]. The medical researches indicated that the consumption of α-linolenic acid might reduce the risks of cardiovascular-related disorders [17, 18]. The scientific evidence obtained from animal studies, epidemiological, and clinical studies in humans have shown that consuming lipids rich in x-3 fatty acids can diminish coronary heart disease. Chia seed is composed of 30-33% fats, 26-41% carbohydrates, 15-25% protein, 18–30% dietary fiber, 4-5% ash, minerals, vitamins, and almost 92% dry matter. High amounts of antioxidants are derived from this seed [19], and also it is reported to be free of mycotoxins and gluten [20, 21].

The seeds of chia are frequently used to improve the omega-3 fatty acids content in poultry products like meat and eggs as well [22]. The important content of chia seeds is a fiber that is studied for its insoluble and soluble fractions, viscosity and water holding capacity [23] and it can be used as a suspending agent, an emulsifier and a foam stabilizer in poultry feed and for pharmaceutical purposes [24]. The fresh matter of chia seed derived from a chia plant has almost 230 g oil/kg [25]. Chia seed is high in proteins and essential amino acids [26] and it also contains some compounds such as quercetin, caffeic acid, myricetin, and kaempferol [27, 28]. Chia seeds and meal do not cause any digestive disorders that are associated with other polyunsaturated fatty acid (PUFA) sources such as marine products or flaxseed, and also do not have fishy flavor [29, 30].

The commercialization of chia seed products as a feed for dogs, horses, cats, pigs, and avian species is quickly developing across the globe. The scientific studies have reported that the nutritional advantages of chia seed in the poultry diet are higher than the other PUFA sources [31, 32]. The chia seed and its valuable components showed that it has great potential to take part in health, animal feed, nutraceuticals, pharmaceuticals, *etc.* [33].

The therapeutic effects of chia seed on controlling diseases, clinical or sub-clinical symptoms, and immune-boosting effects have been studied in humans and different animal models. But, regarding its use in the poultry industry, limited research has been carried out to explore its potential role as an ingredient for poultry diets. So, the aim of this chapter is to gather favorable evidence for poultry researchers to focus on chia seeds as a potential feed ingredient and/or feed additive owing to its toxin and gluten-free property, which makes it a safe feed ingredient in the poultry diet.

DESCRIPTION OF CHIA SEED

The dimension of chia seeds is characterized by almost 0.88 mm thickness, 1.21 mm width and 1.87mm length having an oval shape with tiny dark spots and colors ranging from beige to dark coffee [34]. Ixtaina *et al.* [19], reported that the white seeds are denser and heavier than the darker ones, as shown in Fig. (1). If seeds of this plant are kept clean and dry, they can be usable for a long time because of their antioxidant contents that prevent the degradation of essential oils.

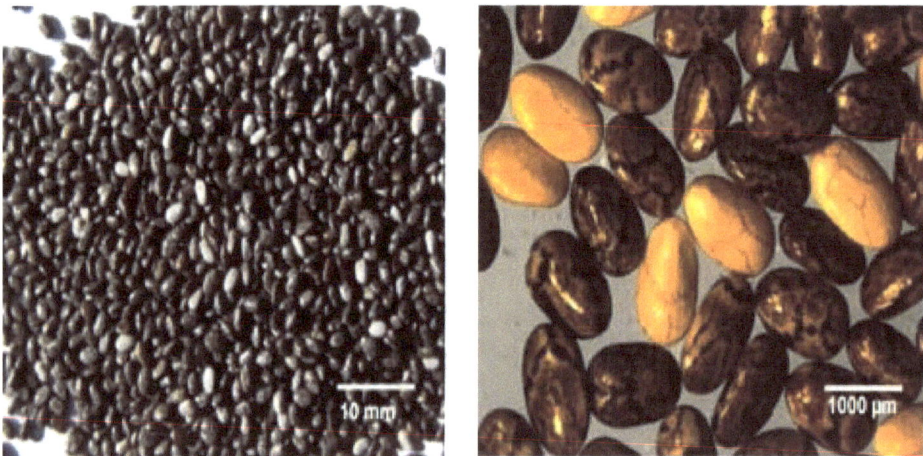

Fig. (1). The form and size of chia seeds.

PHYTOCHEMICALS IN CHIA SEED

As described by Ayerza and Coates [35], the polyphenolic compounds present in chia seeds include; flavonol glycosides, myricetin, chlorogenic acid, quercetin, kaemferol, and caffeic acid. The presence of such components, particularly caffeic acid, chlorogenic acid and quercetin, has been suggested to give antihypertensive, anti-carcinogenic, and neuronal protective properties [36]. Chia seed has also been considered as a durable source of antioxidants [24], which can extremely prevent the lipid peroxidation phenomenon by its phenolic content [37].

NUTRITIONAL COMPOSITION OF CHIA SEED

The chia seeds play prominent roles, both as a functional food and as nutritional ingredients [38]. The nutritional composition of chia seed contains 41% carbohydrate, 30-33% fat, 15-25% protein, 4-5% ash, 18-30% dietary fiber (18–30%) and 90-93% total dry matter. Ting *et al.* [25], guessed that the variation in protein content could be related to climatic, agronomic and soil conditions. Moreover, the high content of fiber in chia seed considered from a healthy outlook increases stool volume, which, in turn, can safeguard against cancer and diverticulosis.

Chia seed is extensively regarded as a part of foods in Japan, Iran, Australia, New Zealand, USA, Canada, Argentina, Chile, and Mexico for different purposes. The high percentage of fiber in chia seed reduced the risk factors of diabetes mellitus by slowing down the process of food digestion and the release of glucose; it also improved the peristaltic movement of intestines and declined cholesterol level of plasma. The biological values of potassium, calcium and magnesium derived from chia seeds are preferable as compared to other cereals [39]. In the United States, the dietary guidelines have suggested that chia seed which is applied in cereals based foods and beverages can be consumed even without being cooked [5]. The nutrient composition of chia seed and fiber contents of different foods have been summarized in Table **1**.

Table 1. Nutrient composition of chia seed and fiber contents of different foods.

Food	Nutrients, USDA [40]		Fiber Content [41]
Chia	Energy (100 g)	486	37.7
Walnuts	Protein %	16.54	5.2
Fava Beans	Fat %	30.47	19
Lentils	Folate µg	49	12–15
Dried Peas	Thiamine mg	0.62	4.4
Figs and Plums	Vitamin C mg	1.6	4
Banana	Niacin mg	883	4
Breakfast Cereals	Riboflavin mg	0.17	17

(Table 1) cont.....

Food	Nutrients, USDA [40]		Fiber Content [41]
Almond	Calcium mg	631	14
Carrots	Potassium	407	2.9
White Bread	Magnesium mg	335	2.2
Cauliflower	Phosphorus mg	860	2.1
Peanut	Selenium (μg)	55.2	8.1
Quince	Iron mg	7.72	6.4
Kiwi	Zinc μg	4.58	1.6

Protein and Amino Acid Contents

The protein profile of chia seed surpasses the protein content of all other cereals that are currently being used in poultry feed (Table **2**). The absence of gluten in chia seed is another exceptional feature of this plant that can be consumed by patients with celiac disease. The scientific results found excellent amounts of 9 essential amino acids (EAA) in chia seed (Table **3**). Protein-rich foods have a great impact on maintaining body weight in human and animal species [42]. The high content of globulin in chia seed caused better thermal stability, even at high temperatures. Sandovaloliveros and Paredes-Lopez [43] reported that chia seed has a notable balance of non-essential amino acids and EAA.

Table 2. Comparison of the protein content of chia seed with other cereals [44].

Cereals	Protein Content %
Chia	20.7
Oats	16.8
Corn	9.42
Rice	6.5
Barley	12.48

Table 3. Amino acid content of chia seed [40, 45].

Amino Acid	Chia (g/100 g)
Aspartic acid	1.69
Serine	1.05
Threonine	0.71
Glycine	0.95
Glutamic acid	3.5
Alanine	1.05

(Table 3) cont.....

Amino Acid	Chia (g/100 g)
Cysteine	0.41
Valine	0.95
Isoleucine	0.8
Leucine	1.37
Methionine	0.59
Leucine	1.37
Tyrosine	0.56
Tryptophane	0.44
Phenylalanine	1.01
Histidine	0.53
Lysine	0.97
Proline	0.77
Arginine	2.14

The Fiber Content of Chia Seed

Many researchers have demonstrated the beneficial impacts of fiber consumption, such as the ability to diminish the risk factors of coronary heart disease [24]. Chia seed is usually composed of almost 370 g/kg of dietary fiber [46]. The fiber content of chia seed is remarkably higher than the other cereals used in poultry feed (Table **4**).

Table 4. Fiber content of some cereal foods in comparison with some dried fruits [40].

Cereals	Fiber g/100 g	Dried Fruits	Fiber g/100 g
Chia	34.4	Dried Plums	7.1
Flax Seed	27.3	Dried Fig	9.8
Quiona	7	Dried Banana	9.9
Amaranth	6.7	Dried Apple	8.7
Peanuts	8.5	Dried Pears	7.5
Amond	12.2	Dried Peaches	8.2
Peanuts	8.5	Dried Pears	7.5

MINERALS CONTENT OF CHIA SEED

Orozco and Romero [47] revealed that the potassium, calcium and phosphorous content of chia is much greater than oats, rice, corn and wheat and also it has 2.4

and 6 times more iron than liver and spinach. The concentration of macronutrient in chia is as follows; phosphorus 860, calcium 631, magnesium 335, and potassium 407mg/100 g. Microelements are as follows ; sodium 16, zinc 4.58, iron 7.72, selenium 55.2, manganese 2.72, copper 0.924 and molybdenum 0.2 μg/100 g .

FATTY ACID COMPOSITION CONTENT OF CHIA SEED

The chia seed, as a great source of omega fatty acids, contains a considerable amount of omega-6 linoleic acid (19%) and omega-3 α-linolenic acid (64%) [48]. Manzella and Paolisso [49] reported that chia seed contains eicosapentaenoic acids and docosahexaenoic acids, which have cardio-protective influences.

THERAPEUTIC PERSPECTIVES OF CHIA SEED

Antioxidant Activity

The polyphenolic compounds of chia seed are potent antioxidants which make it even more valuable in the food industry [50, 51] . The major phenolic compounds found in chia seeds are caffeic acid and chlorogenic acids, followed by kaempferol, myricetin and quercetin [27, 52]. They protect against free radicals and inhibit the peroxidation of fats. Quercetin is a powerful antioxidant with cardio-protective effects [53]. These antioxidants are much more useful than other flavonoid compounds. The composites found in this seed have much stronger antioxidant properties than those of vitamin E, vitamin C and ferulic acid [24, 27, 31]. In a study by Ding *et al.* [54], they concluded that a combination of 0.5% carrageenan and 1% chia raised the production yield of restructured ham-like products and reduced the oxidation of proteins and lipids. The different concentration of antioxidants of chia seed [31] is shown in Table **5**.

Table 5. The concentration of antioxidant compounds in chia seeds.

Compound	Concentration (Mol /kg Seed)
Chlorogenic acid	7.1×10^{-3}
Caffeic acid	6.6×10^{-3}
Hydrolized	
Quercetin	0.2×10^{-3}
Myricetin	3.1×10^{-3}
Caffeic acid	13.5×10^{-3}
Kaempferol	1.1×10^{-3}

EFFECT OF CHIA ON IMMUNE SYSTEM

The protein quality of chia seed is higher than that of common cereals, so that protein quality in chia seed could be valuable in thymus development [55]. Fernandez *et al.* [56], revealed that the diet supplemented with chia seeds (150 g/kg diet) did not reduce the body weight and the Ig E levelwas noticeably higher in the entire experimental period. It is reported that chia in all forms did not cause any clear sign of diseases such as abnormal behaviors, dermatitis, or digestive disorders. Supplementation of animal diets with other sources of omega-3 fatty acids such as marine products or flaxseed can cause fishy flavor, signs of food intolerance, allergy, digestive disorders and diarrhea [44].

CARDIO-PROTECTIVE EFFECTS OF CHIA SEED

Chia seed contains high nutritional values of phytosterols [57], which are known as a valuable nutrient that plays an important role in preventing cardiovascular diseases and possesses bactericidal, antioxidants, and antifungal effects. Currently, the chia seed is considered as a great source of omega-3, which can help diminish the level of triglycerides [58, 59]. Also, the presence of phytosterols as β-sitosterol has the ability to control cholesterol concentration in plasma. Pawlosky *et al.* [60], determined that eicosapentaenoic acids and alpha-linolenic acid are necessary for the formation of vital compounds such as thromboxanes, leukotrienes and prostaglandins, which are involved in multiple physiological functions. The omega-3 fatty acids of chia seeds are efficient in blocking sodium and calcium channel dysfunctions, which can lead to hypertension. Also, omega-3 can improve the parasympathetic tone, protect ventricular arrhythmia and heart rate variability [61].

ANTI-INFLAMMATORY PROPERTIES

Chia seeds possess significant antioxidant and anti-inflammatory properties *in vivo*. Scientific published literature strongly recommends the use of oral chia supplements for inflammatory-related disorders [62]. The dietary intervention studies have elucidated that n-3 PUFA-rich diet alleviates the metabolic syndromes through attenuating the inflammatory status of the system. Hence, it is noteworthy to study the anti-inflammatory properties of Indian chia seeds in an *in vitro* condition [63, 64].

USES OF CHIA SEED IN POULTRY RESEARCH

Chia seeds are considered as one of the highest sources of omega-3 fatty acids among plants. By feeding laying hens with diets enriched in omega-3 fatty acids, it is possible to increase omega-3 fatty acids content in the eggs. Chia seed at 30%

can be incorporated into feed, resulting in higher omega-3 fatty acids content without significantly influencing the sensory quality of poultry eggs. Such eggs will be the best source of omega-3 among consumers [62, 65 - 70].

In another experiment, 10% chia diet significantly lowered the saturated fatty acids as well as the polyunsaturated fatty acid contents and omega-6: omega-3 ratios of the white meats [32, 72]. The compiled literature searched from Google, PubMed, Springer, Science direct, and other published scientific evidence showed that chia seed has been mostly studied on humans and different animal models, but regarding broiler, there is limited research. So it is imperative to perform scientific research on this seed that is a rich source of protein, amino acid and fiber, and also has many therapeutic effects in the control of dyslipidemia, hypertension, and can act as an anti-inflammatory, antioxidant, antidepressant, anti-blood clotting, laxative, antianxietyand antidiabetic agent and as immune booster. Moreover, it provides a good source of B vitamins plus minerals such as calcium, magnesium, phosphorus, zinc, potassium, and others. Also, it is the best source of omega-3 fatty acids, and eggs with abundant omega-3 fatty acids can be produced for patients with cardiovascular disease, as shown in Fig. (**2**).

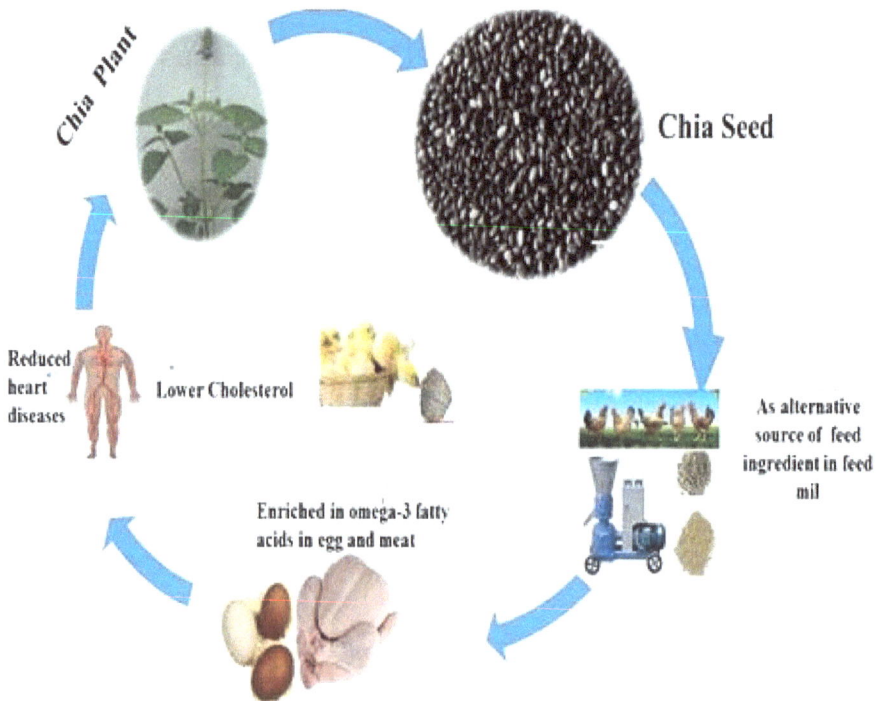

Fig. (2). The chia seed as an alternative feed ingredient can protect the health of consumers.

CONCLUSION

Chia seed (*Salvia hispanica*) is a medicinal and dietary plant species. Chia seed is a natural source of omega-3 fatty acids (α-linolenic acid), soluble and insoluble fibers, and proteins in addition to other important nutritional components, such as minerals, vitamins, phenolic compounds and natural antioxidant. This seed contains high values of phytosterols, which have antioxidants, bactericidal and antifungal effects and can help to prevent cardiovascular diseases. As stated above, the seed is rich in fiber, making it ideal for the proper functioning of the intestine, and contains highly nutritious proteins, more than traditional cereals. It contains vitamins B plus minerals such as calcium, potassium, magnesium, phosphorus, and zinc. This plant does not have any toxic compounds or gluten. Thus it could be used as a safe feed ingredient to reduce the feed cost in the poultry industry. Chia seed is rich in omega-3 fatty acids (α-linolenic acid) so feeding laying hens with chia seed can increase the omega-3 fatty acids content of the eggs. Thereby it would be helpful for consumers that are suffering from heart-related diseases.

CONSENT FOR PUBLICATION

Not applicable.

CONFLICT OF INTEREST

The author declares no conflict of interest, financial or otherwise.

ACKNOWLEDGEMENTS

Declared none.

REFERENCES

[1]   Ayasan T. Effects of dietary inclusion of protexin (probiotic) on hatchability of Japanese quails. Indian J Anim Sci 2013; 83(1): 78-81.

[2]   Hamasalim HJ. Synbiotic as feed additives relating to animal health and performance. Adv Microbiol 2016; 6(4): 288-302.
        [http://dx.doi.org/10.4236/aim.2016.64028]

[3]   Mosihuzzaman M. Herbal medicine in healthcare-an overview. Nat Prod Commun 2012; 7(6): 807-12.
        [http://dx.doi.org/10.1177/1934578X1200700628]

[4]   Elagawany MM. Multiple beneficial applications and modes of action of herbs in poultry health and production-A review. Sci Alert 2015; 11: 152-76.

[5]   Ali A. Productive performance and immune response of broiler chicks as affected by dietary thyme leaves powder. Egypt Poult Sci J 2014; 34(1): 71-84.
        [http://dx.doi.org/10.21608/epsj.2014.5307]

[6]   Gong J, Yin F, Hou Y, Yin Y. Chinese herbs as alternatives to antibiotics in feed for swine and poultry production: potential and challenges in application. Can J Anim Sci 2014; 94(2): 223-41.
[http://dx.doi.org/10.4141/cjas2013-144]

[7]   Saeed M, Baloch AR, Wang M, *et al.* Use of *Cichorium Intybus* Leaf extract as growth promoter, hepatoprotectant and immune modulent in broilers. J Anim Prod Adv 2015; 5(1): 585-91.
[http://dx.doi.org/10.5455/japa.20150118041009]

[8]   Ezzat Abd El-Hack M, Alagawany M, Ragab Farag M, *et al.* Beneficial impacts of thymol essential oil on health and production of animals, fish and poultry: a review. J Essent Oil Res 2016; 28(5): 365-82.
[http://dx.doi.org/10.1080/10412905.2016.1153002]

[9]   Saeed M, Yatao X, Rehman ZU, *et al.* Nutritional and healthical aspects of yacon (smallanthus sonchifolius) for human, animals and poultry. Int J Pharmacol 2017; 13(4): 361-9.
[http://dx.doi.org/10.3923/ijp.2017.361.369]

[10]   Saeed M, Naveed M, Arain MA, *et al.* Quercetin: Nutritional and beneficial effects in poultry. Worlds Poult Sci J 2017; 73(2): 355-64.
[http://dx.doi.org/10.1017/S004393391700023X]

[11]   Saeed M, Abd El-Hack ME, Arif M, *et al.* Impacts of distiller's dried grains with solubles as replacement of soybean meal plus vitamin E supplementation on production, egg quality and blood chemistry of laying hens. Ann Anim Sci 2017; 17(3): 849-62.
[http://dx.doi.org/10.1515/aoas-2016-0091]

[12]   Saeed M, Abd El-Hack ME, Alagawany M, *et al.* Chicory (*Cichorium intybus*) herb: Chemical composition, pharmacology, nutritional and healthical applications. Int J Pharmacol 2017; 13(4): 351-60.
[http://dx.doi.org/10.3923/ijp.2017.351.360]

[13]   Mortensen JZ, Schmidt EB, Nielsen AH, Dyerberg J. The effect of n-6 and n-3 polyunsaturated fatty acids on hemostasis, blood lipids and blood pressure. Throm Heamost 1983; 50: 543-6.

[14]   Dweck AC. The folklore and cosmetic use of various *Salvia species*. Sage The genus Salvia 2000; 14: 1-25.

[15]   Chicco AG, D'Alessandro ME, Hein GJ, Oliva ME, Lombardo YB. Dietary chia seed (*Salvia hispanica* L.) rich in α-linolenic acid improves adiposity and normalises hypertriacylglycerolaemia and insulin resistance in dyslipaemic rats. Br J Nutr 2009; 101(1): 41-50.
[http://dx.doi.org/10.1017/S000711450899053X] [PMID: 18492301]

[16]   Weber CW, Gentry HS, Kohlhepp EA, McCrohan PR. The nutritional and chemical evaluation of chia seeds. Ecol Food Nutr 1991; 26(2): 119-25.
[http://dx.doi.org/10.1080/03670244.1991.9991195]

[17]   Renaud S, Morazain R, Godsey F, *et al.* Nutrients, platelet function and composition in nine groups of French and British farmers. Atherosclerosis 1986; 60(1): 37-48.
[http://dx.doi.org/10.1016/0021-9150(86)90085-7] [PMID: 3707672]

[18]   Baylin A, Kabagambe EK, Ascherio A, Spiegelman D, Campos H. Adipose tissue α-linolenic acid and nonfatal acute myocardial infarction in Costa Rica. Circulation 2003; 107(12): 1586-91.
[http://dx.doi.org/10.1161/01.CIR.0000058165.81208.C6] [PMID: 12668490]

[19]   Ixtaina VY, Nolasco SM, Tomas MC. Physical properties of chia (*Salvia hispanica* L.) seeds. Ind Crops Prod 2008; 28(3): 286-93.
[http://dx.doi.org/10.1016/j.indcrop.2008.03.009]

[20]   Bresson JL, Flynn A, Heinonen M, *et al.* Opinion on the safety of 'Chia seeds (*Salvia hispanica* L.) and ground whole Chia seeds' as a food ingredient [1]. EFSA J 2009; 7: 4.

[21]   Bueno M, Sapio OD, Barolo M, Busilacchi H, Quiroga M, Severin C. Quality tests of *Salvia hispanica* L.(Lamiaceae) fruits marketed in the city of Rosario (Santa Fe province, Argentina). Bol Latinoam

Caribe Plantas Med Aromat 2010; 9(3): 221-7.

[22]	Peiretti PG, Meineri G. Effects on growth performance, carcass characteristics, and the fat and meat fatty acid profile of rabbits fed diets with chia (*Salvia hispanica* L.) seed supplements. Meat Sci 2008; 80(4): 1116-21.
[http://dx.doi.org/10.1016/j.meatsci.2008.05.003] [PMID: 22063845]

[23]	Alfredo VO, Gabriel RR, Luis CG, David BA. Physicochemical properties of a fibrous fraction from chia (*Salvia hispanica* L.). Lebensm Wiss Technol 2009; 42(1): 168-73.
[http://dx.doi.org/10.1016/j.lwt.2008.05.012]

[24]	Reyes-Caudillo E, Tecante A, Valdivia-López MA. Dietary fibre content and antioxidant activity of phenolic compounds present in Mexican chia (*Salvia hispanica* L.) seeds. Food Chem 2008; 107(2): 656-63.
[http://dx.doi.org/10.1016/j.foodchem.2007.08.062]

[25]	Ting IP, Brown JH, Naqvi HH, Kumamoto J, Matsumura M. Chia: A Potential Oil Crop for Arid Zones, in New Industrial Crops and Products, Proceedings of the Association for the Advancement of Industrial Crops. Tucson, Arizona: The University of Arizona, Office of Arid Lands Studies 1990, pp. 197–200.

[26]	Taga MS, Miller EE, Pratt DE. Chia seeds as a source of natural lipid antioxidants. J Am Oil Chem Soc 1984; 61(5): 928-31.
[http://dx.doi.org/10.1007/BF02542169]

[27]	Ayerza R, Coates W. Influence of environment on growing period and yield, protein, oil and α-linolenic content of three chia (*Salvia hispanica* L.) selections. Ind Crop Prod 2009; 30: 321-324.

[28]	Liu SC, Hong PZ, Zhang CH, Ji HW, Gao JL, Zhang L. Cholesterol, lipid content, and fatty acid composition of different tissues of farmed cobia (Rachycentron canadum) from China. J Am Oil Chem Soc 2009; 86(12): 1155-61.
[http://dx.doi.org/10.1007/s11746-009-1458-4]

[29]	Ullah R, Nadeem M, Khalique A, *et al.* Nutritional and therapeutic perspectives of Chia (*Salvia hispanica* L.): a review. J Food Sci Technol 2016; 53(4): 1750-8.
[http://dx.doi.org/10.1007/s13197-015-1967-0] [PMID: 27413203]

[30]	Ayerza R, Coates W. Omega-3 enriched eggs: the influence of dietary α-linolenic fatty acid source on egg production and composition. Can J Anim Sci 2001; 81(3): 355-62.
[http://dx.doi.org/10.4141/A00-094]

[31]	Ayerza R, Coates W, Lauria M. Chia seed (*Salvia hispanica* L.) as an omega-3 fatty acid source for broilers: influence on fatty acid composition, cholesterol and fat content of white and dark meats, growth performance, and sensory characteristics. Poult Sci 2002; 81(6): 826-37.
[http://dx.doi.org/10.1093/ps/81.6.826] [PMID: 12079050]

[32]	Muñoz LA, Cobos A, Diaz O, Aguilera JM. Chia seed (*Salvia hispanica*): an ancient grain and a new functional food. Food Rev Int 2013; 29(4): 394-408.
[http://dx.doi.org/10.1080/87559129.2013.818014]

[33]	Muñoz LA, Cobos A, Diaz O, Aguilera JM. Chia seeds: Microstructure, mucilage extraction and hydration. J Food Eng 2012; 108(1): 216-24.
[http://dx.doi.org/10.1016/j.jfoodeng.2011.06.037]

[34]	Ayerza R, Coates W. Dietary levels of chia: influence on hen weight, egg production and sensory quality, for two strains of hens. Br Poult Sci 2002; 43(2): 283-90.
[http://dx.doi.org/10.1080/00071660120121517] [PMID: 12047094]

[35]	Shahidi F, Naczk M. Phenolic compounds in grains InIn food phenolics Source, chemistry effects, applications. Technomic Publishing Company Inc. 1995; pp. 3-39.

[36]	Tepe B, Sokmen M, Akpulat HA, Sokmen A. Screening of the antioxidant potentials of six *Salvia species* from Turkey. Food Chem 2006; 95(2): 200-4.

[http://dx.doi.org/10.1016/j.foodchem.2004.12.031]

[37]   Coelho MS, Salas-Mellado MD. Chemical characterization of chia (*Salvia hispanica* L.) for use in food products. J Food Nutr Res 2014; 2(5): 263-9.
[http://dx.doi.org/10.12691/jfnr-2-5-9]

[38]   Haytowitz DB, Lemar L, Pehrsson P, *et al.* USDA national nutrient database for standard reference, release 24. Washington, DC, USA: US Department of Agriculture 2011.

[39]   De Tucci J. Chia, la semilla que reduce el colesterol. Magazine Bayres Today 2006; p. 5.

[40]   Fernández I, Ayerza R, Coates W, Vidueiros SM. Nutritional characteristics of chia. Actualización en Nutrición. Tucson, Arizona 85706, USA, Office of Arid Lands Studies. University of Arizona 2006; 7: 23.

[41]   Lejeune MP, Kovacs EM, Westerterp Plantenga MS. Additional protein intake limits weight regain after weight loss in humans. Br J Nutr 2005; 93(2): 281-9.
[http://dx.doi.org/10.1079/BJN20041305] [PMID: 15788122]

[42]   Sandoval-Oliveros MR, Paredes-López O. Isolation and characterization of proteins from chia seeds (*Salvia hispanica* L.). J Agric Food Chem 2013; 61(1): 193-201.
[http://dx.doi.org/10.1021/jf3034978] [PMID: 23240604]

[43]   Beltran-Orozco MC, Romero MR. La Chia, Alimento Milenario, Departamento de Graduados e Investigacion en Alimentos ENCB. Mexico: IPN 2003.

[44]   Altschul AM, Yatsu LY, Ory RL, Engleman EM. Seed proteins. Annu Rev Plant Physiol 1966; 17(1): 113-36.
[http://dx.doi.org/10.1146/annurev.pp.17.060166.000553]

[45]   Mohd Ali N, Yeap SK, Ho WY, Beh BK, Tan SW, Tan SG. The promising future of chia, *Salvia hispanica* L. J Biomed Biotechnol 2012; 2012: 171956.
[http://dx.doi.org/10.1155/2012/171956] [PMID: 3518271]

[46]   Beltrán-Orozco MC, Romero MR. Chía, alimento milenario. In: Técnicos SA, Ed. Alfa Editores Técnicos. México : Revista Industria Alimentaria, Septiembre-Octubre, Iztapalapa 2003; pp. 22-5.

[47]   Reales A, Rivera D, Palazón JA, Obón C. Numerical taxonomy study of *Salvia sect. Salvia (Labiatae)*. Botan J Linn Soc 2004; 145(3): 353-71.

[48]   Manzella D, Paolisso G. Cardiac autonomic activity and Type II diabetes mellitus. Clin Sci (Lond) 2005; 108(2): 93-9.
[http://dx.doi.org/10.1042/CS20040223] [PMID: 15476437]

[49]   da Silva Marineli R, Moraes ÉA, Lenquiste SA, Godoy AT, Eberlin MN, Maróstica Jr MR. Chemical characterization and antioxidant potential of Chilean chia seeds and oil (*Salvia hispanica* L.). Lebensm Wiss Technol 2014; 59(2): 1304-10.
[http://dx.doi.org/10.1016/j.lwt.2014.04.014]

[50]   Scapin G, Schimdt MM, Prestes RC, Ferreira S, Silva AF, Da Rosa CS. Effect of extract of chia seed (*Salvia hispanica*) as an antioxidant in fresh pork sausage. Int Food Res J 2015; 22(3): 1195.

[51]   Ayerza R, Coates W. Chia seeds: new source of omega-3 fatty acids, natural antioxidants, and dietetic fiber. Tucson, Arizona, USA: Southwest Center for Natural Products Research and Commercialization, Office of Arid Lands Studies 2001.

[52]   Pandey KB, Rizvi SI. Plant polyphenols as dietary antioxidants in human health and disease. Oxid Med Cell Longev 2009; 2(5): 270-8.
[http://dx.doi.org/10.4161/oxim.2.5.9498] [PMID: 20716914]

[53]   Ding Y, Lin HW, Lin YL, *et al.* Nutritional composition in the chia seed and its processing properties on restructured ham-like products. J Food Drug Anal 2018; 26(1): 34-124.

[54]   Proceedings of the Nutrition Society , Volume 67 , Issue OCE1: 1st International Immunonutrition

Workshop, Valencia, 3–5 October 2007, Valencia, Spain, May 2008, E12.
[http://dx.doi.org/10.1017/S0029665108006216]

[55]   Ciftci ON, Przybylski R, Rudzińska M. Lipid components of flax, perilla, and chia seeds. Eur J Lipid Sci Technol 2012; 114(7): 794-800.
[http://dx.doi.org/10.1002/ejlt.201100207]

[56]   Jin F, Nieman DC, Sha W, Xie G, Qiu Y, Jia W. Supplementation of milled chia seeds increases plasma ALA and EPA in postmenopausal women. Plant Foods Hum Nutr 2012; 67(2): 105-10.
[http://dx.doi.org/10.1007/s11130-012-0286-0] [PMID: 22538527]

[57]   de Souza Ferreira C, dd Sousa Fomes LdeF, da Silva GE, Rosa G. Effect of chia seed (*Salvia hispanica* L.) consumption on cardiovascular risk factors in humans: a systematic review. Nutr Hosp 2015; 32(5): 1909-18.
[PMID: 26545644]

[58]   Pawlosky R, Hibbeln J, Lin Y, Salem N Jr. n-3 fatty acid metabolism in women. Br J Nutr 2003; 90(5): 993-4.
[http://dx.doi.org/10.1079/BJN2003985] [PMID: 14667193]

[59]   Simopoulos AP. Omega-3 fatty acids and cardiovascular disease: The epidemiological evidence. Environ Health Prev Med 2002; 6(4): 203-9.
[http://dx.doi.org/10.1007/BF02897971]

[60]   Coorey R, Novinda A, Williams H, Jayasena V. Omega-3 fatty acid profile of eggs from laying hens fed diets supplemented with chia, fish oil, and flaxseed. J Food Sci 2015; 80(1): S180-7.
[http://dx.doi.org/10.1111/1750-3841.12735] [PMID: 25557903]

[61]   Gazem RA, Puneeth HR, Madhu CS, Sharada AC. Physicochemical Properties and *in vitro* Anti-Inflammatory Effects of Indian Chia (*Salvia hispanica* L.) Seed Oil. J Pharm Biol Sci 2016; 11: 1-8.

[62]   Simopoulos AP. Omega-3 fatty acids in inflammation and autoimmune diseases. J Am Coll Nutr 2002; 21(6): 495-505.
[http://dx.doi.org/10.1080/07315724.2002.10719248] [PMID: 12480795]

[63]   Segura-Campos MR, Salazar-Vega IM, Chel-Guerrero LA, Betancur-Ancona DA. Biological potential of chia (*Salvia hispanica* L.) protein hydrolysates and their incorporation into functional foods. Lebensm Wiss Technol 2013; 50(2): 723-31.
[http://dx.doi.org/10.1016/j.lwt.2012.07.017]

[64]   Rodea-González DA, Cruz-Olivares J, Román-Guerrero A, Rodríguez-Huezo ME, Vernon-Carter EJ, Pérez-Alonso C. Spray-dried encapsulation of chia essential oil (*Salvia hispanica* L.) in whey protein concentrate-polysaccharide matrices. J Food Eng 2012; 111(1): 102-9.
[http://dx.doi.org/10.1016/j.jfoodeng.2012.01.020]

[65]   Brenna JT, Salem N Jr, Sinclair AJ, Cunnane SC. α-Linolenic acid supplementation and conversion to n-3 long-chain polyunsaturated fatty acids in humans. Prostaglandins Leukot Essent Fatty Acids 2009; 80(2-3): 85-91.
[http://dx.doi.org/10.1016/j.plefa.2009.01.004] [PMID: 19269799]

[66]   Nieman DC, Cayea EJ, Austin MD, Henson DA, McAnulty SR, Jin F. Chia seed does not promote weight loss or alter disease risk factors in overweight adults. Nutr Res 2009; 29(6): 414-8.
[http://dx.doi.org/10.1016/j.nutres.2009.05.011] [PMID: 19628108]

[67]   Wojcikowski K, Johnson DW, Gobe G. Herbs or natural substances as complementary therapies for chronic kidney disease: ideas for future studies. J Lab Clin Med 2006; 147(4): 160-6.
[http://dx.doi.org/10.1016/j.lab.2005.11.011] [PMID: 16581343]

[68]   Jiang RW, Lau KM, Hon PM, Mak TC, Woo KS, Fung KP. Chemistry and biological activities of caffeic acid derivatives from Salvia miltiorrhiza. Curr Med Chem 2005; 12(2): 237-46.
[http://dx.doi.org/10.2174/0929867053363397] [PMID: 15638738]

[69]   Surai PF, Sparks NH. Designer eggs: from improvement of egg composition to functional food.

Trends Food Sci Technol 2001; 12(1): 7-16.
[http://dx.doi.org/10.1016/S0924-2244(01)00048-6]

[70]   Azcona JO, Schang MJ, Garcia PT, Gallinger C, Ayerza R Jr, Coates W. Omega-3 enriched broiler meat: The influence of dietary α-linolenic-ω-3 fatty acid sources on growth, performance and meat fatty acid composition. Can J Anim Sci 2008; 88(2): 257-69.
[http://dx.doi.org/10.4141/CJAS07081]

[71]   Ayerza R, Coates W. Chia: Rediscovering a Forgotten Crop of the Aztecs. University of Arizona Press 2005.

[72]   Bailey CJ, Day C. Traditional plant medicines as treatments for diabetes. Diabetes Care 1989; 12(8): 553-64.
[http://dx.doi.org/10.2337/diacare.12.8.553] [PMID: 2673695]

CHAPTER 10

Cassia Fistula: Potential Health-Promoting Candidate for Livestock and Poultry

Zohaib A. Bhutto[1], Muhammad A. Arain[1,*], Mahmoud Alagawany[2,*], Muhammad Umar[1], Ilahi Bakhash Marghazani[1], Nasrullah[1], Feroza Soomro[3], Mohamed E. Abd El-Hack[2], Muhammad Saeed[4], Mayada R. Farag[5], Ahmed Noreldin[6] and Kuldeep Dhama[7]

[1] *Faculty of Veterinary and Animal Sciences, Lasbela University of Agriculture, Water and Marine Sciences, 3800 Uthal, Balochistan, Pakistan*

[2] *Department of Poultry, Faculty of Agriculture, Zagazig University, 44511Zagazig, Egypt*

[3] *Department of Veterinary Parasitology, Faculty of Animal Husbandry and Veterinary Sciences, Sindh Agriculture University, Tandojam, Pakistan*

[4] *Department of Animal Nutrition, Cholistan University of Veterinary and Animal Sciences Bahawalpur, Pakistan*

[5] *Forensic Medicine and Toxicology Department, Veterinary Medicine Faculty, Zagazig University, Zagazig44511, Egypt*

[6] *Department of Histology and Cytology, Faculty of Veterinary Medicine, Damanhour University, Damanhour 22516, Egypt*

[7] *Division of Pathology, ICAR-Indian Veterinary Research Institute, Izatnagar, Bareilly, 243 122, Uttar Pradesh, India*

Abstract: The beneficial uses of natural herbal plants in medical sciences have achieved great attention due to promising health benefits in comparison with synthetic pharmaceutics. *Cassia fistula* (CF) is one of the most famous medicinal plants due to its broad range of incredible biological functions, such as laxative or purgative, antidiabetic, hypolipidemic, hepatoprotective, antioxidant, anti-inflammatory, antipyretic, antitussive, antimicrobial, anticancer, antiparasitic and wound healing as well. Moreover, flavonoids derived from CF, such as tannins and glycosides, exhibit a broad spectrum of therapeutic activities and low toxic effects. Previously most studies discussed *in vitro*-based models, humans, and rodents. The aim of this review is to highlight the medicinal importance of CF on the production performance of animals. Up to now, there are still many research areas waiting to be explored, such as finding out the metabolic pathway of flavonoids of CF in different animal models, mainly focus on poultry.

* **Corresponding authors Muhammad Arain:** Faculty of Veterinary and Animal Sciences, Lasbela University of Agriculture, Water and Marine Sciences, Uthal - 3800, Balochistan, Pakistan; E-mail: asifarain77@yahoo.com;
Mahmoud Alagawany: Department of Poultry, Faculty of Agriculture, Zagazig University, Zagazig - 44511, Egypt; E-mail: mmalagwany@zu.edu.eg

Therefore, the present chapter aimed to attract attention to health-promoting and medicinal uses of this plant in poultry and animals. The above-mentioned research will provide further medicinal development of this genus.

Keywords: Animals, *Cassia fistula*, Growth promoter, Medicinal properties, Poultry.

INTRODUCTION

According to the World Health Organization (WHO) recommendations, around 70 percent of the world's population utilizes folk medicine to achieve their main health requirements. The developing nations are using ethnomedicine to cure medical problems [1, 2]. The drugs and formulations from the natural origin are commonly believed to be having less toxic and undesirable adverse effects when compared to synthetic origin [1]. In the current century, improving animal and poultry production performance by dietary manipulation is the main target of nutritionists. In the modification of NRC nutrient recommendations [3, 4], using feed additives like enzymes, organic acids and medicinal plants has been reported by many researchers [5 - 9]. *Cassia fistula* (CF) is popularly well known as a golden shower tree and belongs to the *Caesalpiniaceae* family; it is broadly employed for its medicinal qualities. It has purgative effects due to the presence of wax aloin and a tonic [10] and has been documented to treat numerous additional gastrointestinal disorders such as healing ulcers [11]. In traditional/folk medicine, CF is among the important medicinal plant principally used in Unani and Ayurvedic medicines; this plant has been implemented to be useful against skin diseases, liver troubles, tuberculosis glands and its use in the treatment of haematemesis, pruritus, leucoderma and diabetes [12]. Traditionally, the plant is also used as an infusion, decoction, or powder, either singly or along with a mixture of other medicinal plants. Recently, commercial preparations tend to be the standardized extracts of the whole plant. The medicinal plant, its extracts and phytochemicals (extracts from flower, seed, stem barks, fruit and leaf) have been reported for fascinating biological and pharmacological activities, such as antioxidant, anticancer, antidiabetic, anti-inflammatory, hepatoprotective, antiaging, antibacterial, antifungal, analgesic and antidiabetic properties [13 - 19]. In the folk medicine therapeutic system, various diseases and pathological conditions are commonly cured with CF believed to be self-limiting, therefore health-promoting effects require further investigations. Poultry diet is limiting and very expensive for the smallholder resource-poor farmers. Therefore, it is necessary to find cheaper alternative protein sources that sustain productivity and increase protein source options for smallholder poultry farmers. This chapter summarizes the current scientific findings and suggests areas where further research is needed in animal and poultry and also to be the need of time to verify the therapeutic efficacy of *Cassia fistula* in different animals and poultry industries.

PLANT BIOGRAPHY

Cassia fistula is native to the Indian subcontinent and adjacent areas of Southeast Asia. It grows throughout southern Pakistan and eastward throughout India, Bangladesh, China, Hong Kong, Myanmar, Philippines, Malaysia, Indonesia, and Thailand. It is an ornamental plant and is commonly used for traditional herbal medicine. This plant is widely grown in the subcontinent and known by different local names (Fig. **1**). The taxonomical classification of CF is shown in Fig. (**2**). *Cassia fistula* is a modest-sized deciduous tree with 10 m in height, flowers-yellow, leaves swap, pinnate, 30-40 cm long, with 4-8 pairs of ovate leaflets, 7.5-15 cm long and 2-5 cm large. Fruits are pendulous, cylindrical, brown, septate, 25-50 cm long, 1.5-3 cm in diameter, with 25-100 seeds. Seeds are lenticular, light brown, and lustrous.

APPLICATION IN HERBAL MEDICINE

The diverse Cassia species available globally are implemented in herbal medicine. The CF is, no doubt, a modest laxative and can be used safely while treating the children [20]. *Cassia fistula*'s emulsion can be as effective as polyethylene glycol in the treatment of children with functional constipation [21], while the use of leaves and bark with high doses can induce vomiting, nausea, abdominal pain and cramps. *Cassia fistula* is used as a therapy for tumors (abdomen, glands, liver, stomach and throat), burns, cancer, constipation, convulsions, diarrhea, delirium, dysuria, gravel, epilepsy, hematuria, pimples, and glandular tumors. In Ayurvedic medicine systems, the seeds are attributed with antibilious, aperitif, carminative, and laxative properties, while the root is used for burning sensations, adenopathy, leprosy, syphilis, skin diseases and tubercular glands. The leaves are employed there for erysipelas, rheumatism, malaria and ulcers. In Brazil, the seeds are employed as a laxative and the leaves and/or bark as an analgesic and for inflammation [22, 23]. Recently, natural products made from CF plant have been used in an assortment of cosmetic applications as a whitening agent and a source of nutrition.

APPLICATIONS IN AYURVEDIC MEDICINE

A large number of plant species have been used in the traditional Indian Ayurvedic medicine to improve the health status by treating hyperlipidemia like CF, known as Indian Laburnum, commonly found in Pakistan, India, Bangladesh, South America and Tropical Africa as well as the West Indies. In India, the rural people consume the mature pulp of fruit as a purgative and against abdominal pain and cardiac ailments [24]. The Golden Shower Tree is well known as "disease killer" in Ayurvedic medicine practices. Its fruit pulp acts as a mild laxative as well as for stomach and cardiac problems, likewise acid reflux-flowers for pyrexia while rooting for diuresis. The effect of CF in Ayurvedic medicine is known to be involved with treating various disorders, including skin diseases, leprosy, haematemesis, pruritus and diabetes [25]. The skin problems are treated with bark and leaves. The seeds are recognized as aperitif, antibilious, laxative and carminative, while the root is used for burning sensations, curing adenopathy, leprosy, syphilis, skin diseases and tubercular glands [26]. The leaves of the tree are used for erysipelas, rheumatism, malaria, and ulcers, while the buds are used for biliousness, fever, constipation, leprosy, and skin disease and the fruit for abdominal pain, constipation, fever, heart disease and leprosy. Thus, every part of this plant is recognized for its medicinal properties [27, 28]. The plant is being considered as a firewood source in Mexico. The reddish wood, hard and heavy, strong and durable, is suited for cabinetwork and farm implements. The bark has been employed in tanning, often in conjunction with avaram. The drug "*Cassia fistula*", a mild laxative, is obtained from the sweetish pulp around the seed [29].

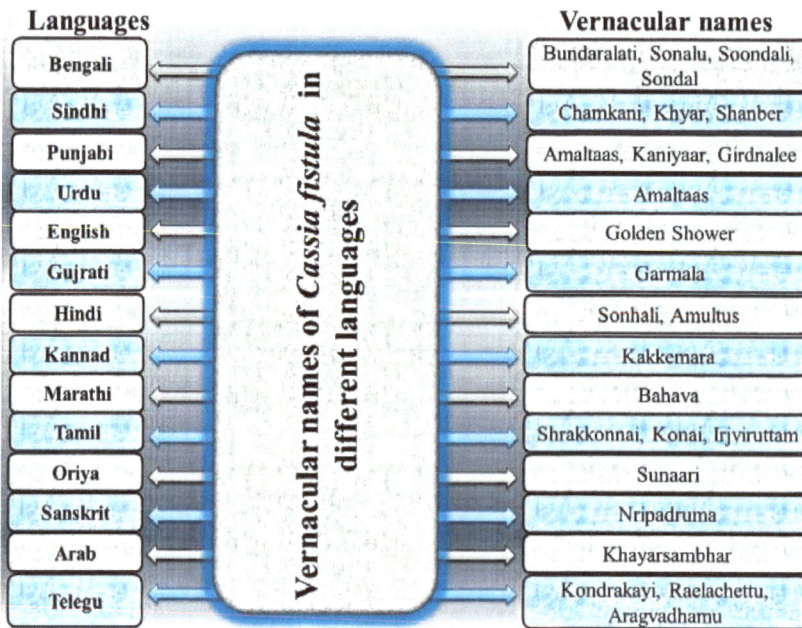

Languages	Vernacular names of *Cassia fistula* in different languages	Vernacular names
Bengali		Bundaralati, Sonalu, Soondali, Sondal
Sindhi		Chamkani, Khyar, Shanber
Punjabi		Amaltaas, Kaniyaar, Girdnalee
Urdu		Amaltaas
English		Golden Shower
Gujrati		Garmala
Hindi		Sonhali, Amultus
Kannad		Kakkemara
Marathi		Bahava
Tamil		Shrakkonnai, Konai, Irjviruttam
Oriya		Sunaari
Sanskrit		Nripadruma
Arab		Khayarsambhar
Telegu		Kondrakayi, Raelachettu, Aragvadhamu

Fig. (1). Vernacular names of *Cassia fistula* in different languages.

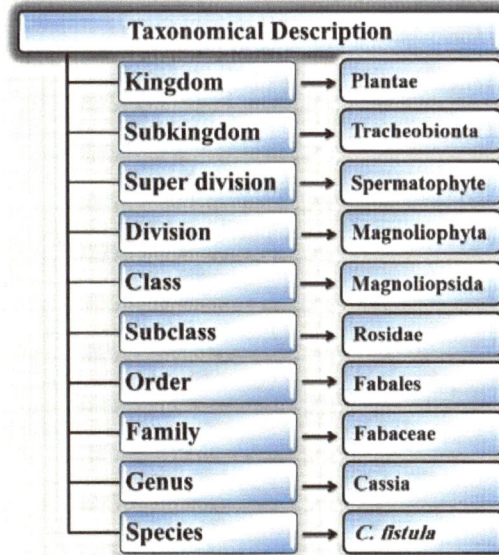

Fig. (2). Taxonomical classification of *Cassia fistula.*

PHYTOCHEMISTRY

The *Cassia fistula* tree is an abundant source of phytochemical phenolic antioxidant agents, likewise flavonoids, flavan-3-ol derivatives and anthraquinones. The presence of other compounds has also been reported, which include terpenoids, alkaloids, reducing sugars, saponins, tannins, carbonyl, phlorotannin, and steroids [30]. The seeds contain approximately 2% anthraquinones, 24% crude protein, 4.5% crude fat, 6.5% crude fiber, and 50% carbohydrates. The stem bark contains two flanol glycosides and xanthone glycosides [31]. The leaves have been documented with 15.88% crude protein, 6.65% crude fat, 20% crude fiber, and 39.86% carbohydrates. Besides, the plant also contains ferulic acid, rhein, rheinglucoside, galactomannan, sennosides A and B, phlobaphenes, oxyanthraquinone substances, emodin, chrysophanic acid, fistuacacidin, barbaloin, lupeol, beta-sitosterol, and hexacosanol [14, 32]. Fig. (3) shows some phytochemicals of *Cassia fistula.*

BIOLOGICAL ACTIVITIES

The CF plant has a wide range of biological activities until now reported in the literature, as depicted in Fig. (4). The CF plant can be used in the future industry for pharmaceutical, cosmeceutical, nutraceutical and functional food. In addition, the components of CF Plant have a positive effect as a growth promoter in the animal and poultry industry. Recently, the extract of CF is used in the synthesis of silver nanoparticles. *Cassia fistula* plant has biological activities as will follow through display all updated information.

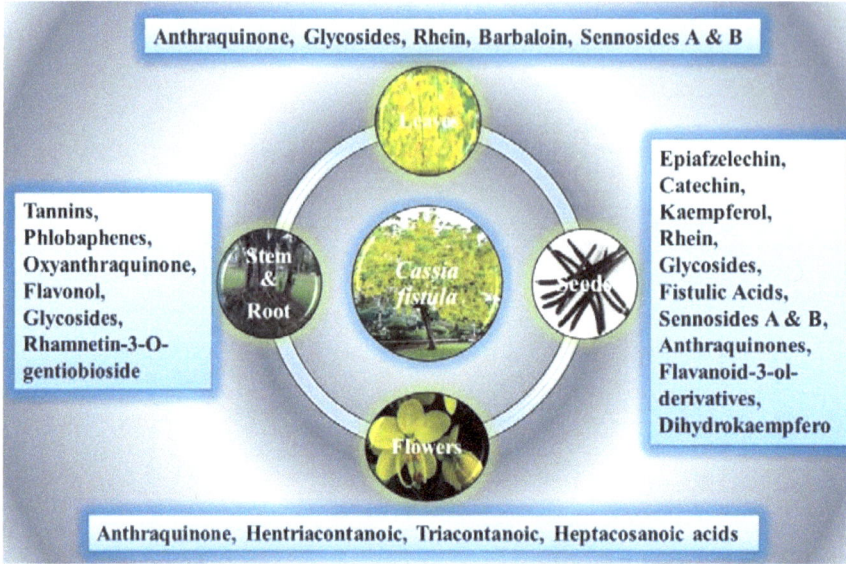

Fig. (3). Some phytochemicals of *Cassia fistula.*

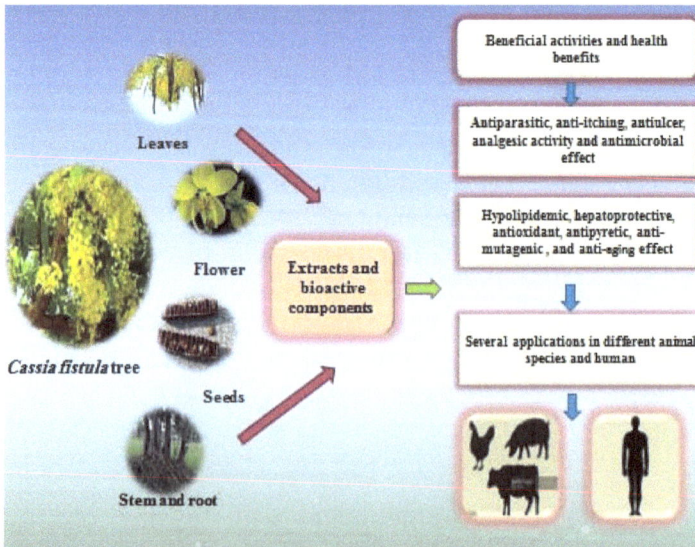

Fig. (4). Biological activities and beneficial applications of *Cassia fistula.*

Antidiabetic activity: The extracts of CF from different parts have hypoglycaemic and antidiabetic effects. For example, the hydroalcoholic extract of CF has been reported to exhibit antidiabetic and hypoglycemic activities in rats [33]. The ethanolic extract from stem bark was investigated for their anti-hyperglycemic activity [34]. The total alcoholic extract of the CF bark and its ethyl acetate fractions showed positive effects on reducing diabetic symptoms in rats exposed to alloxan. The ethyl acetate fraction *vs.* alcohol extract significantly reduced the level of blood glucose, also compared with the standard antidiabetic drug (glibenclamide) [17]. The seed extract produced a hypoglycemic effect on normal rats, while this effect was not be observed for alloxan-induced diabetic rats [35]. The hexane extract from bark produced hypoglycemic activity by decreasing the glucose level of the blood of the streptozotocin experimental rat model [36]. *Cassia* genus has bioactive compounds as bioflavonoids, Roseanne, eugenol, azulene, phenethylamine and dodecatetraenamide [37]. The presence of one of these compounds in the plant extract may help in the uptake of glucose. The transporting molecules of glucose are regulated by myocytes and/or leptocytes in response to great secretion of insulin in blood, resulting in a hypoglycemic effect [38]. We can gain from the above that the bark of CF contains some fractions as alloxan that decrease glucose level in the blood and thus give antidiabetic activity.

Hypolipidemic: The ethanolic extract from CF legume was investigated in rats fed on cholesterol and was found to improve the serum lipid profile. The hexane extract from the bark of CF produced hypolipidemic and hypocholesterolemic effects in the streptozotocin experimental rat model [39]. Oral administration of CF fruit at 100, 300 and 500 mg/kg body weight of mice demonstrated antioxidant and hypolipidemic activities. The findings corroborate the use of CF in traditional medicine for cardiac diseases [40]. The extract of leaf and bark of CF possesses the hypolipidemic property. However, there are no results on the extract of the fruit of CF for the treatment against cardiac diseases and hyperlipidemia [41]. Furthermore, Guruprasad *et al.* [42] stated that the use of aqueous and methanolic leaf extracts of CF at 200 and 400 mg/kg body weight of mice exhibited a significant reduction in TC/HDL-C ratio in animals fed the diet with atherogenic for 21 days. Ethanol extract of CF fruit restored the concentrations of serum lipid and enzyme activities in the heart and liver of hyperlipidemic mice [43]. From these results, it is presumed that the lowering or prevention of hyperlipidemia with *C. fistula* may be attributed to the inhibition of triglycerides and cholesterol biosynthesis [44]. Ultimately, the previous results corroborate the use of CF as hypolipidemic in traditional medicine for cardiac ailments. We think that the hypolipidemic effect of CF might be due to individual and/or synergistic actions of the active constituents at various target sites.

Hepatoprotective: Lipid peroxidation and other oxidative stress damage the liver cell. The extract from different parts of CF also has shown hepatoprotective activity. The liver injury recovered with the treatment of seed ethanolic extract in mice, which were experimentally induced with tetrachloride [45]. The hepatotoxicity was reversed with leaf extracts in bromobenzene-induced mice [46] and in paracetamol-induced rats [13], and ethanolic leaf extracts also produced the same effects in rats, which were experimentally induced with diethylnitrosamine [47, 48]. The leaves and bark extracts treatment has the ability to reverse the CCl_4 induced liver injury in experimental rat models [49]. The methanolic extract of leaves reverse backs the biochemical markers of the liver in paracetamol induced hepatitis in the rat model [50]. We conclude from previous studies that the CF impact as hepatoprotective may be due to the presence of some fraction like alkaloids, flavonoids, saponins, tannin and terpenoids, and through two mechanisms. The first, higher quantities of terpenoids or flavonoids in CF extract give antioxidant activities. The second is the effective blocking of oxidative stress and cytokines production. Thus, CF extracts protected against lipopolysaccharide-induced liver damage by decreasing the TNF- and IL6 level and prevented the cytotoxic effect of cytokines and oxygen-free radicals.

Antioxidant: Earlier study shows that CF is rich in flavonoids and anthraquinones [51]. Compounds like fistulic acid, rhein, chrysophanol, physcion, emodin, 3-formyl-1-hydroxy-8-methoxy anthraquinone, sennoside A and B, kaempferol, epicatechin, catechin, procyanidin B2, epiafzelechin, 5-hydroxymethylfurfural, β-sitosterol, gallic acid, ellagic acid, coumaric acid, rutin, myricetin and quercetin are present in the fruit of CF [8, 52 - 54]. Flavonoids like quercetin, kaempferol, myricetin, rutin, epicatechin, catechin, epiafzelechin and procyanidin B2 have been reported to exert antioxidant activities [55 - 58]. On the other hand, anthraquinones extracted from CF, such as chrysophanol, rhein, physcion and emodin, exhibited antioxidant effects [59 - 62]. It is proved that CF and its extracts have antioxidant properties. The various phytochemicals such as phenolic, proanthocyanidin, and flavonoids in aqueous and methanolic extracts are documented for their antioxidant characteristics [14]. The *in-vitro* study also confirmed that the phytochemical compound in CF has potent antioxidant properties [63]. The flower extract can produce antioxidant activity in rats after alloxan-induced diabetes [25]. The powder of CF fruit pulp showed antioxidant effects *in vivo* and *in vitro* [64]. The hydroalcoholic extract of the fruit pulp of CF shows antioxidant activity by inhibiting hydroxyl radical and reducing power activities [65]. The ethanolic extract of leaf validated for antioxidant effect on diethylnitrosamine-induced rat experimental model [47]. The bark aqueous and methanolic extracts showed antioxidant effects on kidney and liver homogenates [14]. In mice, Guruprasad *et al.* [42], speculated that aqueous and methanolic leaf extracts of CF at 200 and 400 mg/kg BW reduced the level of lipid peroxidation in a dose-dependent manner. The powerful antioxidant action of CF could be attributed to its high contents from flavonoids and phenolics.

Antipyretic: The biomolecules inside methanolic extract from pod possibly have the ability to produce antipyretic activity in rats [66]. Moreover, the ethanolic extract of CF can decline the body temperature in typhoid, paratyphoid A, and paratyphoid B (TAB) vaccine-induced pyrexia. Various kinds of volatile compounds were used for the extraction of CF bark, while methanolic extract showed a significant antipyretic activity [67]. The antipyretic activity of CF is due to the individual or combined impact of the bioactive component present in it. Indeed, the work of any antipyretic is by inhibiting the enzyme cyclooxygenase. The rhein found in CF diminished carrageenan-induced cyclooxygenase. In addition, the impact of CF may be due to its ability to decrease pro-inflammatory mediators and enhance anti-inflammatory signals at injury sites.

Anti-inflammatory: The aqueous extracts from *Cassia fistula* fruits and leaves have been reported to have inflammatory properties [68]. The ethanolic extract of CF investigated in rats proved that its useful effects on inflammatory conditions. The *in-vitro* study reported that the presence of some chemical compounds (alkaloids, saponins, flavonoids, anthraquinone, and phenolic) in the plant might be produced anti-inflammatory action [63]. Flavonoids in CF have shown anti-inflammatory properties by targeting reactive oxygen species [69]. The *Cassia fistula* bark aqueous and methanolic extracts showed anti-inflammatory effects on liver and kidney homogenates [15]. The CF fruit and leave extracts produced an anti-inflammatory effect on experimental rats such as carrageenan-induced oedema [70] and paw edema [71], respectively. In the end, we think that CF pod extracts can use for animals or humans at any age when they are suffering from chronic inflammatory states.

Antileishmanial activity: Hexane extracts of CF fruits showed a powerful antileishmanial effect on the Leishmania L promastigote chagasi [72, 73]. We think that the antileishmanial activity of *Cassia fistula* may be due to some compounds such as terpenoids and eugenol because De-Alencar *et al.* [74], stated that terpenoids have *in vitro* antileishmanial activity. In addition, Teixeira *et al.* [75], illustrated that a series of compounds derived from eugenol and containing 1,2,3-triazolic portions revealed significant antileishmanial activity. Generally, information about the role of CF as an antileishmanial activity is rare.

Nervous system: Natural products play an essential role in the therapy and prevention of various neuronal dysfunctions and neurodegenerative diseases. The methanol extract of the *Cassia fistula* seeds was reported to show antidepressant effects in mice and could modulate their behavioral changes and was concluded to be helpful for novel antidepressant compounds in future drug designing research [76]. Hydroalcoholic extract of CF leaf improved injuries in alcohol-induced peripheral neuropathy rats [77]. *Cassia fistula* contains some compounds such as polyphenolic and alkaloids, and the previous studies indicated that these compounds found in medicinal plants able to delayed neurodegeneration and improve cognitive function and memory. Thus, the positive effect of CF on the nervous system may be due to the presence of these compounds.

Antimicrobial: The *in vitro* studies have been reported for antibacterial and antifungal activity of different volatile and aqueous extracts from the flower [16], leaves, and root extracts [78] and pod extracts of CF plant [79]. The *Staphylococcus aureus* samples were collected from the field, which showed susceptibility to alcoholic extract of CF [80]. The *in-vitro* study reported that the presences of some phytochemicals in the plant are responsible for antimicrobial activity [63]. The methanolic extract from leaves of CF has antifungal activity against *Candida albicans* and antibacterial activity against *Bacillus subtilis*, *Staphylococcus aureus*, *Salmonella typhi*, *Escherichia coli,* and *Pseudomonas aeruginosa* [81]. On the other hand, Irshad *et al.* [82] pointed out that the crude extract of CF (fruit pulp and seed extract) is a good source for anticandidal agents. The anticandidal activity of crude extract of this plant may be due to the presence of phenolic compounds such as rhein and anthraquinone. The antimicrobial activities of these components are already documented [83]. Phytochemical studies presented that ability of CF as antibacterial maybe because it contains components like anthraquinone, saponin, glycosides, flavonoids and steroids that inhibit the growth of the bacterial strains [84, 85]. However, CF extracts must be considered as a new source of antibacterial agents and can be useful to remedy infectious diseases [86].

Antitumor activity: The methanolic extract of CF seed has antitumor effects such as increasing the life span of tumor-bearing mice and inhibiting the growth of *Ehrlich ascites* carcinoma [87]. The extract of CF can reverse the hepatocarcinoma, which was induced with diethylnitrosamine (DENA) and carbon tetrachloride (CCl_4) in experimental model rats [88]. The compound of DENA is hazardous to human health because it causes a wide range of tumors in animal species [89]. The antitumor effects of CF leaf extract may be due to the presence of some components as quercetin and rutin. Quercetin is a bioactive flavonoid, can inhibit the proliferation of cancer cells [90]. Rutin is a natural polyphenolic flavonoid, possesses anticancer activity and has a hepatoprotective effect against CCl_4-induced liver injuries [91].

Larvicidal and ovicidal: The crude extracts of the flower have larvicidal properties, excellent potential to control the population of Culex, Aedes and

Anopheles mosquitoes [92]. The different solvent extracts of leaves have the potential to control the larvae of *Cx. tritaeniorhynchus* and *An. subpictus* mosquito [93]. The methanolic leaf extract has larvicidal and ovicidal properties against *C. quinquefasciatus* and *A. stephensi* [94]. In the last period, the researchers have developed new methods of control, including green synthesis of nanoparticle from aqueous extracts of CF, which may be a suitable alternative vector control approach in this regard.

Antiparasitic: Internal and external parasite infestations cause troubles to animal and human and lead to significant losses in health. The spectroscopical fractionation of the dichloromethane extract of *Cassia fistula* fruits (Leguminosae) resulted in isolation and identification of bioactive components with antileishmanial effects such as isoflavone biochanin A [95]. The extract of seed and fruit pulp of CF produced antihelminthic activity through paralysis and death of adult Pheretimaposthuma worms [96]. At the latest, the antiparasitic activity of CF may be due to some compounds which are responsible for the properties of broad-spectrum antimicrobial and the ability of CF in treating stomach problems as a remedy for intestinal worms.

Anti-itching: *Cassia fistula* has many positive effects on patients of eczema. The rising level of IgE is the commonest sign during eczema, and by application of *Cassia fistula*, the level of IgE decreased [97]. According to the study of Jazani *et al.* [97], used plants in traditional Persian medicine such as CF are anti-itching. Anti-pruritus effects mechanism may be attributed to the suppression of histamine release and the regulation effect for IL-2 and IL-4 [98]. We believe that the anti-itching effects of CF may be due to its ability as an anti-inflammatory. Medical scientists describe anti-inflammatory substances such as creams containing diflorasone diacetate in the treatment of itching.

Antiulcer and analgesic activity: Ulcer is associated with an imbalance between aggressive and protective factors [99]. Many mechanisms like an increase in pepsin activity, acid secretion, reduction in bicarbonate secretion and mucus, as well as reduction in gastric mucosal blood flow, are said to be the leading cause of gastric ulceration [100]. The ethanol leaf extract of CF was reported to treat the rat's ulcer induced by pylorus ligation [101]. The methanolic extract of CF possibly interacted with pain receptors. It reduced the pain response in rats which was caused by thermal, mechanical and writhing stimuli in a dose-dependent manner [19]. Also, this extract has ulcer healing properties that might be due to both reductions in gastric cytoprotection and gastric acid secretion. The bioactivity of the CF extracts as anti-ulcer activities could be attributed to some secondary metabolites as terpenoids, flavonoids, phenolic acids, and saponins [102]. We can provide a summary that the antiulcer activity of CF can be attributed to the presence of some compounds that have the ability to inhibition of acid secretary parameters, strengthening of the gastric mucosal barrier, prevention of lipid peroxidation or inhibition of free radical generation. While general, the analgesic action of CF is supposed to be due to the inhibition of prostaglandin synthesis and a peripheral mechanism of pain inhibition.

Wound healing: The infection is a big problem to treat the injury. Antibiotic resistance by the pathogens makes ineffective drugs. The leave extracts of CF played an important role as antibacterial agents against *Pseudomonas aeruginosa* and *Staphylococcus aureus*. *Cassia fistula* enhanced tissue regeneration at the injury position and showed better wound closure as well as supporting histopathological indices about injury healing, and thus confirming the ability of CF in the treatment of the infected injury [103]. The alcoholic extract of CF leaves has potential wound healing properties in infected albino rats and healthy rat models [104, 105]. Presence Lupeol in CF gives a high potential of wound healing through suppression of CD4+ T helper cell, and reducing the proliferation of pro-inflammatory cytokine (IL4, IL2, TNFα) has exposed anti-inflammatory effect. In addition, Presence Rhein in CF reduces the production of free radicals. Thus, it has shown antioxidant, antimicrobial, besides, its role in inhibit the synthesis of some inflammation factors as leukotriene [106]. So, we can say that the ability of CF to wound healing is due to its impacts as an antioxidant, anti-inflammatory and anti-microbial.

Anti-aging and anti-fertility: The CF flower extract showed anti-aging property when experimented in human skin fibroblasts and might be a suitable option in making cosmeceuticals to provide whitening effects, and designated as anti-aging facial skincare cosmetic [107]. Regarding the anti-fertility effect, the petroleum ether extract of CF seed produced an anti-fertility effect through anti-implantation activity in female rats [108]. The aqueous extract of CF seed produced an estrogen-induced uterotrophic effect, hence behave anti-estrogenic nature in female rats [109]. Another benefit, extracts of CF can inhibit specific enzymes (*e.g.*, α-glycosidase, α-tyrosinase and β-glucuronidase,) involved in the alteration of the skin during aging [110]. So, we urge specialized researchers to study the role of CF in original cosmetic compositions because extracts of CF qualify for avoiding premature skin aging in healthy individuals.

Antimutagenic activity: Antimutagenic activity of plant extracts has been described by several studies [111, 112]. Among all the fractions of *C. fistula* fruits, CaFE fraction showed a promising antimutagenic potential due to its content on a higher quantity of bioactive phytoconstituents, which might be responsible for its efficiency in various assays. The strong antimutagenic potential of this fraction may be attributed to its ability to interact with reactive radical species that are generated during the activation of 2-aminofluorene (2-AF). Wherefore, this fraction can act as a possible source of antimutagenic principles for food and pharmaceutical products [113].

Cassia fistula and synthesis of silver nanoparticles: *Cassia fistula* is hoarding multi-perspective constituents that are used not only as medicines but also in silver nanoparticles synthesizing that are dependably beneficial for its inhibition nature in the microbial growth [114]. Recently, microbial resistant products have gained much significance in many of the emerging fields. Biological materials have been employed for green synthesis of nanoparticles to hegemony the spreading of harmful chemicals into the environment [115]. The presence of carbohydrates, other secondary metabolites, flavonoids, phenolics and phospholipid content in CF parts [116] makes it suitable for the bioreduction of Ag+ to form AgNPs. Several studies on AgNPs synthesis from CF plant parts have been reported [117, 118]. Biogenic AgNPs are considered safe for animals [119]. Priadharsini *et al.* [114] used the extract of CF petal in the synthesis of silver nanoparticles, which acts as evidential biocidal influence against fungal and bacterial isolates. The synthesized AgNPs from CF fruit extract revealed a heightened bactericidal activity against *E. coli* [120]. Indeed, green synthesis of nanoparticle from aqueous extracts of CF provides advantages over chemical and physical methods as it can be easily scaled up for large-scale synthesis

CASSIA FISTULA USE IN ANIMALS AND POULTRY

It was reported that CF wild seeds contain about 31% of crude proteins (CP), chiefly globulin and albumin, and seed is an abundant source of phosphorus in the form of phospholipids (cephalin and lecithin) and also contain 11.8% carbohydrates [121]. The galactomannan is the chief carbohydrate present in the seeds, which is composed up of various types of sugar moieties [122]. The biochemical analysis of pollens of flower indicated 12% of protein with an abundant quantity of free amino acids (phenylalanine, methionine, glutamic acid and proline). Further, more carbohydrate, lipid and free amino acid compositions were 11.75, 12 and 1.42%, correspondingly [123]. The fruits of *Cassia fistula* were also documented for abundant sources of minerals (K, Ca, Fe and Mn), and Fe and Mn concentration was a little higher than apricot, apple, pear, peach and orange. The glutamic acid, aspartic acid and lysine were found in varying percentages in fruit pulp (15.3, 13.0, and 7.8%, respectively) and seed (16.6, 19.5, 6.6%, respectively) [124]. The CF seed is an economical feed ingredient and positively impacts growth performance in broiler chickens [125]. The *Cassia fistula* seed meal was investigated as a replacer of soybean meal (SBM) in feed ration of *Oreochromis niloticus* fingerlings and produced a positive impact on growth parameters [126]. In one study, feed intake and *in vivo* digestibility of nutrients in sheep and goat were evaluated by feeding different plants; the *Cassia fistula* have showed intermediate nutritive values [127] and *in vitro* fermentation experiment also suggested that *Cassia fistula* leaves have nutritive values for browsing ruminants [128]. As the forehead mentioned that the various parts of CF (flowers, fruit and seed) are an abundant source of protein, essential amino acids, carbohydrates and fats; the CF can be included as an economical nutrient source in the poultry and animal feed system.

CONCLUSION

Cassia fistula plant is native to the Subcontinent and Southeast Asian countries and historically employed in herbal. Its various bioactive phytochemicals could be new promising avenues in health application in poultry, animal and human. Based on previously documented literature, the facts were investigated both *in vitro* and *in vivo* based reports and declared that *Cassia fistula* plant has incredible health-promoting effects. Till now, most of the research has been reported in animal models, especially rodents (rat and mice); however gap of knowledge on poultry. *Cassia fistula* seed meal was investigated as a replacer of soybean meal in different animal feed and produced a positive impact on growth parameters, so it could also be considered as an important feed ingredient in poultry. In addition, the extracts of *Cassia fistula* plant displayed a preventive role when designated as a natural antiaging in human skin fibroblasts and which are used as antiaging facial skincare products. As well, the extract of *Cassia fistula* is used in the synthesis of silver nanoparticles. The bioactive compounds in the different parts of *Cassia fistula* can be a novel strategy for future investigation as a therapeutic application in various conditions such as antioxidant, antitumor, anti-inflammatory, antifungal, antibacterial, antiulcer, antipyretic, antimutagenic and anti-parasitic. Finally, CF has widespread use and low toxicity; consequently, it has no limitation in usage. Thus, future research is necessary for the systematic biological and pharmacological effects of *Cassia fistula* and its phytochemicals on a molecular basis in avian species. The meaning of the review will be beneficial for scientists, researchers, veterinary professionals, livestock industry, pharmacists, pharmaceutical industries, and the poultry sector as well as for poultry owners/producers. Wherefore, we recommend more studies to know other useful properties of this multipurpose medicinal plant.

CONSENT FOR PUBLICATION

Not applicable.

CONFLICT OF INTEREST

The author declares no conflict of interest, financial or otherwise.

ACKNOWLEDGEMENTS

Declared none.

REFERENCES

[1]   Bailey CJ, Day C. Traditional plant medicines as treatments for diabetes. Diabetes Care 1989; 12(8): 553-64.
[http://dx.doi.org/10.2337/diacare.12.8.553] [PMID: 2673695]

[2]   Grover JK, Yadav S, Vats V. Medicinal plants of India with anti-diabetic potential. J Ethnopharmacol 2002; 81(1): 81-100.
[http://dx.doi.org/10.1016/S0378-8741(02)00059-4] [PMID: 12020931]

[3]   Elham M, Azhar K, Seyed RH, Loh T, Mohd HB. Change in growth performance and liver function enzymes of broiler chickens challenged with infectious bursal disease virus to dietary supplementation of methionine and threonine. Am J Anim Vet Sci 2010; 5(1): 20-6.
[http://dx.doi.org/10.3844/ajavsp.2010.20.26]

[4]   Fanooci M, Torki M. Effects of qualitative dietary restriction on performance, carcass characteristics, white blood cell count and humoral immune response of broiler chicks. Glob Vet 2010; 4(3): 277-82.

[5]   Ashour EA, Alagawany M, Reda FM, Abd El-Hack ME. Effect of supplementation of Yucca schidigera extract to growing rabbit diets on growth performance, carcass characteristics, serum biochemistry and liver oxidative status. Asian J Anim Vet Adv 2014; 9(11): 732-42.
[http://dx.doi.org/10.3923/ajava.2014.732.742]

[6]   Saeed M, Baloch AR, Wang M, *et al.* Use of Cichorium Intybus Leaf extract as growth promoter, hepatoprotectant and immune modulent in broilers. J Anim Prod Adv 2015; 5(1): 585-91.
[http://dx.doi.org/10.5455/japa.20150118041009]

[7]   Ezzat Abd El-Hack M, Alagawany M, Ragab Farag M, *et al.* Beneficial impacts of thymol essential oil on health and production of animals, fish and poultry: a review. J Essent Oil Res 2016; 28(5): 365-82.
[http://dx.doi.org/10.1080/10412905.2016.1153002]

[8]   Saeed M, Naveed M, Arain MA, *et al.* Quercetin: Nutritional and beneficial effects in poultry. Worlds Poult Sci J 2017; 73(2): 355-64.
[http://dx.doi.org/10.1017/S004393391700023X]

[9]   Arain MA, Mei Z, Hassan FU, *et al.* Lycopene: a natural antioxidant for prevention of heat-induced oxidative stress in poultry. Worlds Poult Sci J 2018; 74(1): 89-100.
[http://dx.doi.org/10.1017/S0043933917001040]

[10]   Biswas K, Ghosh AB. In Bharatia Banawasadhi. Advancement of learning. Calcutta: Calcutta University 1973; p. 336.

[11]   Satyavati G, Sarma M. Medicinal Plant in India. New Delhi: ICMR 1989.

[12]   Dutta A, Bratati DE. Seasonal variation in the content of sennosides and rhein in leaves and pods of *Cassia fistula*. Indian J Pharm Sci 1998; 60(6): 388.

[13]   Bhakta T, Banerjee S, Mandal SC, Maity TK, Saha BP, Pal M. Hepatoprotective activity of *Cassia fistula* leaf extract. Phytomedicine 2001; 8(3): 220-4.
[http://dx.doi.org/10.1078/0944-7113-00029] [PMID: 11417916]

[14]   Luximon-Ramma A, Bahorun T, Soobrattee MA, Aruoma OI. Antioxidant activities of phenolic, proanthocyanidin, and flavonoid components in extracts of *Cassia fistula*. J Agric Food Chem 2002; 50(18): 5042-7.
[http://dx.doi.org/10.1021/jf0201172] [PMID: 12188605]

[15]   Ilavarasan R, Malika M, Venkataraman S. Anti-inflammatory and antioxidant activities of *Cassia fistula* Linn bark extracts. Afr J Tradit Complement Altern Med 2005; 2(1): 70-85.

[16]   Duraipandiyan V, Ignacimuthu S. Antibacterial and antifungal activity of *Cassia fistula* L.: an ethnomedicinal plant. J Ethnopharmacol 2007; 112(3): 590-4.
[http://dx.doi.org/10.1016/j.jep.2007.04.008] [PMID: 17532583]

[17]   Malpani SN, Manjunath KP, Sholapur H, Savadi RV, Akki KS, Darade SS. Antidiabetic activity of *Cassia fistula* Linn. bark in alloxan induced diabetic rats. Int J Pharm Sci Res 2010; 2: 382-5.

[18]   Saeed M, Babazadeh D, Arif M, *et al.* Silymarin: a potent hepatoprotective agent in poultry industry. Worlds Poult Sci J 2017; 73(3): 483-92.
[http://dx.doi.org/10.1017/S0043933917000538]

[19]   Sheikh NW, Patel RD, Upwar NI, Mahobia NK, Seth MV, Panchal UR. Analgesic study of methyl alcohol extract of *Cassia fistula* Pod. J Pharm Res 2010; 3(9): 2218-9.

[20]   Chopra RC. Glossary of Indian medicinal plants. National Institute of Science Communication and Information Resources (CSIR). New Delhi: Council of Scientific and Industrial Research 2000; pp. 1956-92.

[21]   Esmaeilidooki MR, Mozaffarpur SA, Mirzapour M, Shirafkan H, Kamalinejad M, Bijani A. Comparison between the *Cassia fistula*s emulsion with polyethylene glycol (peg4000) in the pediatric functional constipation: a randomized clinical trial. Iran Red Crescent Med J 2016; 18(7): e33998.
[http://dx.doi.org/10.5812/ircmj.33998] [PMID: 27660721]

[22]   Kirtikar KR, Basu BD. Indian Medicinal Plants International Book Distributors. India: Deharadun 1995; pp. 1-456.

[23]   Gupta RK. Medicinal and Aromatic Plants. CBS Publishers and Distributors 2010; pp. 234-499.

[24]   Dhama K, Karthik K, Khandia R, *et al.* Medicinal and therapeutic potential of herbs and plant metabolites/extracts countering viral pathogens-current knowledge and future prospects. Curr Drug Metab 2018; 19(3): 236-63.
[http://dx.doi.org/10.2174/1389200219666180129145252] [PMID: 29380697]

[25]   Yatoo MI, Dimri U, Gopalakrishnan A, *et al.* Beneficial health applications and medicinal values of Pedicularis plants: A review. Biomed Pharmacother 2017; 95: 1301-13.

[26]   Manonmani G, Bhavapriya V, Kalpana S, Govindasamy S, Apparanantham T. Antioxidant activity of *Cassia fistula* (Linn.) flowers in alloxan induced diabetic rats. J Ethnopharmacol 2005; 97(1): 39-42.
[http://dx.doi.org/10.1016/j.jep.2004.09.051] [PMID: 15652272]

[27]   Bhalodia NR, Shukla VJ. Antibacterial and antifungal activities from leaf extracts of *Cassia fistula* l.: An ethnomedicinal plant. J Adv Pharm Technol Res 2011; 2(2): 104-9.
[http://dx.doi.org/10.4103/2231-4040.82956] [PMID: 22171301]

[28]   Danish M, Singh P, Mishra G, Srivastava S, Jha KK, Khosa RL. *Cassia fistula* Linn.(Amulthus)-An important medicinal plant: A review of its traditional uses, phytochemistry and pharmacological properties. J Nat Prod Plant Resour 2011; 1(1): 101-18.

[29]   Agarwal SS. Clinically Useful Herbal Drugs. Ahuja Book Company Pvt. Ltd 2005.

[30]   Rastogi R, Mehrotra B. Compendium of Indian Medicinal Plants published by Central Drug Research Institute. New Delhi: Lucknow and National Institute of Sciences Communication and Information Resources 1994; pp. 8-395.

[31]   Lee CK, Lee PH, Kuo YH. The chemical constituents from the aril of *Cassia fistula* L. J Chin Chem Soc (Taipei) 2001; 48(6A): 1053-8.
[http://dx.doi.org/10.1002/jccs.200100154]

[32]   Kuo YH, Lee PH, Wein YS. Four new compounds from the seeds of *Cassia fistula*. J Nat Prod 2002; 65(8): 1165-7.

[http://dx.doi.org/10.1021/np020003k] [PMID: 12193023]

[33]   Sircar PK, Dey B, Sanyal T, Ganguly SN, Sircar SM. Gibberellic acid in the floral parts of *Cassia fistula*. Phytochemistry 1970; 9(4): 735-6.
[http://dx.doi.org/10.1016/S0031-9422(00)85173-0]

[34]   Silawat N, Jarald EE, Jain N, Yadav A, Deshmukh PT. The mechanism of hypoglycemic and antidiabetic action of hydroalcholic extract of *Cassia fistula* Linn. in rats. J Pharm Res 2009; 1: 82-92.

[35]   Ali MA, Sagar HA, Khatun MC, Azad AK, Begum K, Wahed MI. Antihyperglycemic and analgesic activities of ethanolic extract of *Cassia fistula* (L.) stem bark. Int J Pharm Sci Res 2012; 3(2): 416.

[36]   Singh KN, Bharadwaj UR. Hypoglycaemic activity of Albizzia stipulata, Albizzia moluccana and *Cassia fistula* leguminous seed diets on normal young rats. Indian J Pharmacol 1975; 7(1): 47.

[37]   Bhakta T, Mukherjee PK, Saha K, Pal M, Saha BP. Hypoglycemic activity of *Cassia fistula* Linn.(Leguminosae) leaf (Methanol extract) in alloxan-induced diabetic rats. J Ethnobot 1997; 9: 35-8.

[38]   Rehman G, Hamayun M, Iqbal A, *et al*. In vitro antidiabetic effects and antioxidant potential of *Cassia nemophila* Pods. BioMed Res Int 2018; 2018: 1824790.
[http://dx.doi.org/10.1155/2018/1824790] [PMID: 29607313]

[39]   Rajeswari R, Sriidevi M. Study of *in vitro* glucose uptake activity of isolated compounds from hydro alcoholic leaf extract of Cardiospermum halicacabum linn. Int J Pharm Pharm Sci 2014; 6(11): 181-5.

[40]   Gupta UC, Jain GC. Study on hypolipidemic activity of *Cassia fistula* legume in rats. Asian J Exp Sci 2009; 23(1): 241-8.

[41]   Rahmani AH. *Cassia fistula* Linn: Potential candidate in the health management. Pharmacognosy Res 2015; 7(3): 217-24.
[http://dx.doi.org/10.4103/0974-8490.157956] [PMID: 26130932]

[42]   Reddy NV, Raj GB, Raju G, Anarthe SJ. Antihyperlipidemic activity of *Cassia fistula* bark using high fat diet induced hyperlipidemia. Int J Pharm Pharm Sci 2015; 7(10): 61-4.

[43]   Sutar GV, Dass K, Einstein JW. Screening of different leaf extracts of *Cassia fistula* Linn for investigation of hypolipidemic activity in two different rat models. Int Lett Nat Sci 2015; 3: 30-43.

[44]   Abid R, Mahmood R, Santosh Kumar HS. Hypolipidemic and antioxidant effects of ethanol extract of *Cassia fistula* fruit in hyperlipidemic mice. Pharm Biol 2016; 54(12): 2822-9.
[http://dx.doi.org/10.1080/13880209.2016.1185445] [PMID: 27256804]

[45]   Nanumala SK, Nischal Y, Sarika M, Shravaya SS. Hypolipidemic activity of ethanolic extracts of Cassia angustifolia in Triton X 100 induced hyperlipidemia in rats. Asian J Pharm Clin Res 2014; 7(1): 189-91.

[46]   Xie Q, Guo FF, Zhou W. Protective effects of cassia seed ethanol extract against carbon tetrachloride-induced liver injury in mice. Acta Biochim Pol 2012; 59(2): 265-70.
[http://dx.doi.org/10.18388/abp.2012_2149] [PMID: 22693685]

[47]   Pradeep K, Raj Mohan CV, Gobianand K, Karthikeyan S. Protective effect of *Cassia fistula* Linn. on diethylnitrosamine induced hepatocellular damage and oxidative stress in ethanol pretreated rats. Biol Res 2010; 43(1): 113-25.
[http://dx.doi.org/10.4067/S0716-97602010000100013] [PMID: 21157638]

[48]   Farghali H, Canová NK, Zakhari S. Hepatoprotective properties of extensively studied medicinal plant active constituents: possible common mechanisms. Pharm Biol 2015; 53(6): 781-91.
[http://dx.doi.org/10.3109/13880209.2014.950387] [PMID: 25489628]

[49]   Pradeep K, Mohan CV, Gobianand K, Karthikeyan S. Effect of *Cassia fistula* Linn. leaf extract on diethylnitrosamine induced hepatic injury in rats. Chem Biol Interact 2007; 167(1): 12-8.
[http://dx.doi.org/10.1016/j.cbi.2006.12.011] [PMID: 17289008]

[50]   Wasu SJ, Muley BP. Hepatoprotective Effect of Cassia fistula Linn Ethnobotanical Leaflets 2009;

2009(7): 8.

[51] NB C. Chittam KP, Patil VR. Hepatoprotective activity of *Cassia fistula* seeds against paracetamol-induced hepatic injury in rats. Arch Pharm Sci Res 2009; 2: 218-21.

[52] Chauhan N, Bairwa R, Sharma K, Chauhan N. Review on *Cassia fistula*. Int J Res Ayurveda Pharm 2011; 2: 426-30.

[53] Bahorun T, Neergheen VS, Aruoma OI. Phytochemical constituents of *Cassia fistula*. Afr J Biotechnol 2005; 4(13): 1530-40.

[54] Sumi S, Saj OP. Antibacterial, anthelmintic and phytochemical investigations on the pod extracts of *Cassia fistula* Linn. Int J Med Pharm Sci 2012; 2(1): 6-15.

[55] Abid RI, Mahmood RI, Rajesh KP, Kumara Swamy BE. Potential *in vitro* antioxidant and protective effect of *Cassia fistula* Linn. fruit extracts against induced oxidative damage in human erythrocytes. Int J Pharm Pharm Sci 2014; 6(9): 497-505.

[56] Calderón AI, Wright BJ, Hurst WJ, van Breemen RB. Screening antioxidants using LC-MS: case study with cocoa. J Agric Food Chem 2009; 57(13): 5693-9.
[http://dx.doi.org/10.1021/jf9014203] [PMID: 19489609]

[57] Franiak-Pietryga I, Koter-Michalak M, Broncel M, Duchnowicz P, Chojnowska-Jezierska J. Anti-inflammatory and hypolipemic effects *in vitro* of simvastatin comparing to epicatechin in patients with type-2 hypercholesterolemia. Food Chem Toxicol 2009; 47(2): 393-7.
[http://dx.doi.org/10.1016/j.fct.2008.11.027] [PMID: 19084570]

[58] Chang CJ, Tzeng TF, Liou SS, Chang YS, Liu IM. Kaempferol regulates the lipid-profile in high-fat diet-fed rats through an increase in hepatic PPARα levels. Planta Med 2011; 77(17): 1876-82.
[http://dx.doi.org/10.1055/s-0031-1279992] [PMID: 21728151]

[59] Salvamani S, Gunasekaran B, Shaharuddin NA, Ahmad SA, Shukor MY. Antiartherosclerotic effects of plant flavonoids. BioMed Res Int 2014; 2014: 480258.
[http://dx.doi.org/10.1155/2014/480258] [PMID: 24971331]

[60] Zhao XY, Qiao GF, Li BX, *et al.* Hypoglycaemic and hypolipidaemic effects of emodin and its effect on L-type calcium channels in dyslipidaemic-diabetic rats. Clin Exp Pharmacol Physiol 2009; 36(1): 29-34.
[http://dx.doi.org/10.1111/j.1440-1681.2008.05051.x] [PMID: 18785977]

[61] Rani MS, Emmanuel S, Sreekanth MR, Ignacimuthu S. Evaluation of *in vivo* antioxidant and hepatoprotective activity of Cassia occidentalis Linn against paracetamol-induced liver toxicity in rats. Int J Pharm Pharm Sci 2010; 2(3): 67-70.

[62] Lee W, Yoon G, Hwang YR, Kim YK, Kim SN. Anti-obesity and hypolipidemic effects of Rheum undulatum in high-fat diet-fed C57BL/6 mice through protein tyrosine phosphatase 1B inhibition. BMB Rep 2012; 45(3): 141-6.
[http://dx.doi.org/10.5483/BMBRep.2012.45.3.141] [PMID: 22449699]

[63] Zhou YX, Xia W, Yue W, Peng C, Rahman K, Zhang H. Rhein: a review of pharmacological activities. Evid Based Complement Alternat Med 2015; 2015: 578107.
[http://dx.doi.org/10.1155/2015/578107] [PMID: 26185519]

[64] Kulkarni A, Govindappa M, Chandrappa CP, Ramachandra YL, Koka PS. Phytochemical analysis of *Cassia fistula* and its *in vitro* antimicrobial, antioxidant and anti-inflammatory activities. Adv Med Plant Res 2015; 3(1): 8-17.

[65] Siddhuraju P, Mohan PS, Becker K. Studies on the antioxidant activity of Indian Laburnum (*Cassia fistula* L.): a preliminary assessment of crude extracts from stem bark, leaves, flowers and fruit pulp. Food Chem 2002; 79(1): 61-7.
[http://dx.doi.org/10.1016/S0308-8146(02)00179-6]

[66] Bhalodia NR, Nariya PB, Acharya RN, Shukla VJ. *In vitro* antioxidant activity of hydro alcoholic

extract from the fruit pulp of *Cassia fistula* Linn. Ayu 2013; 34(2): 209-14.
[http://dx.doi.org/10.4103/0974-8520.119684] [PMID: 24250133]

[67]   Singh MP, Singh A, Alam G, Patel R, Datt N. Antipyretic activity of *Cassia fistula* Linn. pods. J Pharm Res 2012; 5: 2593-4.

[68]   Kumar JG, Patel N, Sahoo P, Gupta A, Gunjan M. Antipyretic potential of different extracts of *Cassia fistula* Linn (Fabaceae) bark. Int J Res Ayurveda Pharm 2010; 1(2): 634-6.

[69]   Navanath MS, Naikwade NS, Mule SN, Krishna PP. Evaluation of anti-inflammatory activity of *Cassia fistula* and Ficus benghalensis. J Pharm Res 2009; 2(8): 1304-6.

[70]   Anitha J, Miruthula S. Anti-inflammatory and phytochemicals analysis of *Cassia fistula* Linn. fruit pulp extracts. Int J Pharmscog 2014; 1: 207-15.

[71]   Anwikar S, Bhitre M. Study of the synergistic anti-inflammatory activity of Solanum xanthocarpum Schrad and Wendl and *Cassia fistula* Linn. Int J Ayurveda Res 2010; 1(3): 167-71.
[http://dx.doi.org/10.4103/0974-7788.72489] [PMID: 21170209]

[72]   Bhakta T, Mukherjee PK, Saha K, Pal M, Saha BP, Mandal SC. Evaluation of anti-inflammatory effects of *Cassia fistula* (Leguminosae) leaf extract on rats. J Herbs Spices Med Plants 2000; 6(4): 67-72.
[http://dx.doi.org/10.1300/J044v06n04_08]

[73]   Bhakta T, Mukherjee PK, Mukherjee K, Pal M. Studies on *in vivo* wound healing activity of *Cassia fistula* linn. Leaves (Leguminosae) in rats. Nat Prod Sci 1998; 4(2): 84-7.

[74]   Sartorelli P, Andrade SP, Melhem MS, Prado FO, Tempone AG. Isolation of antileishmanial sterol from the fruits of *Cassia fistula* using bioguided fractionation. Phytother Res 2007; 21(7): 644-7.
[http://dx.doi.org/10.1002/ptr.2131] [PMID: 17397117]

[75]   de Alencar DC, da Silva FM, de Almeida RA, *et al.* Antileishmanial Activity of a New ent-Kaurene Diterpene Glucoside Isolated from Leaves of Xylopia excellens RE Fr.(Annonaceae). Rec Nat Prod 2018; 12(2): 190.
[http://dx.doi.org/10.25135/rnp.16.17.06.111]

[76]   Teixeira RR, Gazolla PAR, da Silva AM, *et al.* Synthesis and leishmanicidal activity of eugenol derivatives bearing 1,2,3-triazole functionalities. Eur J Med Chem 2018; 146: 274-86.
[http://dx.doi.org/10.1016/j.ejmech.2018.01.046] [PMID: 29407957]

[77]   Mazumder UK, Gupta M, Rath N. CNS activities of *Cassia fistula* in mice. Phytotherapy Research. Phytother Res 1998; 12(7): 520-2.

[78]   Sultana R, Ravagna A, Mohmmad-Abdul H, Calabrese V, Butterfield DA. Ferulic acid ethyl ester protects neurons against amyloid β- peptide(1-42)-induced oxidative stress and neurotoxicity: relationship to antioxidant activity. J Neurochem 2005; 92(4): 749-58.
[http://dx.doi.org/10.1111/j.1471-4159.2004.02899.x] [PMID: 15686476]

[79]   Awal MA, Ahsan SM, Haque E, Asghor QH, Ahmed M. *In-vitro* antibacterial activity of leaf and root extract of *Cassia fistula*. Dinajpur Medical College 2010; 3(1): 3-10.

[80]   Abo KA, Lasaki SW, Adeyemi AA. Laxative and antimicrobial properties of Cassia species growing in Ibadan. Niger J Nat Prod Med 1999; 3: 47-50.
[http://dx.doi.org/10.4314/njnpm.v3i1.11758]

[81]   Vimalraj TR, Kumar SS, Vadivel S, Ramesh S, Thejomoorthy P. Antibacterial effect of *Cassia fistula* extract on pathogenic bacteria of veterinary importance. Tamilnadu J Vetern Anim Sci 2009; 5(3): 109-13.

[82]   Negi BS, Dave BP. Evaluation of *in vitro* antimicrobial activity from the leaves extract of *Cassia fistula* Linn. J Pure Appl Microbiol 2010; 4(2): 557-64.

[83]   Irshad M, Shreaz S, Manzoor N, Khan LA, Rizvi MM. Anticandidal activity of *Cassia fistula* and its effect on ergosterol biosynthesis. Pharm Biol 2011; 49(7): 727-33.

[http://dx.doi.org/10.3109/13880209.2010.544318] [PMID: 21591840]

[84] Agarwal SK, Singh SS, Verma S, Kumar S. Antifungal activity of anthraquinone derivatives from Rheum emodi. J Ethnopharmacol 2000; 72(1-2): 43-6.
[http://dx.doi.org/10.1016/S0378-8741(00)00195-1] [PMID: 10967452]

[85] Draughon F. Use of botanicals as biopreservatives in foods. Food Technol (Chicago) 2004; 58(2): 8-20.

[86] Rizvi MM, El Hassadi IM, Younis SB. Bioefficacies of *Cassia fistula*: an Indian labrum. Afr J Pharm Pharmacol 2009; 3(6): 287-92.

[87] Seyyednejad SM, Motamedi H, Vafei M, Bakhtiari A. The antibacterial activity of *Cassia fistula* organic extracts. Jundishapur J Microbiol 2014; 7(1): e8921.
[http://dx.doi.org/10.5812/jjm.8921] [PMID: 25147664]

[88] Gupta M, Mazumder UK, Rath N, Mukhopadhyay DK. Antitumor activity of methanolic extract of *Cassia fistula* L. seed against Ehrlich ascites carcinoma. J Ethnopharmacol 2000; 72(1-2): 151-6.
[http://dx.doi.org/10.1016/S0378-8741(00)00227-0] [PMID: 10967466]

[89] Tawfek NS, Al Azhary DB, Hussien BK, Abd Elgeleel DM. Effects of *Cassia fistula* and Ficus carica leaf extracts on hepatocarcinogenesis in rats. Middle East J Appl Sci 2015; 5(2): 462-79.

[90] Balamurugan K, Karthikeyan J. Evaluation of luteolin in the prevention of N-nitrosodiethylamin--induced hepatocellular carcinoma using animal model system. Indian J Clin Biochem 2012; 27(2): 157-63.
[http://dx.doi.org/10.1007/s12291-011-0166-7] [PMID: 23543260]

[91] Seufi AM, Ibrahim SS, Elmaghraby TK, Hafez EE. Preventive effect of the flavonoid, quercetin, on hepatic cancer in rats *via* oxidant/antioxidant activity: molecular and histological evidences. J Exp Clin Cancer Res 2009; 28(1): 80.
[http://dx.doi.org/10.1186/1756-9966-28-80] [PMID: 19519916]

[92] Khan RA, Khan MR, Sahreen S. CCl$_4$-induced hepatotoxicity: protective effect of rutin on p53, CYP2E1 and the antioxidative status in rat. BMC Complement Altern Med 2012; 12(1): 178.
[http://dx.doi.org/10.1186/1472-6882-12-178] [PMID: 23043521]

[93] Govindarajan M. Larvicidal activity of *Cassia fistula* flower against Culex tritaeniorhynchus giles, Aedes albopictus skuse and Anopheles subpictus grassi (Diptera: Culicidae). Int J Pure Appl Zool 2013; 1: 117-21.

[94] Govindarajan M, Sivakumar R, Rajeswari M. Larvicidal efficacy of *Cassia fistula* Linn. leaf extract against Culex tritaeniorhynchus Giles and Anopheles subpictus Grassi (Diptera: Culicidae). Asian Pac J Trop Dis 2011; 1(4): 295-8.
[http://dx.doi.org/10.1016/S2222-1808(11)60070-4]

[95] Govindarajan M, Jebanesan A, Pushpanathan T. Larvicidal and ovicidal activity of *Cassia fistula* Linn. leaf extract against filarial and malarial vector mosquitoes. Parasitol Res 2008; 102(2): 289-92.
[http://dx.doi.org/10.1007/s00436-007-0761-y] [PMID: 17989995]

[96] Sartorelli P, Carvalho CS, Reimão JQ, Ferreira MJ, Tempone AG. Antiparasitic activity of biochanin A, an isolated isoflavone from fruits of *Cassia fistula* (Leguminosae). Parasitol Res 2009; 104(2): 311-4.
[http://dx.doi.org/10.1007/s00436-008-1193-z] [PMID: 18810492]

[97] Irshad M, Man S, Rizvi MA. Assessment of anthelmintic activity of *Cassia fistula* L. Middle East J Sci Res 2010; 5(5): 346-9.

[98] Jazani AM, Azgomi RN, Shirbeigi L. Pruritus treatment in viewpoints of traditional persian medicine. Iran J Med Sci 2016; 41(3) (Suppl.): S53.
[PMID: 27840519]

[99] Liu JH, You GF, Li YP. Study on the anti-pruritus mechanism of Qindai Keyin pills for psoriasis [J].

West China J Pharm Sci 2011; 4.

[100] Yuan Y, Padol IT, Hunt RH. Peptic ulcer disease today. Nat Clin Pract Gastroenterol Hepatol 2006; 3(2): 80-9.
[http://dx.doi.org/10.1038/ncpgasthep0393] [PMID: 16456574]

[101] Galunska B, Marazova K, Tankova T, *et al.* Effects of paracetamol and propacetamol on gastric mucosal damage and gastric lipid peroxidation caused by acetylsalicylic acid (ASA) in rats. Pharmacol Res 2002; 46(2): 141-7.
[http://dx.doi.org/10.1016/S1043-6618(02)00083-X] [PMID: 12220953]

[102] Karthikeyan S, Gobianand K. Antiulcer activity of ethanol leaf extract of *Cassia fistula*. Pharm Biol 2010; 48(8): 869-77.
[http://dx.doi.org/10.3109/13880200903302838] [PMID: 20673173]

[103] Borrelli F, Izzo AA. The plant kingdom as a source of anti-ulcer remedies. Phytother Res 2000; 14(8): 581-91.
[http://dx.doi.org/10.1002/1099-1573(200012)14:8<581::AID-PTR776>3.0.CO;2-S] [PMID: 11113992]

[104] Vasudevan K, Manoharan S, Panjamurthy K, Vellaichamy L, Chellammal A. Evaluation of antihyperglycemic effect of *Cassia fistula* (linn.) leaves in streptozotocin induced diabetic rats. Electron J Pharmacol Ther 2008; 1: 57-60.

[105] Bhakta T, Mukherjee PK, Saha K, Pal M, Saha BP. Studies on antitussive activity of *Cassia fistula* (Leguminosae) leaf extract. Pharm Biol 1998; 36(2): 140-3.
[http://dx.doi.org/10.1076/phbi.36.2.140.4598]

[106] Senthil Kumar M, Sripriya R, Vijaya Raghavan H, Sehgal PK. Wound healing potential of *Cassia fistula* on infected albino rat model. J Surg Res 2006; 131(2): 283-9.
[http://dx.doi.org/10.1016/j.jss.2005.08.025] [PMID: 16242721]

[107] Atarzadeh F, Kamalinejad M, Dastgheib L, Amin G, Jaladat AM, Nimrouzi M. *Cassia fistula*· A remedy from Traditional Persian Medicine for treatment of cutaneous lesions of pemphigus vulgaris. Avicenna J Phytomed 2017; 7(2): 107-15.
[PMID: 28348966]

[108] Limtrakul P, Yodkeeree S, Thippraphan P, Punfa W, Srisomboon J. Anti-aging and tyrosinase inhibition effects of *Cassia fistula* flower butanolic extract. BMC Complement Altern Med 2016; 16(1): 497.
[http://dx.doi.org/10.1186/s12906-016-1484-3] [PMID: 27912751]

[109] Yadav R, Jain GC. Antifertility effect of aqueous extract of seeds of *Cassia fistula* in female rats. Adv Contracept 1999; 15(4): 293-301.
[http://dx.doi.org/10.1023/A:1006784224191] [PMID: 11145371]

[110] Khan BA, Akhtar N, Menaa B, Menaa A, Braga VA, Menaa F. Relative free radicals scavenging and enzymatic activities of Hippophae rhamnoides and *Cassia fistula* extracts: Importance for cosmetic, food and medicinal applications. Cosmetics 2017; 4(1): 3.
[http://dx.doi.org/10.3390/cosmetics4010003]

[111] Negi PS, Jayaprakasha GK, Jena BS. Antioxidant and antimutagenic activities of pomegranate peel extracts. Food Chem 2003; 80(3): 393-7.
[http://dx.doi.org/10.1016/S0308-8146(02)00279-0]

[112] Chandel M, Sharma U, Kumar N, Singh B, Kaur S. *In vitro* studies on the antioxidant/antigenotoxic potential of aqueous fraction from Anthocephalus cadamba bark. In: Perspectives in Cancer Prevention-Translational Cancer Research. New Delhi: Springer 2014; pp. 61-72.

[113] Kaur S, Kumar M, Kaur P, Kaur V, Kaur S. Modulatory effects of *Cassia fistula* fruits against free radicals and genotoxicity of mutagens. Food Chem Toxicol 2016; 98(Pt B): 220-31.
[http://dx.doi.org/10.1016/j.fct.2016.10.027] [PMID: 27984161]

[114] Priadharsini K, Sulthana AS, Shree CG, Palani P. Florisynthesis and characterisation of silver nanoparticles-a paradigm as antimicrobial functionalized PLA matrix. In: 2016 IEEE 16th International Conference on Nanotechnology (IEEE-NANO) 2016; 435-9.

[115] Narayanan KB, Sakthivel N. Biological synthesis of metal nanoparticles by microbes. Adv Colloid Interface Sci 2010; 156(1-2): 1-13.
[http://dx.doi.org/10.1016/j.cis.2010.02.001] [PMID: 20181326]

[116] Anitha J, Miruthula S. Traditional medicinal uses, phytochemical profile and pharmacological activities of luffa acutangula linn. Int J Pharmacog 2014; 1(3): 174-83.

[117] Indhumathy J, Gurupavithra S, Ravishankar K, Jayachitra A. Green synthesis of silver nanoparticles using *Cassia fistula* leaf extract and its applications. MJPMS2014 2014; 3: 5-20.

[118] Remya RR, Rajasree SR, Aranganathan L, Suman TY. An investigation on cytotoxic effect of bioactive AgNPs synthesized using *Cassia fistula* flower extract on breast cancer cell MCF-7. Biotechnol Rep (Amst) 2015; 8: 110-5.
[http://dx.doi.org/10.1016/j.btre.2015.10.004] [PMID: 28352579]

[119] Rashid MI, Mujawar LH, Rehan ZA, *et al.* One-step synthesis of silver nanoparticles using Phoenix dactylifera leaves extract and their enhanced bactericidal activity. J Mol Liq 2016; 223: 1114-22.
[http://dx.doi.org/10.1016/j.molliq.2016.09.030]

[120] Rashid MI, Mujawar LH, Mujallid MI, *et al.* Potent bactericidal activity of silver nanoparticles synthesized from *Cassia fistula* fruit. Microb Pathog 2017; 107: 354-60.
[http://dx.doi.org/10.1016/j.micpath.2017.03.048] [PMID: 28416381]

[121] Balogun IO, Olatidoye OP. Chemical Composition and Nutritional Evaluation of Velvet Bean Seeds (*Mucuna utilis*) For Domestic Consumption and Industrial Utilization in Nigeria. Pak J Nutr 2012; 11(2): 116-22.

[122] Lal J, Gupta PC. Partial hydrolysis and the structure of the galactomannan from *Cassia fistula* seeds. Planta Med 1976; 30(08): 378-83.
[http://dx.doi.org/10.1055/s-0028-1097747]

[123] Mondal AK, Parui S, Mandal S. Biochemical analysis of four species of *Cassia L.* pollen. Aerobiologia 1998; 14(1): 45-50.
[http://dx.doi.org/10.1007/BF02694594]

[124] Barthakur NN, Arnold NP, Alli I. The Indian laburnum (*Cassia fistula* L.) fruit: an analysis of its chemical constituents. Plant Foods Hum Nutr 1995; 47(1): 55-62.
[http://dx.doi.org/10.1007/BF01088167] [PMID: 7784398]

[125] Augustine C, Igwebuike JU, Salome S, *et al.* Evaluation of Economic Performance of Broiler Chickens Fed Graded Levels of Processed Cassia obtusifolia Seed Meal. Intern J Sustain Agricult 2010; 2(3): 47-50.

[126] Adebayo OT, Fagbenro OA, Jegede T. Evaluation of *Cassia fistula* meal as a replacement for soybean meal in practical diets of Oreochromis niloticus fingerlings. Aquacult Nutr 2004; 10(2): 99-104.
[http://dx.doi.org/10.1111/j.1365-2095.2003.00286.x]

[127] Salem AZ, Salem MZ, El-Adawy MM, Robinson PH. Nutritive evaluations of some browse tree foliages during the dry season: secondary compounds, feed intake and *in vivo* digestibility in sheep and goats. Anim Feed Sci Technol 2006; 127(3-4): 251-67.
[http://dx.doi.org/10.1016/j.anifeedsci.2005.09.005]

[128] Salem AZ, Robinson PH, El-Adawy MM, Hassan AA. *In vitro* fermentation and microbial protein synthesis of some browse tree leaves with or without addition of polyethylene glycol. Anim Feed Sci Technol 2007; 138(3-4): 318-30.
[http://dx.doi.org/10.1016/j.anifeedsci.2006.11.026]

CHAPTER 11

Moringa (*Moringa oleifera*) and its Role in Poultry Nutrition

Ahmed Noreldin[1], Mohamed E. Abd El-Hack[2], Shaaban S. Elnesr[3], Mayada R. Farag[4], Hamada A. M. Elwan[5] and Mahmoud Alagawany[2,*]

[1] *Department of Histology and Cytology, Faculty of Veterinary Medicine, Damanhour University, Damanhour 22516, Egypt*

[2] *Department of Poultry, Faculty of Agriculture, Zagazig University, 44511Zagazig, Egypt*

[3] *Poultry Production Department, Faculty of Agriculture, Fayoum University, Fayoum 63514, Egypt*

[4] *Forensic Medicine and Toxicology Department, Veterinary Medicine Faculty, Zagazig University, Zagazig 44511, Egypt*

[5] *Animal and Poultry Production Department, Faculty of Agriculture, Minia University, El-Minya 61519, Egypt*

Abstract: Utilizing novel rations in chicken feeding in developing countries has drawn considerable interest in the recent few years. *Moringa oleifera* is originally planted in India. It is cultivated in tropical and subtropical regions all over the world. It is famous as 'drumstick tree' or 'horseradish tree'. *Moringa* can bear both aridity rime and intense moderate conditions. Thus, it is vastly planted in numerous soils. Each part of this tree is convenient for either nutritional or merchant targets. In general, it has elevated nutritious values. Leaves contain a high amount of minerals, essential phytochemicals and vitamins. Leaves can be utilized to cure undernourishment. In addition, it could be utilized as a prospective antioxidant, an anticancer, antidiabetic, anti-inflammatory and antimicrobial agent. Moringa contains a crude protein that varies from 71.2 to 391.7 g/kg, and varying parts of this plant are the reason for this variation. But *Moringa* holds anti-nutritional factors like phytates, trypsin inhibitors, oxalates, tannins, saponins and cyanide that negatively influence the metabolism of protein and mineral, as well its bioavailability to the chick. Phosphorus bioavailability can be boosted by adding phytase to the diet, which breaks down phytate that binds phosphorus. Previous studies demonstrated that the integration of *Moringa* in poultry diets could enhance productive performance traits and chickens' growth. Thus, this chapter compiles the usage and possible toxicity of *Moringa oleifera* and its characterization. In addition, the nutritional composition, phytochemicals, antioxidants of *Moringa oleifera* leaf meal and its application in poultry diets are also outlined.

* **Corresponding author M. Alagawany:** Department of Poultry, Faculty of Agriculture, Zagazig University, Zagazig - 44511, Egypt; E-mail: mmalagwany@zu.edu.eg

Keywords: Antioxidants, Leafs, *Moringa oleifera*, Phytochemicals, Poultry, Productive performance.

INTRODUCTION

In past years, various phytogenic fodder inclusions, *i.e.*, aromatic plants or their essential oil, have been studied in chickens [1 - 3]. Even their various species with different inclusion levels have been investigated to detect a safe, natural and cheap feed additive with the high frugal product [4]. The feed inclusion level of aromatic plant parts varied from 0.01 to 30 g/kg diet, *e.g.*, rosemary powder at 0.4 to 0.5 g/kg feed [5], anise seeds at 0.25 to 1.5 g/kg diet [6], yarrow, rosemary and marjoram at 10 g/kg feed [4], oregano addition at 10 to 30 g/kg feed [7] and rosemary at 5 to10 g/kg feed [4, 8], were shown for respectable positive influences in terms of poultry output and health. Essential oil feed inclusion levels are relatively lower than other plant parts but show an analogous level of influences. Examples comprise Essential oils from herbs such as thyme, marjoram, rosemary and yarrow at 1000 mg/kg feed [4], rosemary and sage extracts at 500 mg/kg of feed [9], anise oil at 100 to 400 mg/kg feed [2], thymol and cinnamaldehyde at 100 mg/kg feed [10] while oregano essential oil at 50 to 300 mg/kg of feed [11 - 13].

The usage of phytogenic compounds in fodder could be the perfect feed quality. Firstly, their antioxidative and antibacterial properties (*e.g.*, rosmarinic acid, carvacrol, and thymol) engage together to enhance the overall fineness of mash [14]. Secondly, they have the capability to delay the development of mycotoxigenic fungi [15]. Phytogenic extracts/essential oils have antimycotic characteristics, which could be beneficial in prohibiting mycotoxin production in stored wheat grains. The development of toxigenic fungi, *e.g.*, *Fusarium moniliforme*, *Aspergillus ochraceus*, *Aspergillus parasiticus* and *Aspergillus flavus* could be mitigated by cinnamon, thyme and anise [16, 17]. The current chapter proposed to allow more information about uses, nutritional values and nature of *Moringa oleifera* as a hopeful material for poultry.

DESCRIPTION OF *MORINGA OLEIFERA*

Moringa oleifera was generally known as the "drumstick tree." Other popular names include ben oil tree, horseradish tree or benzoyl tree. The tree is 'multi-purpose' as all of its parts (the pods, leaves, flowers, seeds, roots, and fruits) are eaten [18] (Fig. **1**).

Moringa oleifera is a deciduous, fast-growing tree. Its top most elevation could be 10-12, and its trunk could accomplish a diameter of 45 cm. The flowers are around 2.0 cm wide and 1.0-1.5 cm in length. Flowering begins through the first six months after cultivation. The fruit is a three-sided brown capsule of 20-45 cm size, pendulous, consists of spherical, dark brown seeds of about 1 cm diameter. The seeds possess three thin whitish wings, which are in charge of the smooth distribution of seed by the wind and water [19]. The tree needs an annual rainfall of 250 mm and 3000 mm and qualified for remaining alive at a temperature of 25-40°C, which makes it favorable for equatorial climates.

Kingdom:	Plantae
Subkingdom:	Viridiplantae
Infrakingdom:	Streptophyta
Superdivision:	Embryophyta
Division:	Tracheophyta
Subdivision:	Spermatophytina
Class:	Magnoliopsida
Superorder:	Rosanae
Order:	Brassicales
Family:	Moringaceae
Scientific name:	*Moringa oleifera* Lam.

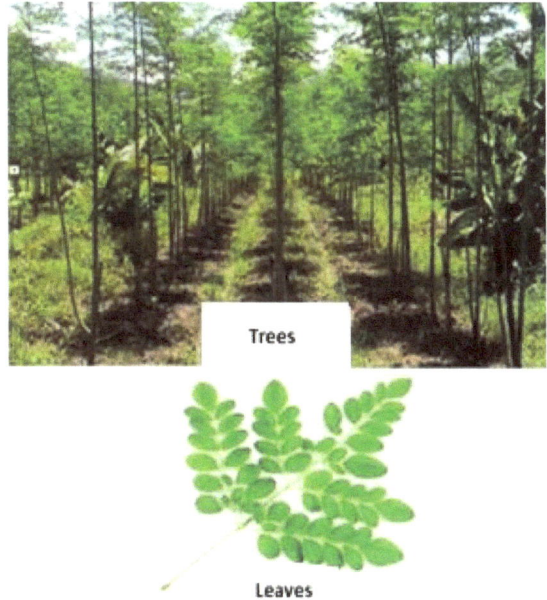

Fig. (1). Taxonomy of *Moringa Oliefera*.

USES OF *MORINGA OLEIFERA*

The most favorable character of *Moringa oleifera* is that all parts are treated as food. Through the drought period, its leaves could be utilized as a feed or food [20]. In Africa and Asia, *Moringa oleifera* flowers, pods, leaves, and roots are cooked as an alternate of vegetables [21]. Due to the perfect mineral profile, high protein and existence of vitamins, especially A, B, and C in leaves, make them quixotic for vegetarians, especially children, nursing mothers and pregnant [20]. *Moringa oleifera* seeds are eaten and roasted or cooked. They consist of 30 to 40 percent of edible oil (ben oil) [21]. Ben oil provides perfect amounts of tocopherols, sterols, and oleic acid, which stop rancidity [20]. It has medicinal characteristics depicted in Fig. (**2**) (antioxidant, antiviral, cardioprotective, anti-inflammatory, anticancer, and antiasthmatic). Terygospermin found in seeds of

Moringa oleifera possesses both fungicide and antibiotic action *versus Bacillus subtilis, Fusarium solani, Pseudomonas aeruginosa* and *Staphylococcus aureus* [6, 22]. Anemic patients are cured with their leaves because they are rich in iron. Cardiac diseases are treated by utilizing its bark and roots [18]. According to Ogbe and Affiku [23], the performance could be enhanced by the addition *Moringa oleifera* leaves. In a similar way, Price [6] observed that soybean meal (SBM) inserted of *Moringa oleifera* leaves considerably influenced growth performance (weight, body, and body weight gain) in chickens. Also, feed conversion ratio (FCR) and health status were improved with *Moringa. Moringa oleifera* seeds could be utilized for th e refining of water and production of biodiesel [18]. Aruna and Srilatha [24] reported that *Moringa oleifera* seed powder has antibacterial characteristics when utilized it for water clarification and refining of fish ponds. Egbuikwem and Sangodoyin [25] also observed that turbidity elimination.

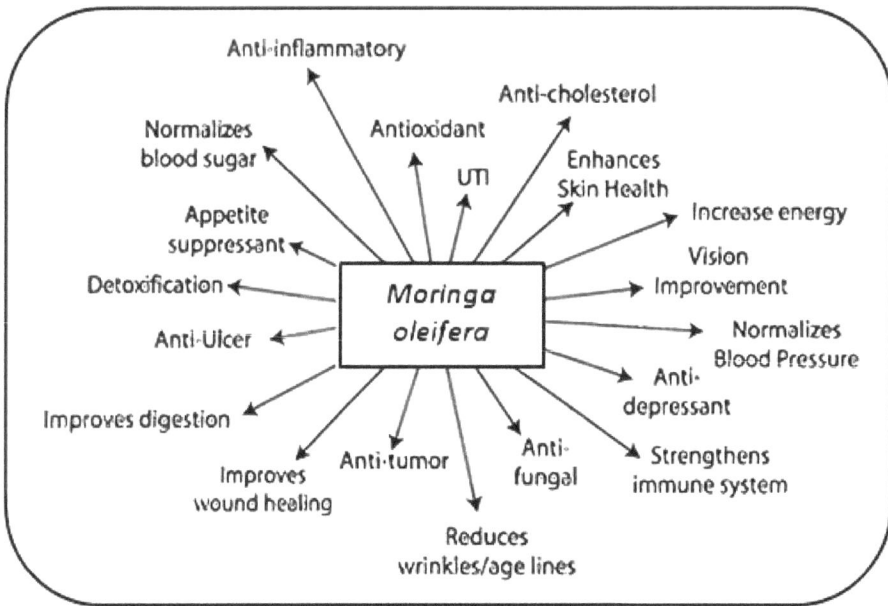

Fig. (2). Medicinal characteristics of *Moringa Oliefera.*

Competences of the best levels of *Moringa oleifera* seed extract for the pond, stream and well water samples were more than 90%. They exhibited efficient *versus E. coli* of the stream water. Rashid, Anwar [26] mentioned that it has wonderful fineness necessary for biodiesel. The existence of 1% of flocculant proteins in its oil cakes restrict organics and mineral particles in the cleaning of drinking water and so could be utilized for water treating. Thus, it could also be efficiently utilized for precipitation fibers in the juice and beer industries. Even though the influences on turbidity eliminating are not as perfect as alum, *Moringa oleifera* seeds have also been deemed as a probable recompense to some traditional synthetic chemical coagulants such as alum, which could elevate the hazard of cancer, because it is the biodegradable, natural, safe and friendly substance [24, 25, 27]. According to Foidl [28] and Pandey, Pandey [21], *Moringa oleifera* oil holds an aroma and might be utilized in perfume manufacture.

Furthermore, it does not undergo rancidity, which makes it a good oil. *Moringa oleifera* lumber is not convenient for heavy building, but its bark can be utilized in dyeing manufacture [21]. Splash *Moringa oleifera* leaf extract on leaves of soybean, peanut, black gram, coffee, and sugarcane elevated plant production by 20-35% [28]. According to Chollom, Agada [29], *Moringa oleifera* leaf extract has powerful antiviral effectiveness *versus* Newcastle disease virus (NDV).

PROSPECTIVE TOXICITY OF *MORINGA OLEIFERA*

To our awareness, few investigations have been detected to authenticate the sorely ill influences of *Moringa oleifera* as medicine or food in humans. In an investigation to estimate the probable toxicity of seeds from *Moringa Stenopetala* and *Moringa oleifera*, no toxic leverages were detected through the investigation period, and no changes were observed in the histologic images of twenty-eight organs in the outbred Sprague-Dawley rats [30]. In a safety evaluation investigation, it was mentioned that the safety of repeated doses of *Moringa oleifera* aqueous leaf extracts till 2000 mg/kg to rats for 21 days [31]. This investigation also mentioned that the level of packed cell volume (PCV) was increased markedly by 400 mg/kg dose of the extract. In comparison, a marked lowering of the levels of red blood cell counts and hemoglobin resulted from 800 mg/kg dose. Asare, Gyan [32] reported similar observations that confirmed the safe intake at levels less than 1000 mg/kg body weight. The roasted *Moringa oleifera* seeds contained chemically and biosynthetically related compounds such as 4-hydroxyphenyl-acetamide, 4-hydroxyphenyl acetonitrile, and phenyl acetonitrile, which have mutagenic action [33]. Another study mentioned that violent uterine contraction caused by the bark of the *Moringa oleifera* that results in fetal death [34]. Moreover, the biochemical and hematological parameters of fish had been changed badly by *Moringa oleifera* seed powder [35]. Fahey [36] mentioned that the presence of isothiocyanate that produces glycosides could be the cause of the various effects of extracts of *Moringa oleifera* on the different hematological parameters. Another study mentioned a decrease in serum protein levels because of using *Moringa oleifera* [37]. The authors suggested that glycoside cyanides and isothiocyanate could make stress-mediated mobilization of protein. Gao *et al.* [38] used mice animal models to detect the toxic effect of increasing doses of *Moringa oleifera*. They explained the toxic effects of *Moringa oleifera* by a significant reduction of liver triglycerides content led to increasing serum lipopolysaccharide level and activated inflammatory responses in the intestine and liver, which resulted in the alteration of the specific gut bacteria. Moreover, another study observed the dangerous influences of monthly intake of dietary tannic acid, which is an important component of *Moringa oleifera*, on the growth performance of common carp (*Cypriinus Carpio L.*) [39]. Therefore, the products of *Moringa oleifera* should be used carefully in the diets of fish. The toxicity of *Moringa oleifera* might be useful as it was revealed by Pontual, Pires-Neto [40] who isolated a trypsin inhibitor for the flowers of *Moringa oleifera* and found a significant selective effect against *Trypanosoma cruzi* with low adverse effects on the mammelian cells.

NUTRITIONAL COMPOSITION OF *MORINGA OLEIFERA* LEAF

Fahey [36] reported that *Moringa oleifera* leaves are suitable to be used as a highly digestible nutrient in many developing regions which its intake can be as dried powder, cooked or fresh. Moreover, *Moringa oleifera* leaves might be utilized as a feed additive for enhancing growth performance and feed efficiency or be utilized for getting more environmentally friendly and economically sustainable by replacing the conventional crops [41, 42]. Furthermore, better ADF, NDF, GE, CP, amino acids and EE of *Moringa oleifera* leaves lead to better digestibility for nutrients [43]. However, other anti-nutritional factors and certain toxins are included in some parts of *Moringa oleifera* tree that restrict their utilizing as a safe food for animals or humans. Saponins, tannins, alkaloids and some inhibitors are present in the bark of *Moringa oleifera* tree [28]. So, Becker and Makkar [39] suggested more precautions must be considered before including *Moringa oleifera* in diets, especially in carp diets.

PHYTOCHEMICALS OF *MORINGA OLEIFERA* LEAF

Bennett, Mellon [44] investigated the phytochemical properties of *Moringa oleifera* leaves and detected the presence of glycosylates, isothiocyanate and rhamnose (*i.e.*, simple sugar). Moreover, benzyl glucosinolates, 4-(4'-Oacetyl-a-L-rhamnopyranosyloxy)-benzylthiocyanate and 4-(a-L-rhamnopyranosyloxy)-benzylisothiocyanate are found which have antibacterial, hypotensive and anticancer activity [45]. Moreover, Bennett, Mellon [44] detected the presence of isoquercitrin, flavonoid pigments like kaempferitrin, kaempferol, rhamnetin and quercetin in *Moringa oleifera* flowers. Furthermore, Foidl, Makkar [28] and Pandey *et al.* [21] observed the presence of cytokine type hormones in the *Moringa oleifera* leaves extract in 80% ethanol. In addition, Al-Asmari, Albalawi [46] proved that *Moringa oleifera* leaves extract had cancer-preventive effects. Moringine and Moringinine, two types of alkaloids, reported being found in *Moringa oleifera* root bark [47].

ANTIOXIDANTS IN *MORINGA OLEIFERA* LEAF

Moringa oleifera species are the ideal resource of quercetin and flavonoids like kaempferol, which are wide spectrum dietary antioxidants [48]. Moreover, authors detected some natural antioxidants in three different agroclimatic origins of *Moringa oleifera* [49]. On a dry weight basis, ascorbate (Vit C) = 70-100 μmol/g, β-carotene = 1.1-2.8 μmol/g, phenolics = 74-210 μmol/g and α-tocopherol 0.7-1.1 μmol/g. Interestingly, *Moringa oleifera* species have higher antioxidant contents than vegetables and fruits, which have excessive antioxidant contents [50]. Moreover, *Moringa oleifera* leaves possess important flavonoids like quercetin and kaempferol, which have more antioxidant activity than ascorbic acid [49, 51]. Furthermore, Siddhuraju and Becker [49] detected the presence of a considerable amount of ascorbic acid in *Moringa oleifera* leaves. The antioxidants trap free radicals that cause excessive oxidative DNA damage. Therefore, they protect animals from infections and degenerative diseases [52].

INCLUSION OF *MORINGA OLEIFERA* LEAF IN POULTRY DIETS

Donkor, Glover [53] mentioned that heavy metals like mercury, arsenic, and cadmium are absent in *Moringa oleifera* leaves, but *Moringa oleifera* leaves had considerable amounts of vitamins (A, B and C). Therefore, they could be included safely into poultry ration and could improve the performance of poultry. But Price [6] observed lower palatability of *Moringa oleifera* leaf powder or leaves when feeding poultry.

Gaia [54] suggested the supplementing of feed containing *Moringa oleifera* leaves by different enzymes like phytase for increasing the availability of phosphorus. Supplementing enough level of *Moringa oleifera* leaves in poultry diets could result in positive influences on the growth performances of poultry. It is safe to include *Moringa oleifera* leaf meal in cassava-based layer diets to 10%. Ayssiwede, Zanmenou [55] suggested that perfect antimicrobial properties of *Moringa oleifera* leave against gut pathogens and enhanced digestibility lead to improved feed efficiency. Moreover, *Moringa oleifera* could easily decrease egg cholesterol content because it has hypocholesterolemic properties, so it is preferable to be supplemented in poultry diets [56]. Furthermore, *Moringa oleifera* leaves in poultry diets (up to 10%) have good effects on the yolk color and did not have bad influences on the egg-laying rate [57]. Therefore, the authors recommended 10% *Moringa oleifera* leaf meal of laying hen diets. It was reported that internal egg quality *versus* the control was markedly improved by poultry ration supplemented 2.5% *Moringa oleifera* leaf meal [58]. Egg laying and egg mass percentage were linearly lowered by supplementing different levels of *Moringa oleifera* leaf meal (0%, 5%, 10%, and 15%) in layer diets. Still, with the increment levels of *Moringa oleifera* leaf meal, egg weight exposed a quadratic trend [56]. Kakengi, Kaijage [59] and Abou-Elezz, Sarmiento-Franco [57] observed the good influences of 5% *Moringa oleifera* leaf meal on birds, but dietary levels up to 15% and 20% showed bad influences.

The extra addition of Moringa was reported to have bad influences on egg-laying performance. Kakengi, Kaijage [59] observed that total egg weight and egg production percentage markedly lowered by supplementing of *Moringa oleifera* leaf meal at 20% to the layer diet. Similarly, other authors mentioned that adding 20% *Moringa oleifera* leaf meal badly influenced the egg-laying rate and egg mass production, but there was no bad influence by adding 5% *Moringa oleifera* leaf meal [60]. In agreement with previous authors, Tesfaye, Animut [61] mentioned that *Moringa oleifera* leaf meal was treated as a probable alternative for soybean meal in broiler feed. A high dietary level of *Moringa oleifera* leaf meal lowered the growth rate. Olugbemi, Mutayoba [56] explained the bad influences of an elevated level of the leaf meals in diets by the low digestibility of protein. Similar to this result, Kakengi, Kaijage [59] detected the increment in dry matter intake and feed intake in laying hens when fed diets containing 10% and 20% *Moringa oleifera* leaf meal, but, feed efficiency was badly influenced by the higher levels.

Supplementing of the low level of *Moringa oleifera* leaf meal has no bad influences on the growth performance and nutrient digestibility. Juniar, Widodo [62] supplemented *Moringa oleifera* leaf meal to 10% and did not observe any bad influences on feed conversion ratio, feed consumption, and body weight. El-Tazi [63] observed an improvement in body weight and total feed intake, and feed conversion ratio in broilers rations containing 5% *Moringa oleifera* leaf meal for 7 weeks. The *Moringa oleifera* leaf meal could be included in the diets of grower rabbits instead of the groundnut cake, also the percentage of *Moringa oleifera* leaf meal could reach 60% to achieve feed cost efficiency [64]. Moreover, Gadzirayi, Masamha [65] observed the increment of dry matter intake (DMI) by the inclusion of *Moringa oleifera* leaf meal in broilers ration. The authors explained their result by increasing metabolizable concentration. Nkukwana, Muchenje [66] investigated the effect of *Moringa oleifera* leaf meal on the pH of the broiler chickens and intestinal morphology and detected the improvement of the villi length and increasing pH, which is a good indication of the healthy gut. Similar results were reported by Khan, Zaneb [67], who concluded that the addition of 1.2% of *Moringa oleifera* improved the acidic mucin production and the intestinal morphology without any apparent influence on the growth parameters.

Moringa oleifera leaf meal had perfect influences on shell thickness and egg shape index and was considered a perfect resource for yolk pigments [68]. Tesfaye, Animut [61] recorded the perfect effects of *Moringa oleifera* on the yolk to high carotene content when birds fed *Moringa oleifera* leaf meal. Kaijage, Sarwatt [68] reported that the quality of good eggs for consumers contains lower yolk index and higher albumens, which lead to lower concentrations of cholesterol. Abou-Elezz, Sarmiento-Franco [57] observed that supplementation of *Moringa oleifera* at higher levels led to lower productivity; however, lower levels of inclusion improved egg quality. Kakengi, Kaijage [59] reported the perfect influence of a mixture of *Moringa oleifera* leaf meal with a sunflower on egg weight. Lu, Wang [69] mentioned that a high percentage of *Moringa oleifera* leaf meal resulted in decreased egg weight, this result may be attributed to lower crude fiber (CF) digestibility, energy availability and lower protein retention. Olugbemi, Mutayoba [56] detected hypocholesterolemic properties of *Moringa oleifera* leaf meal and observed the reduction of egg cholesterol content by its adding to layer diets. Similar results were observed by Helmy *et al.* [70], who detected the hypocholesterolemic influence of *Moringa oleifera* leaf powder on rat. Briones, Leung [71] reported the high impact of fresh, meal and extract of *Moringa oleifera* on feed conversion ratio (FCR), egg weight, egg production, yolk color and percentage of broken eggs in layer chickens and quail.

Ahmad, Ejaz [72] reported that ethanolic extract of the leaves of *Moringa oleifera* has a significant antiviral effect against infectious bursal disease by the concentration of 50 µg ml^{-1}, but above 100 µg ml^{-1} had been reported to have toxic effects [73]. Moreover, Raza, Muhammad [74] recorded the perfect effect of aqueous seed extract *of Moringa oleifera* against the Newcastle disease virus. Liaqat, Mahmood [75] reported the high impact of the replacement of canola meal with *Moringa oleifera* leaf powder on the enhancement of the vaccination against Newcastle disease and infectious bursal disease without any adverse effect on blood hematology and weight gain in broilers.

It was reported that *Moringa oleifera* is characterized by high contents of phytochemicals, antioxidant activity, stability, and palatability of poultry products [50, 76]. Flavonols are the most important antioxidants in *Moringa* [21]. Pennington and Fisher [77] suggested the utilizing of *Moringa* to extend the shelf life of poultry products due to their significantly higher antioxidant activity than vitamin C. These results indicated the optimal use of *Moringa oleifera* leaves as a good feedstuff in poultry, but great care should be paid to their percentages in poultry diets.

CONCLUSION

In a severe drought frost environment, a highly valuable tree, *Moringa oleifera* tree, can be cultivated. *Moringa* includes crude protein ranged from 71.2 to 391.7 g/kg, which is different between various parts of *Moringa* plant. From the previous results, *Moringa* leaf meal could be partially used as a protein source in chickens diets instead of soybean meal and sunflower seed cake. The most suitable inclusion levels of *Moringa oleifera* leaf meal are 5 to 10% in broiler diets and 10% in diets of laying hens, which have been mentioned to achieve a high economic profit with perfect productive performance and enhanced growth. But, the high inclusion of *Moringa oleifera* leaf meal in rations (80% in rabbits and 20% in laying hens or broiler) might lead to bad influences due to the high level of tannin in moringa, which affects nutrient digestibility or feed intake.

CONSENT FOR PUBLICATION

Not applicable.

CONFLICT OF INTEREST

The author declares no conflict of interest, financial or otherwise.

ACKNOWLEDGEMENTS

Declared none.

REFERENCES

[1]   Ahossi P, Dougnon J, Kiki P, Houessionon J. Effects of Tridax procumbens powder on zootechnical, biochemical parameters and carcass characteristics of Hubbard broiler chicken. J Anim Health Prod 2016; 4: 15-21.

[2]   Ciftci M, Güler T, Dalkiliç B, Ertas ON. The effect of anise oil (Pimpinella an¡ sum L.) on broiler performance. Int J Poult Sci 2005; 4(11): 851-5.
       [http://dx.doi.org/10.3923/ijps.2005.851.855]

[3]   Nghonjuyi N, Tiambo C, Kimbi H, Manka'a C, Juliano R, Lisita F. Efficacy of ethanolic extract of Carica papaya leaves as a substitute of sulphanomide for the control of coccidiosis in KABIR chickens in Cameroon. J Anim Health Prod 2015; 3(1): 21-7.
       [http://dx.doi.org/10.14737/journal.jahp/2015/3.1.21.27]

[4]   Cross DE, McDevitt RM, Hillman K, Acamovic T. The effect of herbs and their associated essential oils on performance, dietary digestibility and gut microflora in chickens from 7 to 28 days of age. Br Poult Sci 2007; 48(4): 496-506.
       [http://dx.doi.org/10.1080/00071660701463221] [PMID: 17701503]

[5]   Botsoglou N, Florou-Paneri P, Botsoglou E, *et al.* The effect of feeding rosemary, oregano, saffron and a-tocopheryl acetate on hen performance and oxidative stability of eggs. S Afr J Anim Sci 2005; 35(3): 143-51.

[6]   Price M. The Moringa Tree ECHO Technical Note Educational Concerns for Hunger Organization, N. FL: Ft. Meyers 1985.

[7]   Christaki E, Bonos E, Florou-Paneri P. Comparative evaluation of dietary oregano, anise and olive leaves in laying Japanese quails. Rev Bras Cienc Avic 2011; 13(2): 97-101.
[http://dx.doi.org/10.1590/S1516-635X2011000200003]

[8]   Govaris A, Florou-Paneri P, Botsoglou E, Giannenas I, Amvrosiadis I, Botsoglou N. The inhibitory potential of feed supplementation with rosemary and/or α-tocopheryl acetate on microbial growth and lipid oxidation of turkey breast during refrigerated storage. Lebensm Wiss Technol 2007; 40(2): 331-7.
[http://dx.doi.org/10.1016/j.lwt.2005.10.006]

[9]   Lopez-Bote CJ, Gray JI, Gomaa EA, Flegal CJ. Effect of dietary administration of oil extracts from rosemary and sage on lipid oxidation in broiler meat. Br Poult Sci 1998; 39(2): 235-40.
[http://dx.doi.org/10.1080/00071669889187] [PMID: 9649877]

[10]   Amerah AM, Péron A, Zaefarian F, Ravindran V. Influence of whole wheat inclusion and a blend of essential oils on the performance, nutrient utilisation, digestive tract development and ileal microbiota profile of broiler chickens. Br Poult Sci 2011; 52(1): 124-32.
[http://dx.doi.org/10.1080/00071668.2010.548791] [PMID: 21337207]

[11]   Govaris A, Botsoglou E, Florou-Paneri P, Moulas A, Papageorgiou G. Dietary supplementation of oregano essential oil and-tocopheryl acetate on microbial growth and lipid oxidation of turkey breast fillets during storage. Int J Poult Sci 2005; 4(12): 969-75.
[http://dx.doi.org/10.3923/ijps.2005.969.975]

[12]   Giannenas I, Florou-Paneri P, Papazahariadou M, Christaki E, Botsoglou NA, Spais AB. Effect of dietary supplementation with oregano essential oil on performance of broilers after experimental infection with *Eimeria* tenella. Arch Tierernahr 2003; 57(2): 99-106.
[PMID: 12866780]

[13]   Botsoglou NA, Christaki E, Fletouris DJ, Florou-Paneri P, Spais AB. The effect of dietary oregano essential oil on lipid oxidation in raw and cooked chicken during refrigerated storage. Meat Sci 2002; 62(2): 259-65.
[http://dx.doi.org/10.1016/S0309-1740(01)00256-X] [PMID: 22061420]

[14]   Burits M, Bucar F. Antioxidant activity of *Nigella sativa* essential oil. Phytother Res 2000; 14(5): 323-8.
[http://dx.doi.org/10.1002/1099-1573(200008)14:5<323::AID-PTR621>3.0.CO;2-Q]   [PMID: 10925395]

[15]   Soliman KM, Badeaa RI. Effect of oil extracted from some medicinal plants on different mycotoxigenic fungi. Food Chem Toxicol 2002; 40(11): 1669-75.
[http://dx.doi.org/10.1016/S0278-6915(02)00120-5] [PMID: 12176092]

[16]   Abd El-Hack M, Alagawany M. Performance, egg quality, blood profile, immune function, and antioxidant enzyme activities in laying hens fed diets with thyme powder. J Anim Feed Sci 2015; 24(2)
[http://dx.doi.org/10.22358/jafs/65638/2015]

[17]   Abd El-Hack ME, Alagawany M, Ragab Farag M, *et al.* Beneficial impacts of thymol essential oil on health and production of animals, fish and poultry: a review. J Essent Oil Res 2016; 28(5): 365-82.
[http://dx.doi.org/10.1080/10412905.2016.1153002]

[18]   Orwa C, Mutua A, Kindt R, Jamnadass R, Simons A. Agroforestree database: a tree species reference and selection guide version 40. Nairobi, Kenya: World Agroforestry Centre ICRAF 2009; pp. 335-6.

[19]   Olson M, Carlquist S. Stem and root anatomical correlations with life form diversity, ecology, and systematics in Moringa (Moringaceae). Bot J Linn Soc 2001; 135(4): 315-48. [http://dx.doi.org/10.1111/j.1095-8339.2001.tb00786.x]

[20]   Moringa FAO Traditional crop of the month 2014. [Available from: http://www.fao.org/traditional-crops/moringa/en/]

[21]   Pandey A, Pandey R, Tripathi P, *et al. Moringa oleifera* Lam. sahijan)- a plant with a plethora of diverse therapeutic benefits: an updated retrospection. Med Aromat Plants 2012; 1(1): 1-8. [http://dx.doi.org/10.4172/2167-0412.1000101]

[22]   Jabeen R, Shahid M, Jamil A, Ashraf M. Microscopic evaluation of the antimicrobial activity of seed extracts of *Moringa oleifera*. Pak J Bot 2008; 40(4): 1349-58.

[23]   Ogbe A, Affiku JP. Proximate study, mineral and anti-nutrient composition of *Moringa oleifera* leaves harvested from Lafia, Nigeria: potential benefits in poultry nutrition and health. J Microbiol Biotechnol Food Sci 2011; 1(3): 296.

[24]   Aruna M, Srilatha N. Water clarification using *Moringa oleifera* Lam. seed as a natural coagulant. Curr Biot 2012; 5(4): 472-86.

[25]   Egbuikwem P, Sangodoyin A. Coagulation efficacy of *Moringa oleifera* seed extract compared to alum for removal of turbidity and *E. coli* in three different water sources. Eur Int J Sci Tech 2013; 2(7): 13-20.

[26]   Rashid U, Anwar F, Moser BR, Knothe G. *Moringa oleifera* oil: a possible source of biodiesel. Bioresour Technol 2008; 99(17): 8175-9. [http://dx.doi.org/10.1016/j.biortech.2008.03.066] [PMID: 18474424]

[27]   Preston K, Lantagne D, Kotlarz N, Jellison K. Turbidity and chlorine demand reduction using alum and moringa flocculation before household chlorination in developing countries. J Water Health 2010; 8(1): 60-70. [http://dx.doi.org/10.2166/wh.2009.210] [PMID: 20009248]

[28]   Foidl N, Makkar H, Becker K. The potential of Moringa oleifera for agricultural and industrial uses. What development potential for Moringa products?; October 20th - November 2nd Dar Es Salaam. 2011.

[29]   Chollom S, Agada G, Gotep J, *et al.* Investigation of aqueous extract of *Moringa oleifera* lam seed for antiviral activity against newcastle disease virus *in ovo*. J Med Plants Res 2012; 6(22): 3870-5. [http://dx.doi.org/10.5897/JMPR12.394]

[30]   Berger MR, Habs M, Jahn SAA, Schmahl D. Toxicological assessment of seeds from *Moringa oleifera* and Moringa stenopetala, two highly efficient primary coagulants for domestic water treatment of tropical raw waters. East Afr Med J 1984; 61(9): 712-6. [PMID: 6535725]

[31]   Adedapo A, Mogbojuri O, Emikpe B. Safety evaluations of the aqueous extract of the leaves of *Moringa oleifera* in rats. J Med Plants Res 2009; 3(8): 586-91.

[32]   Asare GA, Gyan B, Bugyei K, *et al.* Toxicity potentials of the nutraceutical *Moringa oleifera* at supra-supplementation levels. J Ethnopharmacol 2012; 139(1): 265-72. [http://dx.doi.org/10.1016/j.jep.2011.11.009] [PMID: 22101359]

[33]   Villasenor IM, Finch P, Lim-Sylianco CY, Dayrit F. Structure of a mutagen from roasted seeds of *Moringa oleifera*. Carcinogenesis 1989; 10(6): 1085-7. [http://dx.doi.org/10.1093/carcin/10.6.1085] [PMID: 2720902]

[34]   Bhattacharya J, Guha G, Bhattacharya B. Powder microscopy of bark--poison used for abortion: moringa pterygosperma gaertn. J Indian Forensic Sci 1978; 17(1): 47-50. [PMID: 12262404]

[35]   Kavitha C, Ramesh M, Kumaran SS, Lakshmi SA. Toxicity of *Moringa oleifera* seed extract on some

hematological and biochemical profiles in a freshwater fish, *Cyprinus carpio.* Exp Toxicol Pathol 2012; 64(7-8): 681-7.
[http://dx.doi.org/10.1016/j.etp.2011.01.001] [PMID: 21282048]

[36]   Fahey JW. *Moringa oleifera*: a review of the medical evidence for its nutritional, therapeutic, and prophylactic properties. Trees Life J 2005; 1: 5.

[37]   Das B, Mukherjee S. Sublethal effect of quinalphos on selected blood parameters of Labeo rohita (Ham.) fingerlings. Asian Fish Sci 2000; 13: 225-33.

[38]   Gao X, Xie Q, Liu L, Kong P, Sheng J, Xiang H. Metabolic adaptation to the aqueous leaf extract of *Moringa oleifera* Lam.-supplemented diet is related to the modulation of gut microbiota in mice. Appl Microbiol Biotechnol 2017; 101(12): 5115-30.
[http://dx.doi.org/10.1007/s00253-017-8233-5] [PMID: 28382453]

[39]   Becker K, Makkar H. Effects of dietary tannic acid and quebracho tannin on growth performance and metabolic rates of common carp (*Cyprinus carpio* L.). Aquaculture 1999; 175(3): 327-35.
[http://dx.doi.org/10.1016/S0044-8486(99)00106-4]

[40]   Pontual E, Pires-Neto D, Fraige K, *et al.* A trypsin inhibitor from *Moringa oleifera* flower extract is cytotoxic to Trypanosoma cruzi with high selectivity over mammalian cells. Nat Prod Res 2017; 1-5.
[PMID: 29047320]

[41]   Aregheore E. Intake and digestibility of *Moringa oleifera*–batiki grass mixtures by growing goats. Small Rumin Res 2002; 46(1): 23-8.
[http://dx.doi.org/10.1016/S0921-4488(02)00178-5]

[42]   Richter N, Siddhuraju P, Becker K. Evaluation of nutritional quality of moringa (*Moringa oleifera* Lam.) leaves as an alternative protein source for Nile tilapia (Oreochromis niloticus L.). Aquaculture 2003; 217(1): 599-611.
[http://dx.doi.org/10.1016/S0044-8486(02)00497-0]

[43]   Rubanza C, Shem M, Otsyina R, Bakengesa S, Ichinohe T, Fujihara T. Polyphenolics and tannins effect on *in vitro* digestibility of selected Acacia species leaves. Anim Feed Sci Technol 2005; 119(1): 129-42.
[http://dx.doi.org/10.1016/j.anifeedsci.2004.12.004]

[44]   Bennett RN, Mellon FA, Foidl N, *et al.* Profiling glucosinolates and phenolics in vegetative and reproductive tissues of the multi-purpose trees *Moringa oleifera* L. (horseradish tree) and Moringa stenopetala L. J Agric Food Chem 2003; 51(12): 3546-53.
[http://dx.doi.org/10.1021/jf0211480] [PMID: 12769522]

[45]   Fahey JW, Zalcmann AT, Talalay P. The chemical diversity and distribution of glucosinolates and isothiocyanates among plants. Phytochemistry 2001; 56(1): 5-51.
[http://dx.doi.org/10.1016/S0031-9422(00)00316-2] [PMID: 11198818]

[46]   Al-Asmari AK, Albalawi SM, Athar MT, Khan AQ, Al-Shahrani H, Islam M. *Moringa oleifera* as an anti-cancer agent against breast and colorectal cancer cell lines. PLoS One 2015; 10(8): e0135814.
[http://dx.doi.org/10.1371/journal.pone.0135814] [PMID: 26288313]

[47]   Grubben G, Denton O. Plant Resources of Tropical Africa. PROTA 2004.

[48]   Yaméogo CW, Bengaly MD, Savadogo A, Nikiema PA, Traore SA. Determination of chemical composition and nutritional values of *Moringa oleifera* leaves. Pak J Nutr 2011; 10(3): 264-8.
[http://dx.doi.org/10.3923/pjn.2011.264.268]

[49]   Siddhuraju P, Becker K. Antioxidant properties of various solvent extracts of total phenolic constituents from three different agroclimatic origins of drumstick tree (*Moringa oleifera* Lam.) leaves. J Agric Food Chem 2003; 51(8): 2144-55.
[http://dx.doi.org/10.1021/jf020444+] [PMID: 12670148]

[50]   Abbas T, Ahmed M. Use of *Moringa oleifera* seeds in broilers diet and its effects on the performance and carcass characteristics. Int J Appl Poult Res 2012; 1: 1-4.

[51]   Anwar F, Bhanger MI. Analytical characterization of *Moringa oleifera* seed oil grown in temperate regions of Pakistan. J Agric Food Chem 2003; 51(22): 6558-63.
        [http://dx.doi.org/10.1021/jf0209894] [PMID: 14558778]

[52]   Verma AR, Vijayakumar M, Mathela CS, Rao CV. *In vitro* and *in vivo* antioxidant properties of different fractions of *Moringa oleifera* leaves. Food Chem Toxicol 2009; 47(9): 2196-201.
        [http://dx.doi.org/10.1016/j.fct.2009.06.005] [PMID: 19520138]

[53]   Donkor A, Glover RL, Addae D, Kubi KA. Estimating the nutritional value of the leaves of *Moringa oleifera* on poultry. Food Chem Toxicol 2013; 4(11): 1077.

[54]   Gaia S. Wonder tree 100 facts moringa fact 04 exceptional animal feed moringa as livestock feed & pet food: Moringa Mission Trust 2005. [Available from: http://gaiathelivingplanet.blogspot.com/2005/06/wondertree-100-facts-moringa-fact-04.html]

[55]   Ayssiwede SB, Zanmenou J, Issa Y, *et al.* Nutrient composition of some unconventional and local feed resources available in Senegal and recoverable in indigenous chickens or animal feeding. Pak J Nutr 2011; 10(8): 707-17.
        [http://dx.doi.org/10.3923/pjn.2011.707.717]

[56]   Olugbemi T, Mutayoba S, Lekule F. *Moringa oleifera* leaf meal as a hypocholesterolemic agent in laying hen diets. Bone 2010; 8(8.00): 8.00.

[57]   Abou-Elezz F, Sarmiento-Franco L, Santos-Ricalde R, Solorio-Sanchez F. Nutritional effects of dietary inclusion of Leucaena leucocephala and *Moringa oleifera* leaf meal on Rhode Island Red hens' performance. Cuban J Agr Sci 2011; 45(2): 163-9.

[58]   Ebenebe CI, Anizoba MA, Ufele AN. Effect of various levels of Moringa leaf meal on the egg quality of Isa brown breed of layers. Adv Life Sci Technol 2013; 14: 1-6.

[59]   Kakengi A, Kaijage J, Sarwatt S, Mutayoba S, Shem M, Fujihara T. Effect of *Moringa oleifera* leaf meal as a substitute for sunflower seed meal on performance of laying hens in Tanzania. Bone 2007; 1(9.4): 446.

[60]   Mutayoba S, Mutayoba B, Okot P. The performance of growing pullets fed diets with varying energy and leucaena leaf meal levels. Livest Res Rural Dev 2003; 15: 139-48.

[61]   Tesfaye E, Animut G, Urge M, Dessie T. Moringa olifera leaf meal as an alternative protein feed ingredient in broiler ration. Int J Poult Sci 2013; 12(5): 289.
        [http://dx.doi.org/10.3923/ijps.2013.289.297]

[62]   Juniar I, Widodo E, Sjofjan O. Effect of *Moringa oleifera* leaf meal in feed on broiler production performance. Jurnal Ilmu-Ilmu Peternakan 2010; 18(3): 63-6.

[63]   El-Tazi SM. Effect of feeding different levels of *Moringa oleifera* leaf meal on the performance and carcass quality of broiler chicks. Int J Sci Res (Ahmedabad) 2014; 3: 147-51.

[64]   Adeniji A, Lawal M. Effects of replacing groundnut cake with *Moringa oleifera* leaf meal in the diets of grower rabbits. Int J Mol Vet Res 2012; 2: 1.

[65]   Gadzirayi C, Masamha B, Mupangwa J, Washaya S. Performance of broiler chickens fed on mature *Moringa oleifera* leaf meal as a protein supplement to soyabean meal. Int J Poult Sci 2012; 11(1): 5-10.
        [http://dx.doi.org/10.3923/ijps.2012.5.10]

[66]   Nkukwana T, Muchenje V, Masika P, Mushonga B. Intestinal morphology, digestive organ size and digesta pH of broiler chickens fed diets supplemented with or without *Moringa oleifera* leaf meal. S Afr J Anim Sci 2015; 45(4): 362-70.
        [http://dx.doi.org/10.4314/sajas.v45i4.2]

[67]   Khan I, Zaneb H, Masood S, Yousaf MS, Rehman HF, Rehman H. Effect of *Moringa oleifera* leaf powder supplementation on growth performance and intestinal morphology in broiler chickens. J Anim Physiol Anim Nutr (Berl) 2017; 101(S1) (Suppl. 1): 114-21.

[http://dx.doi.org/10.1111/jpn.12634] [PMID: 28627054]

[68]   Kaijage J, Sarwatt S, Mutayoba S. *Moringa oleifera* Leaf Meal can Improve Quality Characteristics and Consumer Preference of Marketable Eggs. Numerical Proceedings Papers 2003.

[69]   Lu W, Wang J, Zhang H, Wu S, Qi G. Evaluation of *Moringa oleifera* leaf in laying hens: effects on laying performance, egg quality, plasma biochemistry and organ histopathological indices. Ital J Anim Sci 2016; 15(4): 658-65.
[http://dx.doi.org/10.1080/1828051X.2016.1249967]

[70]   Helmy SA, Morsy NFS, Elaby SM, Ghaly MAA. Hypolipidemic Effect of *Moringa oleifera* Lam Leaf Powder and its Extract in Diet-Induced Hypercholesterolemic Rats. J Med Food 2017; 20(8): 755-62.
[http://dx.doi.org/10.1089/jmf.2016.0155] [PMID: 28459609]

[71]   Briones J, Leung A, Bautista N, *et al.* Utilization of *Moringa oleifera* Lam. in animal production. Acta Hortic. 1158: 467-74.

[72]   Ahmad W, Ejaz S, Anwar K, Ashraf M. Exploration of the *in vitro* cytotoxic and antiviral activities of different medicinal plants against infectious bursal disease (IBD) virus. Open Life Sci 2014; 9(5): 531-42.
[http://dx.doi.org/10.2478/s11535-013-0276-8]

[73]   Saetung A, Itharat A, Dechsukum C, Wattanapiromsakul C, Keawpradub N, Ratanasuwan P. Cytotoxic activity of Thai medicinal plants for cancer treatment. Songklanakarin J Sci Technol 2005; 27(Sup 2): 78-469.

[74]   Raza A, Muhammad F, Bashir S, *et al.* Antiviral and immune boosting activities of different medicinal plants against Newcastle disease virus in poultry. Worlds Poult Sci J 2015; 71(3): 523-32.
[http://dx.doi.org/10.1017/S0043933915002147]

[75]   Liaqat S, Mahmood S, Ahmad S, Kamran Z, Koutoulis K. Replacement of canola meal with *Moringa oleifera* leaf powder affects performance and immune response in broilers. J Appl Poult Res 2016; 25(3): 352-8.
[http://dx.doi.org/10.3382/japr/pfw018]

[76]   Jung S, Choe JH, Kim B, Yun H, Kruk ZA, Jo C. Effect of dietary mixture of gallic acid and linoleic acid on antioxidative potential and quality of breast meat from broilers. Meat Sci 2010; 86(2): 520-6.
[http://dx.doi.org/10.1016/j.meatsci.2010.06.007] [PMID: 20609528]

[77]   Pennington JA, Fisher RA. Classification of fruits and vegetables. J Food Compos Anal 2009; 22: S23-31.
[http://dx.doi.org/10.1016/j.jfca.2008.11.012]

CHAPTER 12

Green Tea (*Camellia sinensis*) and its Beneficial Role in Poultry Nutrition

Mahmoud Alagawany[1,*], Mohammad Mehedi Hasan Khan[2], Rashed Chowdhury[2], Mayada R. Farag[3], Rana M. Bilal[4] and Mohamed E. Abd El-Hack[1,*]

[1] *Department of Poultry, Faculty of Agriculture, Zagazig University, 44511Zagazig, Egypt*

[2] *Department of Biochemistry and Chemistry Sylhet Agricultural University, Bangladesh*

[3] *Forensic Medicine and Toxicology Department, Veterinary Medicine Faculty, Zagazig University, Zagazig 44511, Egypt*

[4] *University College of Veterinary and Animal Sciences, The Islamia University of Bahawalpur, Pakistan*

Abstract: Green tea (*Camellia sinensis*) is a famous herbal plant used as a potent antioxidant since ancient times with abundant health benefits. Numerous studies have shown the health benefits of green tea for many diseases. The objective of this article is to know the importance and various uses of green tea and its important constituents in poultry for safeguarding various health issues. The present review article also focuses on several beneficial health applications and salient medicinal properties of green tea that have not been comprehensively reviewed previously. Owing to the bioactive constituents, including caffeine, amino acids (AA), L-theanine, polyphenols/ flavonoids and carbohydrates, among other potent molecules, green tea has many pharmacological and physiological characteristics. Moreover, *Camellia sinensis* possesses essential biological compounds such as alkaloids, carotenoids, minerals, amino acids, carbohydrates, lipids, and volatile compounds. Based on scientific literature evidence, green tea has multifunctional applications in livestock animal sectors of dairy, goat and poultry industry. Green tea active ingredients have been shown to possess many health benefits with various mechanisms like antioxidative, anti-inflammatory, antiarthritic, antistress, hypolipidemic, hypocholesterolemic, skin/collagen protective, hepatoprotective, antidiabetic, antimicrobial, anti-infective, anti-parasitic, anti-cancerous, inhibition of tumorigenesis and angiogenesis, and improving memory and bone health. The findings presented would be useful for poultry researchers and farmers and would help to propagate the multidimensional health benefits of green tea.

* **Corresponding authors Mahmoud Alagawany and Mohamed E. Abd El-Hack:** Department of Poultry, Faculty of Agriculture, Zagazig University, Zagazig - 44511, Egypt; E-mails: mmalagwany@zu.edu.eg and m.ezzat@zu.edu.eg

Keywords: Animal, Applications, Green tea, Health, L-theanine, Poultry.

INTRODUCTION

Tea was first used in China as a medicinal drink and later became a popular beverage next to water throughout the world [1]. A Chinese king Shen Nung, in 2737 BC for the first time, proposed the concept of using tea when accidentally, some tea leaves were boiled in water, and a lovely smell was produced [2]. Tea is cultivated in more than 45 countries throughout the world [3]. There are various kinds of tea available in the world tea market, like black (fully fermented), green(non-fermented), flavored, oolong (semi-fermented), white tea, *etc.*, based on the manufacturing process [4]. In Europe, South Asia, and North America, the most popular is black tea, whereas oolong and green teas are consumed mainly in East Asian countries [5]. Green tea is basically made from the leaves of a plant scientifically known as *Camellia sinensis*, which has been used in different parts of the world. Green tea is thought to contain higher polyphenols and and flavonoids due to being non-fermented and therefore has greater antioxidant potential and health benefits than black tea [5, 6]. The major polyphenolic compounds found in green tea are catechins, epicatechin, epicatechin-3-gallate, and epigallocatechin-3-gallate [7]. Besides human consumption, low-grade green tea and green tea byproducts or spent tea has been used as an ingredient for animal feeds. Supplementation of green tea has been studied by several authors in fish [8], quails [9], ruminants [10], broilers [11, 12] and layer chickens [13, 14]. Green tea, the derivatives, and byproducts of green tea such as green tea extracts, green tea leaves, spent tea, green tea flowers and green tea polyphenols have been used as feed ingredients for improving the performance of poultry [13 - 15]. Recently, green tea powder supplementation in poultry diet showed a positive response for production parameters, immunity, growth and carcass characteristics [16, 17]. There are other plant secondary metabolites such as alkaloids and saponins found in green tea leaves. However, in comparison to black tea, the most important metabolites after catechin are theanine. In 1949, L-theanine was discovered in the leaves of green tea. This caramel-flavored attractive aromatic amino acid is a unique taste constituent of tea and helps to alleviate tea polyphenols astringency and caffeine bitterness [18]. L-theanine as a safe and non-toxic photogenic food supplement was suggested through different technical, safety and toxicological evaluations. L-theanine was synthesized chemically for the first time from aqueous ethylamine and pyrrolidone carboxylic acid [19].

The non-protein L-theanine (γ-Glutamylethylamide) is found mostly in the leaves of tea plants [20]. Dietary supplementation of L-theanine mitigated the damage induced by reactive oxygen species (ROS) [21]. Catechins of green tea can bind with many minerals and hence affect their metabolism [22]. Excess uptake reduces zinc and iron level; enhances manganese; however, the final blood plasma concentration of copper is not altered greatly [23, 24]. Wen [25] demonstrated that adding 400 mg L-theanine/kg daily in the diet increases the level of secretory IgA in the jejunum and the levels of IL-2 and IFN- γ in the serum of chickens. Theanine can reduce the toxic side impacts stimulated by anticancer drugs and can relieve lipid peroxidation and oxidative stress [26].

HEALTH BENEFITS ON POULTRY SPECIES

Green tea has a beneficial effect on poultry due to its polyphenolic contents having strong antioxidant properties [27]. *Camellia sinensis* contains natural flavonoids that have anti-coccidial properties [28]. The recent investigations assured that supplementing of green tea by-products to broilers and layers diets can enhance performance and decline the amount of cholesterol in egg yolk and blood serum, besides its impact on the criteria of egg quality. Supplementation of by-products derived from green tea minimizes the numbers of all microflora in caecum as a result of its antimicrobial impact [14].

Broilers Chickens

A limited number of studies in broiler chicken nutrition describing the supplementation of green tea leaves, extracts or powder have been published. However, the results are very inconsistent amongst studies. Supplementing green tea extracts at a rate of 200 mg kg^{-1} diet showed a positive response on the growth performance of broiler chicken [29]. Khalaji *et al.* [30] did not find any significant effect of green tea on broiler growth at a rate of 300 mg kg^{-1}. Growth parameters and feed intake level also were declined in treated broiler chicken fed with green tea extracts at 500 mg kg^{-1} [30]. Uuganbayar [31] claimed that 1% to 1.50% green tea supplementation in broiler diet reduced chicks body weight gain [32].

Farahat *et al.* [11] and Cao *et al.* [12] did not find any significant differences in body weight, daily gain, daily feed intake and feed conversion ratio of broiler chickens after supplementation of different concentrations of green tea extract (125 to 2000mg kg^{-1}). They also added that birds fed diets supplemented with graded concentrations of green extract tea had improved antioxidant and immunostimulant traits. Furthermore, the antibody titer against Newcastle disease virus vaccines was increased in chicks fed diets supplemented with green tea [11].

Yang *et al.* [33] showed insignificant improvement in feed efficiency percent and growth performance of broiler chickens by green tea by-product. The authors added that supplementing diets with powdered green tea by-product decreased blood LDL cholesterol comparing to the control group while increased HDL levels docosahexaenoic acid (DHA) in the blood. Moreover, cholesterol content in meat tended to decline due to dietary supplementation with green tea by-product. Shomali *et al.* [34] studied impacts of higher doses of powdered green tea (1.00%, 2.00%, or 4.00%) on the growth of broiler and found insignificant differences in weight gain, consumed feed and feed efficiency. El-Deek *et al.* [35] concluded that the dietary addition of green tea (1.50 and 3.00 g/kg diet) did not affect the performance and meat quality of broiler; however, environmental pollution *via* excreted nitrogen was reduced with green treatments. Live body weight, feed intake and ideal digestibility of nutrients were not remarkably influenced by green tea supplementation (10 g^{-1} kg diet) in broiler chickens as compared with the control. While plasma cholesterol and triglyceride were lowered with supplemental green tea compared to control birds [36].

On the contrary, Kaneko *et al.* [37] reported favorable effects of green tea powder on broiler growth performance when fed at levels up to 1000 mg kg^{-1}. Using liquid extract (hydro alcoholic) of green tea, at the level of 0.10 g/kg or 0.20 g/kg of broiler diets improved values of live body weight, feed conversion, dressing percentage, and carcass weight probably due to the caecal microflora [38].

Green tea polyphenols (TP) have been proven to have varieties of biological properties, including antimicrobial [39], antioxidative [40, 41] and anti-inflammatory activities [40]. Zhao *et al.* [42] claimed that green tea polyphenols are responsible for lower drip loss, which causes muscle tenderness. Zou *et al.* [43] reported similar findings in another experiment with broiler chick, suggesting that TP may degrade the myofibrillar protein myosin that could be involved in tenderness as well. Moreover, in layers, a concentration of 0.1 or 0.3% green tea extract reduced low-density lipoprotein and serum total cholesterol contents [44].

Recently, green tea has been used as an immunomodulatory agent against coccidiosis in broiler chicken. Supplementing green tea in a powder form in broiler diet improved cellular and humoral immunity against coccidiosis in a dose-dependent manner by increasing lymphoproliferative immune response [17, 45]. They also found enhanced immunoglobulin levels (Total immunoglobulin, IgG, and IgM) in blood serum of treated broilers.. Furthermore, *in vitro,* results showed that high doses of green tea extracts had more antimicrobial activity [46]. Jang *et al.* [28] reported that the immunomodulatory and anticoccidial potential of green tea might be due to the actions of its antioxidant compounds however, the actual mode of action aganist parasites is still unknown. Farahat *et al.* [11] concluded that the optimum inclusion levels of green tea extracts in broiler diets ranged from 125 to 500 mg kg^{-1}. Further studies are warranted to find out the actual dose level of green tea powder for improving the immune status of broiler chicken as recommended [16].

Laying Hens

Uuganbayar *et al.* [47] examined the impact of dietary supplementation with green tea powder in layers up to 2.00% and found no adverse impact on egg yield as well as egg weight compared with control. Kojima and Yoshida [48] did not find any significant differences in the rate of egg yield, egg output or egg weight between laying hens consumed rations enriched by 1% green tea powder and the control, however increasing the level up to 5.00% and 10.00% produced the lowest values. Biswas *et al.* [49] also observed that supplementing the layer rations with 0.6% Japanese green tea did not affect egg yield for long-term trials. Enriching layer rations with 1.5% green tea powder as well as 0.5% green tea extract did not affect egg mass, feed consumption, or egg production [50]. Layers fed with green tea powder at levels of 1 or 2% reduced yolk cholesterol as compared to control treatment [51].

On the other hand, supplementation of 0.2% green tea produced statistically the best egg mass as well as egg production compared with control [52]. Uuganbayar *et al.* [53] found that egg yield of hens consumed diets supplemented with 1% or 2% green tea (Japanese, Chinese and Korean) were statistically improved in comparison to the control group. The influences of supplementing leaves of green tea (1% to 5%) and its extract (0.50 L to 2.50 L 100 kg^{-1} diet) for layers showed improvement of egg yield and egg output compared with the control [54]. Concerning quality egg criteria, using a low level (0.3%) of powdered green tea as a dietary supplementation improved the albumen percentage and Haugh unit score [32]. Improvement in the egg quality traits (internal and external) was also recorded with green tea powder supplementation [55].

The phenolic contents of green tea can prevent the adverse effects of vanadium on egg quality, liver, and antioxidants and make the recovery time in laying hen shorter [13, 56]. They reported that dietary supplementation of tea polyphenols (1000 mg kg^{-1}) improved the short-chain fatty acid production that affects the caecum microbiota ecology and protects duodenal cells from excess apoptosis caused by vanadium in laying hens. The production performance of layers mainly depends on daily intake levels, including feed nutrition. Though green tea powder and its extracts or essential oil have potential health benefits on poultry, however, the average intake levels may vary due to different taste and essence of green tea leaves. The reduced feed intake in laying birds was observed due to supplementation of either 10 to 50 mg kg^{-1} or 5 to 25 mg kg^{-1} of green tea essential oil (EO) when compared to the non-supplemented control diet [54]. The authors also reported reduced FCR by approximately 11% and by 12% when green tea was included in the form of EO at 25 mg kg^{-1}. Also, 50 mg kg^{-1} green tea leaves or 25 mg kg^{-1} green tea EO did not affect body weight gain which was consistent with another finding by Xu *et al.* [57] where authors reported green tea as an antiobesity factor.

CONCLUSION

The beneficial aspects of green tea have been proved, and it could be advisable to encourage its regular consumption as an alternative to other beverage drinks. In conclusion, this literature review highlights that green tea and L-theanine have various health-improving effects, including anti-carcinogenic, anti-oxidative, anti-inflammatory, antimutagenic, antimicrobial, hypolipidemic, antiviral, antifungal and anti-parasitic effects in addition to improving memory and bone health. The use of green tea and its products tends to improve the growth and productive performance of animals and poultry. Based on the above findings, L-theanine could be utilized in the diets of pigs, goats, mice, and poultry but at limited quantity. Hitherto, there are yet no more investigations on L-theanine amino acid in the poultry industry, so it needs to be studied more by involving it in poultry diet as a natural anti-stressor to alleviate the environmental stress problem which is a big blatantly impediment in the poultry industry and to improve the health status and productivity as well.

CONSENT FOR PUBLICATION

Not applicable.

CONFLICT OF INTEREST

The author declares no conflict of interest, financial or otherwise.

ACKNOWLEDGEMENTS

Declared none.

REFERENCES

[1]   Tea (*Camellia sinensis* (L.)): a putative anticancer agent in bladder carcinoma?. Anti-Cancer Agents in Medicinal Chemistry (Formerly Current Medicinal Chemistry-Anti-Cancer Agents). 1 Jan 2015; 15(1): 26-36.

[2]   Wheeler DS, Wheeler WJ. The medicinal chemistry of tea. Drug Dev Res 2004; 61(2): 45-65.
       [http://dx.doi.org/10.1002/ddr.10341]

[3]   Pastoriza S, Mesías M, Cabrera C, Rufián-Henares JA. Healthy properties of green and white teas: an update. Food Funct 2017; 8(8): 2650-62.
       [http://dx.doi.org/10.1039/C7FO00611J] [PMID: 28640307]

[4]   Lee LS, Kim SH, Kim YB, Kim YC. Quantitative analysis of major constituents in green tea with different plucking periods and their antioxidant activity. Molecules 2014; 19(7): 9173-86.
       [http://dx.doi.org/10.3390/molecules19079173] [PMID: 24988187]

[5]   Nibir YM, Sumit AF, Akhand AA, Ahsan N, Hossain MS. Comparative assessment of total polyphenols, antioxidant and antimicrobial activity of different tea varieties of Bangladesh. Asian Pac J Trop Biomed 2017; 7(4): 352-7.
[http://dx.doi.org/10.1016/j.apjtb.2017.01.005]

[6]   Delwing-Dal Magro D, Roecker R, Junges GM, *et al.* Protective effect of green tea extract against proline-induced oxidative damage in the rat kidney. Biomed Pharmacother 2016; 83: 1422-7.
[http://dx.doi.org/10.1016/j.biopha.2016.08.057] [PMID: 27589827]

[7]   Singh BN, Shankar S, Srivastava RK. Green tea catechin, epigallocatechin-3-gallate (EGCG): mechanisms, perspectives and clinical applications. Biochem Pharmacol 2011; 82(12): 1807-21.
[http://dx.doi.org/10.1016/j.bcp.2011.07.093] [PMID: 21827739]

[8]   Hasanpour S, Salati AP, Falahatkar B, Azarm HM. Effects of dietary green tea (*Camellia sinensis* L.) supplementation on growth performance, lipid metabolism, and antioxidant status in a sturgeon hybrid of Sterlet (Huso huso ♂ × Acipenser ruthenus ♀) fed oxidized fish oil. Fish Physiol Biochem 2017; 43(5): 1315-23.
[http://dx.doi.org/10.1007/s10695-017-0374-z] [PMID: 28488192]

[9]   Abdel-Azeem FA. Green tea flowers (*Camellia sinensis*) as natural anti-oxidants feed additives in growing Japanese quail diets. Egypt Poult Sci J 2005; 25(3): 569-88.

[10]   Ramdani D, Chaudhry AS, Seal CJ. Chemical composition, plant secondary metabolites, and minerals of green and black teas and the effect of different tea-to-water ratios during their extraction on the composition of their spent leaves as potential additives for ruminants. J Agric Food Chem 2013; 61(20): 4961-7.
[http://dx.doi.org/10.1021/jf4002439] [PMID: 23621359]

[11]   Farahat M, Abdallah F, Abdel-Hamid T, Hernandez-Santana A. Effect of supplementing broiler chicken diets with green tea extract on the growth performance, lipid profile, antioxidant status and immune response. Br Poult Sci 2016; 57(5): 714-22.
[http://dx.doi.org/10.1080/00071668.2016.1196339] [PMID: 27302855]

[12]   Cao BH, Karasawa Y, Guo YM. Effects of green tea polyphenols and fructo-oligosaccharides in semi-purified diets on broilersPerformance and caecal microflora and their metabolites. Asian-Australas J Anim Sci 2005; 18(1): 85-9.
[http://dx.doi.org/10.5713/ajas.2005.85]

[13]   Yuan ZH, Zhang KY, Ding XM, *et al.* Effect of tea polyphenols on production performance, egg quality, and hepatic antioxidant status of laying hens in vanadium-containing diets. Poult Sci 2016; 95(7): 1709-17.
[http://dx.doi.org/10.3382/ps/pew097] [PMID: 27044874]

[14]   Khan SH. The use of green tea (*Camellia sinensis*) as a phytogenic substance in poultry diets. Onderstepoort J Vet Res 2014; 81(1): 1-8.

[15]   Saraee MH, Seidavi A, Dadashbeiki M, Laudadio V, Tufarelli V. Supplementing fish oil and green tea (*Camellia sinensis*) powder in broiler diet: effects on productive performance. Res Opin Anim Vet Sci 2015; 5(2): 99-104.

[16]   Seidavi A, Dadashbeiki M, Asadpour L, *et al.* Dietary green tea powder affects the immunologic parameters of broiler chicks. Ital J Anim Sci 2017; 16(1): 108-14.
[http://dx.doi.org/10.1080/1828051X.2016.1261007]

[17]   Seidavi A, Asadpour L, Dadashbeiki M, Payan-Carreira R. Effects of dietary fish oil and green tea powder supplementation on broiler chickens immunity. Acta Sci Vet 2014; 42(1): 1-3.

[18]   Eschenauer G, Sweet BV. Pharmacology and therapeutic uses of theanine. Am J Health Syst Pharm 2006; 63(1): 26-30, 28-30.
[http://dx.doi.org/10.2146/ajhp050148] [PMID: 16373462]

[19]   White DJ, de Klerk S, Woods W, Gondalia S, Noonan C, Scholey AB. Anti-stress, behavioural and

magnetoencephalography effects of an L-theanine-based nutrient drink: a randomised, double-blind, placebo-controlled, crossover trial. Nutrients 2016; 8(1): 53.
[http://dx.doi.org/10.3390/nu8010053] [PMID: 26797633]

[20]   Deng WW, Ogita S, Ashihara H. Distribution and biosynthesis of theanine in Theaceae plants. Plant Physiol Biochem 2010; 48(1): 70-2.
[http://dx.doi.org/10.1016/j.plaphy.2009.09.009] [PMID: 19828327]

[21]   Cooper R. Green tea and theanine: health benefits. Int J Food Sci Nutr 2012; 63(sup1): 7-90.
[http://dx.doi.org/10.3109/09637486.2011.629180]

[22]   Saeed M, El-Hack ME, Alagawany M, *et al.* Phytochemistry, modes of action and beneficial health applications of green tea (*Camellia sinensis*) in humans and animals. Int J Pharmacol 2017; 13(7): 698-708.
[http://dx.doi.org/10.3923/ijp.2017.698.708]

[23]   Mira L, Fernandez MT, Santos M, Rocha R, Florêncio MH, Jennings KR. Interactions of flavonoids with iron and copper ions: a mechanism for their antioxidant activity. Free Radic Res 2002; 36(11): 1199-208.
[http://dx.doi.org/10.1080/1071576021000016463] [PMID: 12592672]

[24]   Nelson M, Poulter J. Impact of tea drinking on iron status in the UK: a review. J Hum Nutr Diet 2004; 17(1): 43-54.
[http://dx.doi.org/10.1046/j.1365-277X.2003.00497.x] [PMID: 14718031]

[25]   Wen H, Wei S, Zhang S, Hou D, Xiao W, He X. Effects of L-theanine on performance and immune function of yellow-feathered broilers. Chin J Anim Nutr 2012; 24(10): 1946-54.

[26]   Saeed M, Naveed M, Arif M, *et al.* Green tea (*Camellia sinensis*) and l-theanine: Medicinal values and beneficial applications in humans-A comprehensive review. Biomed Pharmacother 2017; 95: 1260-75.
[http://dx.doi.org/10.1016/j.biopha.2017.09.024] [PMID: 28938517]

[27]   Izzreen NQ, Mohd Fadzelly AB. Phytochemicals and antioxidant properties of different parts of *Camellia sinensis* leaves from Sabah Tea Plantation in Sabah, Malaysia. Int Food Res J 2013; 20(1): 307 12.

[28]   Jang SI, Jun MH, Lillehoj HS, *et al.* Anticoccidial effect of green tea-based diets against *Eimeria maxima*. Vet Parasitol 2007; 144(1-2): 172-5.
[http://dx.doi.org/10.1016/j.vetpar.2006.09.005] [PMID: 17027157]

[29]   Shahid W, Ahmad A, Mangaiyarkarasi R, *et al.* Effect of polyphenolic rich green tea extract as antioxidant on broiler performance during 0–4 weeks. Int J Adv Res (Indore) 2013; 1(9): 177-81.

[30]   Khalaji S, Zaghari M, Hatami K, Hedari-Dastjerdi S, Lotfi L, Nazarian H. Black cumin seeds, Artemisia leaves (Artemisia sieberi), and Camellia L. plant extract as phytogenic products in broiler diets and their effects on performance, blood constituents, immunity, and cecal microbial population. Poult Sci 2011; 90(11): 2500-10.
[http://dx.doi.org/10.3382/ps.2011-01393] [PMID: 22010235]

[31]   Uuganbayar D. A study on the utilization of green tea for laying hens and broiler chicks. A Dissertation for the degree of doctor of philosophy, Sunchon National University. Sunchon 2004.

[32]   Biswas AH, Wakita M. Effect of dietary Japanese green tea powder supplementation on feed utilization and carcass profiles in broilers. J Poult Sci 2001; 38(1): 50-7.
[http://dx.doi.org/10.2141/jpsa.38.50]

[33]   Yang CJ, Yang IY, Oh DH, *et al.* Effect of green tea by-product on performance and body composition in broiler chicks. Asian-Australas J Anim Sci 2003; 16(6): 867-72.
[http://dx.doi.org/10.5713/ajas.2003.867]

[34]   Shomali T, Mosleh N, Nazifi S. Two weeks of dietary supplementation with green tea powder does not affect performance, D-xylose absorption, and selected serum parameters in broiler chickens. Comp Clin Pathol 2012; 21(5): 1023-7.

[http://dx.doi.org/10.1007/s00580-011-1220-9]

[35] El-Deek AA, Al-Harthi MA, Osman M, Al-Jassas F, Nassar R. Effect of different levels of green tea (*Camellia sinensis*) as a substitute for oxytetracycline as a growth promoter in broilers diets containing two crude protein levels. Arch Geflugelkd 2012; 76(2): 88-98.

[36] Afsharmanesh M, Sadaghi B. Effects of dietary alternatives (probiotic, green tea powder, and Kombucha tea) as antimicrobial growth promoters on growth, ileal nutrient digestibility, blood parameters, and immune response of broiler chickens. Comp Clin Pathol 2014; 23(3): 717-24.
[http://dx.doi.org/10.1007/s00580-013-1676-x]

[37] Kaneko K, Yamasaki K, Tagawa Y, Tokunaga M, Tobisa M, Furuse M. Effects of dietary Japanese green tea powder on growth, meat ingredient and lipid accumulation in broilers. Jpn Poult Sci 2001; 38(5): J77-85.
[http://dx.doi.org/10.2141/jpsa.38.J77]

[38] Erener G, Ocak N, Altop A, Cankaya S, Aksoy HM, Ozturk E. Growth performance, meat quality and caecal coliform bacteria count of broiler chicks fed diet with green tea extract. Asian-Australas J Anim Sci 2011; 24(8): 1128-35.
[http://dx.doi.org/10.5713/ajas.2011.10434]

[39] Koech KR, Wachira FN, Ngure RM, *et al.* Antioxidant, antimicrobial and synergistic activities of tea polyphenols. Afr Crop Sci J 2014; 22. Supplement.
[http://dx.doi.org/10.1016/j.ijid.2014.03.631]

[40] Li HL, Li ZJ, Wei ZS, *et al.* Long-term effects of oral tea polyphenols and Lactobacillus brevis M8 on biochemical parameters, digestive enzymes, and cytokines expression in broilers. J Zhejiang Univ Sci B 2015; 16(12): 1019-26.
[http://dx.doi.org/10.1631/jzus.B1500160] [PMID: 26642185]

[41] Klimczak I, Gliszczyńska-Świgło A. Green tea extract as an anti-browning agent for cloudy apple juice. J Sci Food Agric 2017; 97(5): 1420-6.
[http://dx.doi.org/10.1002/jsfa.7880] [PMID: 27378649]

[42] Zhao J, Lv W, Wang J, Li J, Liu X, Zhu J. Effects of tea polyphenols on the post-mortem integrity of large yellow croaker (Pseudosciaena crocea) fillet proteins. Food Chem 2013; 141(3): 2666-74.
[http://dx.doi.org/10.1016/j.foodchem.2013.04.126] [PMID: 23871009]

[43] Zou X, Xiao R, Li H, *et al.* Effect of a novel strain of Lactobacillus brevis M8 and tea polyphenol diets on performance, meat quality and intestinal microbiota in broilers. Ital J Anim Sci 2018; 17(2): 396-407.
[http://dx.doi.org/10.1080/1828051X.2017.1365260]

[44] Huang J, Hao Q, Wang Q, Wang Y, Wan X, Zhou Y. Supplementation with green tea extract affects lipid metabolism and egg yolk lipid composition in laying hens. J Appl Poult Res 2019; 28(4): 881-91.
[http://dx.doi.org/10.3382/japr/pfz046]

[45] Abbas A, Iqbal Z, Abbas RZ, *et al.* Immunomodulatory effects of *Camellia sinensis* against coccidiosis in chickens. J Anim Plant Sci 2017; 27: 415-21.

[46] Neyestani TR, Khalaji N, Gharavi AA. Black and green teas may have selective synergistic or antagonistic effects on certain antibiotics against Streptococcus pyogenes *in vitro.* J Nutr Environ Med 2007; 16(3-4): 258-66.
[http://dx.doi.org/10.1080/13590840701703934]

[47] Uuganbayar D, Bae IH, Choi KS, Shin IS, Firman JD, Yang CJ. Effects of green tea powder on laying performance and egg quality in laying hens. Asian-Australas J Anim Sci 2005; 18(12): 1769-74.
[http://dx.doi.org/10.5713/ajas.2005.1769]

[48] Kojima S, Yoshida Y. Effects of green tea powder feed supplement on performance of hens in the late stage of laying. Int J Poult Sci 2008; 7(5): 491-6.
[http://dx.doi.org/10.3923/ijps.2008.491.496]

[49]   Biswas MA, Miyazaki Y, Nomura K, Wakita M. Influences of long-term feeding of Japanese green tea powder on laying performance and egg quality in hens. Asian-Australas J Anim Sci 2000; 13(7): 980-5.
[http://dx.doi.org/10.5713/ajas.2000.980]

[50]   Ariana M, Samie A, Edriss MA, Jahanian R. Effects of powder and extract form of green tea and marigold, and-tocopheryl acetate on performance, egg quality and egg yolk cholesterol levels of laying hens in late phase of production. J Med Plants Res 2011; 5(13): 2710-6.

[51]   Panja P. The effects of China tea (*Camellia sinensis*) supplementation in laying hen diets on production, quality and cholesterol content of egg. Songklanakarin J Sci Technol 2007; 29(6): 636-8.

[52]   Al-Harthi MA. Responses of laying hens to different levels of amoxicillin, hot pepper or green tea and their effects on productive performance, egg quality and chemical composition of yolk and blood plasma constituents. Egypt Poult Sci J 2004; 24(4): 845-68.

[53]   Uuganbayar D, Shin IS, Yang CJ. Comparative performance of hens fed diets containing Korean, Japanese and Chinese green tea. Asian-Australas J Anim Sci 2006; 19(8): 1190-6.
[http://dx.doi.org/10.5713/ajas.2006.1190]

[54]   Abdo ZM, Hassan RA, El-Salam AA, Helmy SA. Effect of adding green tea and its aqueous extract as natural antioxidants to laying hen diet on productive, reproductive performance and egg quality during storage and its content of cholesterol. Egypt Poult Sci J 2010; 30(4): 1121-49.

[55]   Xia B, Liu Y, Sun D, Liu J, Zhu Y, Lu L. Effects of green tea powder supplementation on egg production and egg quality in laying hens. J Appl Anim Res 2018; 46(1): 927-31.
[http://dx.doi.org/10.1080/09712119.2018.1431240]

[56]   Zhang R, Dong X, Zhou M, *et al.* Oral administration of Lactobacillus plantarum and Bacillus subtilis on rumen fermentation and the bacterial community in calves. Anim Sci J 2017; 88(5): 755-62.
[http://dx.doi.org/10.1111/asj.12691] [PMID: 27628956]

[57]   Xu J, Hu FL, Wang W, Wan XC, Bao GH. Investigation on biochemical compositional changes during the microbial fermentation process of Fu brick tea by LC-MS based metabolomics. Food Chem 2015; 186: 176-84.
[http://dx.doi.org/10.1016/j.foodchem.2014.12.045] [PMID: 25976808]

CHAPTER 13

Beneficial Impacts of Essential Oils on Poultry Health and Production

Mohamed E. Abd El-Hack[1,*], **Mohamed T. El-saadony**[2], **Nahed Yehia**[3], **Asmaa F. Khafaga**[4], **Mayada R. Farag**[5] and **Mahmoud Alagawany**[1,*]

[1] *Department of Poultry, Faculty of Agriculture, Zagazig University, Zagazig 44511, Egypt*

[2] *Department of Agricultural Microbiology, Faculty of Agriculture, Zagazig University, Zagazig 44511, Egypt*

[3] *Reference Laboratory for Veterinary Quality Control on Poultry Production, Animal Health Research Institute, Agricultural Research Center, Egypt*

[4] *Department of Pathology, Faculty of Veterinary Medicine, Alexandria University, Edfina 22758, Egypt*

[5] *Forensic Medicine and Toxicology Department, Veterinary Medicine Faculty, Zagazig University, Zagazig 44511, Egypt*

Abstract: With the rapid growth of the poultry sector, a major human health concern is noticed relating to the excessive and uncontrolled abuse of antibiotics, which leads to the development of antibiotic-resistant bacteria. Antibiotics are used in sub-therapeutic doses as antimicrobial agents for rapid growth performance in poultry and for prevention of diseases. For this reason, there is a need to develop alternatives to antibiotics. The beneficial effects of plants and plant extracts that have traditional use are evaluated in many studies. The most common beneficial effects of these plants and their extracts are stimulating endogenous digestive enzymes and antioxidants. Essential oils (EOs) have a wide variety of effects, including antimicrobial, antioxidants, and digestive stimulant activities. Essential oils have been demonstrated to positively affect growth performance, gut health, and meat quality, but the responses are inconsistent. The inconsistencies have been related to the species/subspecies of the plant, harvest time, geographical location, and plant part used that can affect the EOs structure. The oils undergo a patented micro fusion process that creates a surface area of oil droplets that is 20 times greater than other commercially available oilsthus increasing the stability and effectiveness of the oils. The EOs exhibit high antioxidant activity, which is attributed to its two main phenols, carvacrol, and thymol. Conclusively, essential oils can be used in poultry nutrition, but still need more studies, especially metabolism, and the optimum dose in various poultry species.

* **Corresponding authors Mahmoud Alagawany and Mohamed E. Abd El-Hack:** Poultry Department, Faculty of Agriculture, Zagazig University, Zagazig, Egypt; E-mails: mmalagwany@zu.edu.eg and m.ezzat@zu.edu.eg

Keywords: Antibiotics, Carvacrol, Essential oils, Growth, Poultry, Resveratrol, Thymol.

INTRODUCTION

Generally, feed additives enhanced the poultry growth capacity, but some may be added to replace antibiotics for the prevention of diseases. However, there is a large difference in the efficacy of feed additives. Of the alternatives listed, phytochemicals, specifically essential oils (EOs), have been shown to have the most inconsistent results [1 - 3]. Essential oils are aromatic oils that can be extracted from plant material, typically by distillation. There are about 300 EOs that are commercially available, and the inconsistency in results may be due to this wide variety of oils, or the fact that the chemical compounds in oils can be affected by species, climatic conditions, harvest time, and plant part [4, 5]. The EOs have been shown to impact growth efficiency and gut health of poultry. Mathlouthi *et al.* [6] reported that broilers fed avilamycin (0.04/kg), rosemary, and oregano (0.1 g/kg), or a blend of EOs (1g/kg) had significantly increased weight compared to control groups. Alp *et al.* [7] concluded that broilers fed an anticoccidial (100 mg/kg) or oregano essential oil (0.3 g/kg) had improved feed conversion ratio (FCR) over broilers on a control diet, but there were no differences in the final weight on day 42. While, other research indicates that EOs showed a negative or minimal effect on growth performance [8].

Although the exact mechanism of EOs in enhancing growth performance is not known, Jang *et al.* [9] reported that broilers that were fed a blend of EOs had increased pancreatic amylase, trypsin, and maltase activity in the small intestine as compared to control birds. The increased digestive secretions, which could result in increased nutrient absorption may assist in the antimicrobial activity of EOs. EOs can affect gut health in two major ways: shifts in gut microbiota and changes in the microscopic anatomy of the small intestine [1, 10, 11]. The combination of these two effects leads to an increased ability of the poultry to combat disease caused by pathogenic organisms.

However, research on the impact of EOs on the histology of the intestine in poultry is limited, especially research on broilers that are under a coccidiosis disease challenge. Basmacioğlu *et al.* [10] investigated the impact of EOs blend on the ileum histology and found that broilers that were fed on the EOs mixture had increased villus height and lower crypt depth at 42 days of age over compared to control birds.. OviedoRondón *et al.* [12] found that feeding EOs to coccidiosis-infected broilers impacted the microbial community in infected broilers by preventing drastic shifts in the microbial populations after the infection. Shifts in microbial populations can stimulate an immune response because new antigens were developed [4]. Furthermore, Evans *et al.* [13] observed a decrease in the oocyst excretion from chickens after feeding on a blend of EOs. Essential oils are also known to decrease the lipid oxidation of meat due to their antioxidant activity [11]. Essential oils, particularly oregano, sage, and rosemary, are known to have a high antioxidant activity [1]. Oregano is derived from *Origanum vulgare* and both carvacrol and thymol give it its antioxidant effect [8]. The present chapter summarizes the beneficial impacts of different EOs on poultry health and production.

SOME TYPES OF ESSENTIAL OILS

Thymol

Sources of Thymol

Thymol is a component of several medicinal plants, such as *Thymus zygis*, *Thymus vulgaris*, *Origanum compactum*, *Origanum onites*, *Origanum dictamnus*, *Monarda fistulosa*, *Thymus hyemalis*, a *Thymus glandulosus*, and *Origanum vulgare,* as recorded by Lee *et al.* [14] also, the North American wildflowers and bee balms *Monarda didyma* are considered as natural sources of thymol [15].

CHEMICAL AND PHYSICAL CHARACTERISTICS

Thymol is a white crystalline substance and is similar in taste to carvacrol. The melting range of thymol is 49 to 51°C, while the boiling point is 232°C. Due to the deprotonating of the phenol, it is soluble in alcohol and alkaline solutions but less soluble in water at neutral pH [16]. It absorbs the UV radiation until 274 nm. The structural formula of thymol is shown in Fig. (**1**).

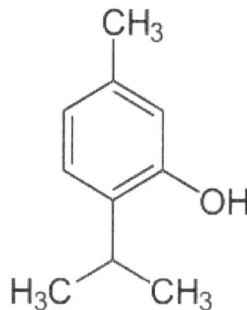

Fig. (1). Basic structural formula of Thymol.

BENEFICIAL ASPECTS OF THYMOL

Thymol showed antioxidant, antiviral and antibacterial activities *in vitro*, where it decreased the secretion of α-hemolysin and enterotoxins A, B generated by methicillin-resistant *Staphylococcus aureus*. It also could act as coccidiostat, anti-inflammatory, antileishmanial, antispasmodic and anthelmintic *in vivo*. Moreover, it had endocrine and immune stimulation activities. Thymol showed anti-inflammatory effect by inhibiting the release of elastase enzyme from neutrophils [17 - 19]. Additionally, thymol decreased the bacterial resistance to antibiotics as penicillin as reported by Palaniappan *et al.* [20]. Aijaz *et al.* [21] recorded a high antifungal action of thymol, specifically against fluconazole-resistant strains of *Candida albicans* [22]. Mezzoug *et al.* [23] mentioned that carvacrol and thymol, as essential oils were detected to have a powerful antimutagenic effect. Furthermore, Andersen [24], assured that thymol has antitumor activity.

Several studies have reported a large variety of beneficial thymol nutritional and physiological effects. It would accelerate the secretions of digestive enzymes *e.g.*, amylase, proteases, and lipase, salivary amylase, and bile acids [4, 25]. Lee *et al.* [26] recorded increased pancreatic amylase, trypsin, and maltase in broiler chickens. Cross *et al.* [27] detected an increase in body weight of broiler chickens when supplied by thyme essential oil 1,000 mg/kg. Similarly, poultry performance and activities of digestive enzymes were improved with the thymol EO [26 - 28]. Moreover, Hashemipour *et al.* [29] detected that mixed supplementation of carvacrol and thymol 0.2, 0.1, 0.06 g per kg of diet, accelerated the growth parameter, and activated digestive enzymes in chicks. In addition, the IgG level in the blood was enhanced by the diet supplemented by extracts of oregano and thyme comparing with the control diet in mice and pigs [2, 30].

Immunomodulatory Effect

The key goals of poultry production are to increase immunity to limit infectious diseases, failure in vaccination, immunosuppressive diseases, and misuse of antibiotics by using natural immune-stimulators [31]. The humoral, cellular immunity, and phagocyte system of the host. The oregano EO and thymol phenolic compounds could accelerate the cellular and humoral immune responses of broiler chickens which play an important role in resistance to multiple infections [32]. Botsoglou *et al.* [28] suggested that carvacrol and thymol had antiviral, antibacterial, and antioxidant properties that would increase the immune responses of chicks. Al-Kassie [33], also stated that thyme and cinnamon oil extract improved the broilers' performance.

Scavenging Effect

Botsoglou *et al*. [28] added 0.05 to 0.1g/kg of oregano extract in broiler chicken feed and record a high antioxidant impact in the broiler tissues. Yanishlieva *et al*. [34] recorded that thymol had the highest antioxidant effect than other active compounds at the tough condition of temperatures and during lipids oxidation. Youdim and Deans [35] found that thymol supplemented in the feed of aging rats significantly increased the effects of antioxidant enzymes GSH-Px and SOD in the brain. Likewise, Lin *et al*. [36] noticed that chickens fed on diets supplied by herbal extracts had activated antioxidant enzymes (SOD and GSH PX) and a decreased MDA concentration. Hydroxyl group in phenolic compounds of herbal extract decreased the proxy radicals and which is formed during lipid oxidation. In this regard, Luna *et al*. [37] noticed that thymol or carvacrol inhibits lipid oxidation in the diet supplied with them than any other synthetic compounds. In addition to such beneficial effects, thymol has been suggested to have anticancer activity *in vitro* on leukemia cell line HL-60 [38].

Antimicrobial Activity

The thyme EO and thymol had an antimicrobial impact *in vivo* and *in vitro* against a wide spectrum of bacteria [3]. Several essential oils and their effective compounds, such as resveratrol carvacrol, eugenol, and thymol, had no risk on the health of the consumer, and they have been registered by the European Commission [31, 39, 40]. The antimicrobial activity of effective EOs maybe because of the phenolic content, *e.g*., resveratrol, eugenol cinnamaldehyde, curcumin, thymol, and carvacrol which were extracted from the following thyme, oregano, turmeric, clove and cinnamon and other herbs [31, 41 - 44].

Nevas *et al*. [45] recorded that oregano, savory, and thyme EOs with high concentrations of carvacrol and thymol, generally inhibit gram positive (G+) more than gram negative (G-) pathogenic bacteria ex. *Salmonella typhimurium* and *Listeria monocytogenes* [46]. As previously described, Johny *et al*. [47] recorded that thymol molecule diminished *C. jejuni* and *Salmonella enteritidis* in the cecum of broiler chicks. In addition, Arsi *et al*. [48] noted that campylobacter numbers were decreased by adding thymol and carvacrol by 0.5%. Sokovic *et al*. [49, 50] and Lu and Wu [51] reported the thymol's antimicrobial activity against many species of harmful microorganisms such as *Pseudomonas, Aspergillus, Streptococci, Bacillus, Fusarium Listeria*, and *Salmonella*. Pinto *et al*. [52] noticed that thymol EO acted as an antifungal agent by inducing a major reduction of the ergosterol concentration in the cytoplasmic membrane.

Antiviral Activity

Herbal plants and extracts as cold-pressed essential oils have been reported to possess antiviral activities [49]. *Carum copticum* oil was found to inhibit virus particles and protect the host cells. Also, monoterpenes and thymol EO inhibited herpes simplex virus (HSV) [53]. Also, antiviral drugs and essential oils had low toxicity with their antiviral activities as they could decrease the production of the virus *via* decreasing the synthesis of viral DNA or RNA [46].

RESVERATROL

Natural Sources

Resveratrol is found in grapevines, mulberries, strawberry raspberries, red grapes (*Vitis* spp.), and in other fruits as Japanese knotweed (*Polygonumcuspidatum*) berries (blueberries, cranberries, and lingonberries, all *Vaccinium*spp.), yucca (*yucca shidigera*) peanuts (*Arachis* spp.), and turmeric (*Curcuma longa*) [54]. Also, Yao *et al.* [55] stated that resveratrol is present in *Gnetumcleistostachyum*, *Dracaena loureiro, Cassia* spp., mulberry (*Morus* spp., *Maclurapomifera*, *Nothofagusfusca* spp.), and red sandalwood (*Pterocarpus* spp., a major source of pterostilbene). In addition to natural sources, resveratrol can be produced by chemical synthesis [56] and by biotechnological synthesis (metabolic engineered microorganisms) [57, 58]. Resveratrol is highly lipophilic and hydrophilic, causing antioxidant action more than vitamins C and E [59]. The structural formula of resveratrol is shown in Fig. (2).

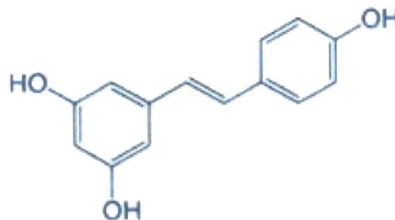

Fig. (2). The basic structural formula of resveratrol.

BIOLOGICAL ACTIVITIES AND MECHANISMS

The mode of action is not clear, but it was shown to be similar to the biochemical effects of calorie restriction. Some researchers noticed that resveratrol activated Sirtuin1 (a protein functions in the cellular response to inflammatory, metabolic, and oxidative stressors), peroxisome proliferator-activated receptor-gamma coactivator-1-alpha (PGC-1α; a master regulator of mitochondrial biogenesis), and improved the function of the mitochondria [60]. It could increase the activity of MnSOD (SOD_2) that converted superoxide O_2 (a respiration residue in complexes 1 and 3 of the electron chain reaction) into H_2O_2. SOD_2 can reduce the superoxides caused by pancreatic cancer, mitochondrial dysfunction, permeability transition, and apoptotic death in various diseases [61] and can provide resistance to irradiation damage and reperfusion injury [62]. It has been reported to up-regulate antioxidant enzymes such as (GSH-Px, SOD, and CAT) with a slight change in CAT or GSH-Px; these activities resulted in H_2O_2 accumulation in mitochondria that stimulate cancer cell apoptosis [2]. Resveratrol stopped the carcinogenesis at the different stages (initiation, promotion, and progression) in addition to the modulation of the NF-kB transcription factor [63]. *In vitro*, resveratrol has been shown to cause apoptosis in some lines of the cancer cell cultures and had a beneficial effect against neuronal cell death, and maybe effective against diseases such as Alzheimer's disease and Huntington in addition to its inhibitory effect on cardiac fibroblasts and cardiac fibrosis progression [64, 65].

Moreover, resveratrol can increase the secretion of natural testosterone by acting as a modulator of estrogen receptors [66] and an aromatase inhibitor [67, 68]. Olas and Wachowicz [69] reported that resveratrol can inhibit ROS production and lipid peroxidation better than vitamin E [4].

METABOLISM, BIOSYNTHESIS, AND BIOAVAILABILITY

Resveratrol existed in small amounts in plants. Resveratrol is one of the protective molecules called phytoalexin, which could protect against infection and ultraviolet irradiation damaging [70, 71]. Resveratrol is toxic to many plant pathogens, but fungi overcome this toxicity by their cell membranes which can expel the compound outside the cell [72]. Resveratrol is vulnerable to oxidative deprivation, but its association with glycosyl formed glycosylated resveratrol that could maintain its biological activity to be more stable and soluble, therefore, be easily absorbed by the intestine and metabolized in the liver and lungs. To discover the metabolic pathway and the bioavailability of resveratrol, several research strategies, including *in vivo* and laboratory methods, were used. Approximately 75 percent of this polyphenol is excreted through urinary excretion. Resveratrol's oral bioavailability is nearly negligible due to the quick and extensive metabolism which produced resveratrol glucuronides and resveratrol sulfates metabolites [73]. In future investigations, the possible biological activity of resveratrol conjugates should be considered. Resveratrol's oral bioavailability is independent of dosage and aqueous solubility [74].

Antioxidant Activity and Role in Poultry Nutrition

Previously, several trials were performed to assess resveratrol's dependence and functionality in poultry and animal foods. Pisoschi *et al.* [68] vaccinated mice with an extreme dose (20 mg/kg for 20 d) of resveratrol and various herbal extracts such as thyme, oregano; and cinnamon and they noticed no inverse effects on diet consumption, growth rate, biochemical and hematological parameters as well as histological changes. On the other hand, the MDA levels in the liver were decreased after vaccination with different concentrations of resveratrol (0.005,0.02,0.05 g/kg of diet), while the IgG, GSH-Px, and SOD levels were increased in the serum of mice and pigs compared to the control [75, 76]. Alexander *et al.* [77] reported that diet with resveratrol decreased the weight by a simultaneous decrease in energy consumption by13% and a 29% increase in the metabolic rest rate. Resveratrol (200 mg/kg/day) could prevent the depth of daily inactivity, which is an important energy-saving process.

Changes in FCR were observed with the application of resveratrol to the diets of pigs [78]. In the same sense, Viveros *et al.* [79] reported that grapes' phenolic compounds succeeded in raising the ideal populations of useful bacteria and crypt depth: villus height ratio at the broiler jejunum. Such details may have a principle influence on intestinal physiology and biochemistry.

The supplementation of resveratrol to diet (0.2 or 0.4 g/kg diets) did not affect food intake, egg development or outdoor and indoor egg quality standards related to the shell, yolk, and albumen in quail layers excluding yolk widths during the period from 4 to 16 weeks of age [80]. Conversely, resveratrol-supplemented quail diets resulted in lower levels of liver heat shock protein (Hsp70), blood and yolk malondialdehyde (MDA), and higher concentrations of blood vitamin E than diets without resveratrol.

Poultry feed supplemented with pure antioxidants significantly decreased MDA levels in meat, egg yolk, and blood serum, thereby enhancing the oxidative stability of eggs and meat [81 - 83]. Sgambato *et al.* [84], indicated that resveratrol plays a defensive role against different stressors especially oxidative stress. The scavenging activity of resveratrol could increase several antioxidant enzymes activities, such as SOD and GSH-Px to cope with the metal-induced hydroxyl and superoxide radicals [85]. It also can activate erythroid-derived nuclear factor, a major transcription factor that regulates antioxidant response [86]. Similarly, earlier research suggested that dietary resveratrol decreased the MDA levels and increased the activity of serum antioxidant enzymes [87]. Das [74]; Sahin *et al.* [87]; Liu *et al.* [83], reported that resveratrol has been reported to protect the organism from the stress of oxidation by enhancing antioxidant capacity to resist thermal stress, UV radiation, lipopolysaccharide, and ethanol-induced oxidative stresses by inhibiting reactive oxygen species [74, 87]. Moreover, chicken supported with resveratrol (0.2, 0.4, or 0.6 mg/kg diet) showed increased meat quality and quantity and increased antioxidant enzymes, insulin growth factor 1, growth hormone, concentration and the growth of immune organs (fabricius spleen, thymus) compared to the control during heat stress but the feed conversion rate and MDA levels were decreased [83, 88].. Sridhar *et al.* [89] reported that reseveratrol at 0.5 and 1.0% of birds' diet decreased the feed intake during 4-5 weeks of age without affecting the feed conversion ratio.. The broiler diets supplemented with resveratrol improved the birds' antioxidant status and reduced liver damage. Pisoschi *et al.* [68]; Moon *et al.* [78] The supplementation of piglets diet with resveratrol (0.2%) increased the FCR and serum IgG concentration but, the amount of TNF-α was reduced against control and enhanced the immunity, growth efficiency, and fecal microbial shedding of tiny piglets [68, 78].

Momchilova *et al.* [90] found that resveratrol supplementation decreased unsaturated: saturated fatty acids ratio in glycerophospholipids membrane, reduced the ROS and lipid peroxide concentration without affecting the GSH content in hepatocytes. Kucinska *et al.* [91] found that the activity of anti-apoptotic proteins, caspase 3 and 9, was increased with increasing the resveratrol level in the diet, indicating the ability of resveratrol to act as anti-apoptosis factor during stress such as oxidative stress, deficiency of glutathione, as well as the loss of mRNA.

The supplementation with resveratrol (700 µg/kg) improved bone mineral density and reduced the loss of femur calcium associated with an estrogen deficiency [75]. Zhai *et al.* [2] stated that resveratrol inhibited Fe^{++} activated lipid peroxidation primarily through the lipid peroxyl radicals' reduction. Aburjai [92] suggested that rhaponticin and trans-resveratrol-3-O-β-D-glucopyranoside from *Rheum palaestinum* exhibited antiplatelet activity; however, the inhibitory effects of both compounds on platelet aggregation were lower compared with resveratrol. Resveratrol has been found to be able to reserve the cardiovascular damage caused by obesity and chronic hypertension and can provide a protection against congestive heart failure [87, 93].

CARVACROL

Carvacrol Origin

Carvacrol is found in medical plants, such as *Monarda didyma, Satureja hortensis, Origanum dictamnus, Origanum compactum, Nigella sativa, Origanum onites, Origanum scabrum, Origanum vulgare and thyme Origanum microphyllum* [94, 95]. Besides, cymophenol which is chemically synthesized by the metabolism of microorganisms [4, 96].

Carvacrol's Chemical Formula and Properties

Carvacrol is lyophilic thymol with a density ranged from 0.975 to 0.976g/ml at 20° C to 25° C and its melting point is 1 [97]. Carvacrol (cymophenol) is a monoterpenoid phenoliccompound, with the chemical structure $C_6H_3CH_3$ (OH) (C_3H_7), [78, 94]. According to IUPAC is so-called 5-isopropyl-2-methyl phenol or 2-Methyl-5-(1-methyl ethyl)-phenol. The structural formula of carvacrol is shown in Fig. (**3**).

BIOLOGICAL ACTIVITIES' MECHANISMS

The use of plant additives in feed showed good effects, improved the secretion of digestive enzymes, and increased the digestive system motilityand served as an antioxidant, antimicrobial, immune-stimulator, anti-worming, anti-coccidiosis and anti-provocative [18]. Basmacioğlu-Malayoğlu *et al.* [98] confirmed the efficacy of plant extracts or EOs active compounds as antimicrobial and antioxidants *in vitro* or *in vivo*, but the mechanics of these additives, the optimal dose, and their nutritional demonstration are still unknown in poultry. In addition, carvacrol can be added to non-alcoholic drinks (0.028g/kg), baked goods (0.015g/kg), chewing gum (0.0084g/kg) *etc.* [3]. Nevertheless, this compound's mode of action has been unknown to researchers. Therefore, increasing the knowledge about the carvacrol mechanism is very important to be applicable in nutrition modes of action. Some of the reported carvacrol's modes of action and beneficial aspects are shown in Fig. (**4**).

METABOLISM AND EXCRETION

Carvacrol's main metabolic pathway is associated with the esterification of the glucuronic acid $(C_6H_{10}O_7)$ and sulfuric acid (H_2SO_4) phenolic group. Additionally, converting the end methyl groups into primary alcohols is a minor route of carvacrol metabolism. Austgulen *et al.* [99] reported that rats excreted a significant percentage (0.001mol/kg) of carvacrol conjugated with glucuronide in urine and resulting in benzyl alcohol derivatives. A small metabolite was also found resulting from ring hydroxylation. However, after just one day, carvacrol residue in urine was very small; this finding is a good indication of carvacrol metabolism at a high rate and also the excretion of it began from day one.

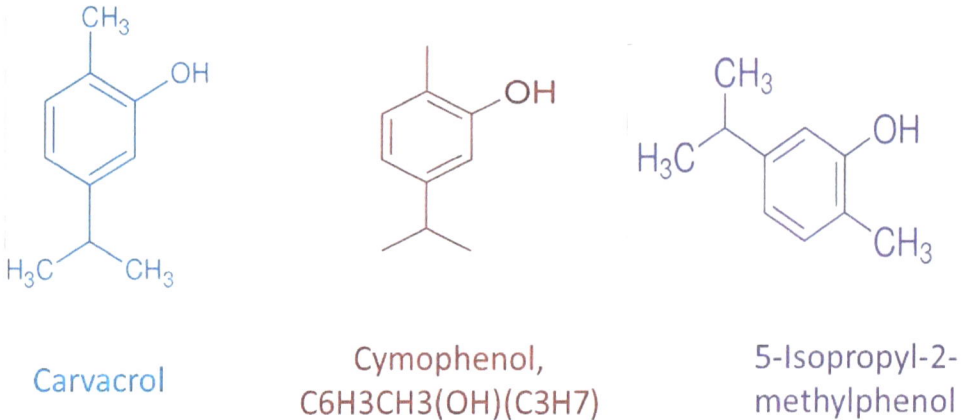

Carvacrol

Cymophenol,
C6H3CH3(OH)(C3H7)

5-Isopropyl-2-
methylphenol

Fig. (3). Basic structural formula of carvacrol and its derivative.

Several experiments with pig showed that carvacrol was degraded in cecum at 29%, whereas jejunum was not affected. When piglets feed with 12.5, 12.7, 13.0, and 13.2 mg carvacrol/kg body weight, showed half the amounts in the entire digestive tract between 1.84 and 2.05 hours. Carvacrol was easily absorbed in the stomach and intestine. The plasma concentrations (conjugated and free compounds) reached the maximum at 1.39 hours then urine concentrations were increased [100].

BENEFICIAL CHARACTERISTICS OF CARVACROL

Growth Performance and Nutrients Bioavailability

The thymol and carvacrol mixture in the broiler chicks at 0.06, 0.1, and 0.2 g/kg increased the efficiency of the growth and the activities of and antioxidants enzymes [29]. Jamroz and Kamel [101], daily observation of reported that supplementation of carvacrol at 0.3 g/kg in poultry feed improved the feed conversion (%) and body weight ratio by 8.1 and 7.7%, respectively. Lee *et al.* [26] stated that using carvacrol and thymol improved feed efficiency and growth performance due to their beneficial effects on digestion.

Jaafari *et al.* [102] observed an increase in the weight of broilers fed on raw or cholesterol-rich food supplemented with carvacrol (200 ppm) but feed intake, feed conversion and triglycerides levels in the plasma were decreased with no effect on the cholesterol content. When carvacrol (200 ppm/kg) was supplemented to a soy and corn diet containing methyl carboxyl cellulose, the cholesterol production or its plasma content was not significantly affected, while a negative effect on the body weight of broilers was reported [103]. Umaya and Manpal [104] found that supplementation of broilers diet with carvacrol at five ppm for seven days increased the body weight, and decreased the intestinal lesions significantly. The carvacrol supplementation in broilers regulated estrogen, fat, and androgen in intestinal lymphocytes. Nutritional supplement with carvacrol at five ppm/kg to chickens changes 74 genes expression in the lymphocytes. Carvacrol led to increased regulation of many metabolisms and endocrine genes, such as Celine Protein X (SEPX1) and Protein Serene 3 (PRSS3) [100] however more studies must be done to explain and simplify the carvacrol molecular mechanism in the chicken's gastrointestinal system.

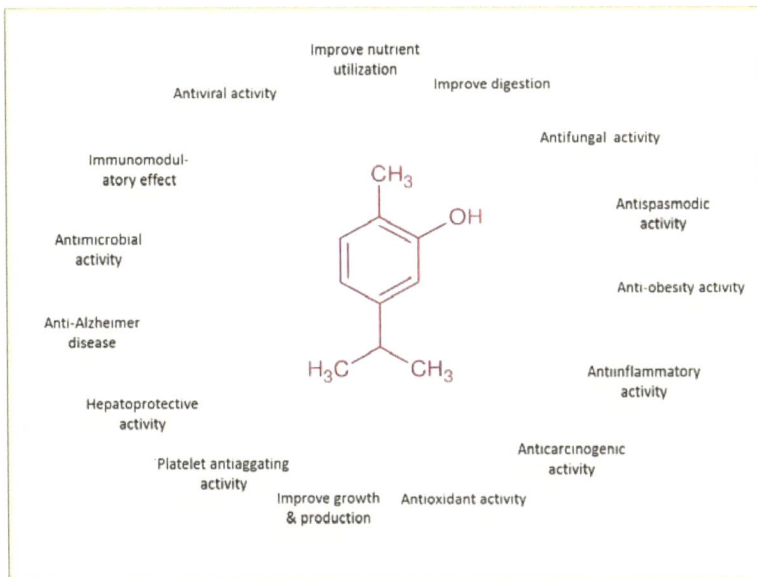

Fig. (4). Modes of action and biological activities of carvacrol.

Over recent decades, public concern has been raised about the meat quality and quantity. Poultry meat is high in soft lipids; therefore, it is vulnerable to oxidative degradation that adversely affects the quality of meat. Broilers chicken fed a diet with carvacrol (150 ppm) for 42 days, induced a decrease the development of thiobarbituric acid (the indicator of lipid oxidation) in the meat samples after 5-10 days of storage. Similar findings were obtained by Yanishlieva *et al.* [34]; Hu *et al.* [95] showed that carvacrol fortification reduced microbial load and lipid oxidation in cold preserved chicken patties, as well as improved the poultry meat consistency. Therefore, carvacrol can be recommended to be used as a natural anti-oxidant.

Antiviral Activity

Sokovic *et al*. [49] stated that the EOs and herbal extracts including carvacrol showed antiviral activity against human respiratory syncytial virus (HRSV) and rotavirus (RV). Also, the extract and oil from Mexican oregano (*Lippia graveolens*) can reduce/inhibit animal viral diseases. . Pisoschi *et al*. [68] reported that phenolic compounds in carvacrol and oregano EOs showed antiviral activity against multiple viral diseases, such as RV, norovirus, and H1N1 and other influenza viruses [68, 95].

Antimicrobial Activity

The thyme, clove, turmeric, cinnamon, and oregano EOs have antimicrobial properties due to phenolic compounds content, such as eugenol, thymol, curcumin, cinnamaldehyde, and carvacrol. Alagawany *et al*. [31], Veldhuizen *et al*. [105], Hu *et al*. [95] explained that the antimicrobial mechanism of phenolic compounds is mainly due to the hydrophobicity of these compounds when interacting with the cell membrane of microorganism.

Arsi *et al*. [48] reported a reduction in campylobacter numbers with carvacrol supplementation of 1 percent or the mixing of carvacrol and thymol at 0.5 percent. Sokovic *et al*. [50] and Baser [106], observed carvacrol's antimicrobial effects against multiple microbial species such as *Listeria, Bacillus, Salmonella, Aspergillus, Pseudomonas, Streptococci*, and others. Burt *et al*. [107, 108] found that cymophenol supplements could extremely inhibit the growth of various harmful bacteria like *Escherichia coli* and salmonella, which infect chickens due to the carvacrol vapor.

Cymophenol Scavenging Activity

Cells produce reactive oxygen intermediates or free radicals during normal metabolism. The excessive accumulation of free radicals as (H_2O_2 $O_2^{\cdot-}$, OH) resulted in tissue damage and the loss of many cellular functions. The antioxidant carvacrol can scavenge free radicals from the cells in addition to inhibiting the synthesis of prostaglandin and inducing drug-metabolizing enzymes [109].

Carvacrol's efficacy in ripping free radicals, *i.e.*, peroxyl radicals' hydrogen peroxide, superoxide radicals, and nitric oxide has been also reported by Aristatile *et al*. [110].

Immunomodulatory Effect

Improving the poultry immunity is important aim for combating any infectious diseases. Acamovic and Brooker [32] reported that thyme and carvacrol (flavonoid-rich herbs) could boost immunity because of their antioxidant activities and enhancing the vitamin C activity. Similarly, Botsoglou *et al.* [28] suggested that carvacrol could increase the chicks' immunity due to its antiviral, antibacterial, and antioxidant activities. Stevanovic *et al.* [100] noted that supplementing the bird's diets with phenol-derivatives such as thymol, carvacrol, capsicum, oleoresin, and cinnamaldehyde significantly increased the resistant of chickens aganist infectious diseases of poultry. Moreover, Hashemipour *et al.* [29] stated that poultry fed on diets containing carvacrol, and thymol showed improved primary and secondary responses to antigen IgG and sheep red blood cells (SRBC).

Anti-Tumor Effects

Plant antioxidants like carvacrol have anti-carcinogenic and anti-aggregating effects on platelets [111]. Also, Karkabounas *et al.* [112] confirmed the carvacrol anticancer and antiplatelet impacts both *in vivo* and *in vitro* as in case of pulmonary tumors, and hepatocellular carcinoma. Yin *et al.* [113] reported that the supplementation by carvacrol induced the expression of caspase-3, -6, or-9 proteins and genomic DNA fragmentations.

Hepatoprotective Effect

Aristatile *et al.* [114] observed that the addition of carvacrol (0.08 mg/kg) to rats' diet reduced lipid peroxidation in liver, kidney and blood plasma and restored the level of liver enzymes to their common value. Researchers also reported that the carvacrol treatment fixed the DNA damage and the reduction in D-galactosamin- -induced mitochondrial enzymes, and enhanced liver antioxidants and by reducing the lipid oxidation [115].

ANTI-HYPERNOCICEPTIVE AND ANTI-INFLAMMATORY PROPERTIES

The hypernociception is the hypersensitivity of nociceptive pathways that causing inflammatory hyperalgesia.. Trabace *et al.* [116] suggested that regular administration of carvacrol (0.05 and 0.1g/kg) against indomethacin increased the threshold response of mice exposed to carrageenan. Marchand *et al.* [117] described that the carvacrol can prevent the migration of single neutrophil cells resulting from the development of cellular inflammation and reduce prostaglandins and nitric oxide. Cell morphology was not affected by carvacrol treatment except for a decrease in the levels of tumor necrosis factor alpha (TNF-α) in pleura. Guimaraes *et al*. [118] found that reducing the activation of nitric oxide synthase and, in turn, the nitric oxide macrophages lead to the anti-hypernociceptive effect of carvacrol. However, Marchand *et al*. [117] had conflicting reports about including carvacrol's antioxidant role in reducing lipid peroxidation and nitric oxides within hypernociception. Carvacrol decreased gene expression of inflammatory cytokines in birds affected *Eimeria acervulina* [3].

Anti-Obesity Effect

Overweightness is a disease of accumulating extra fat of the body to the point that it can have a detrimental impact on the physical condition, contributing to bigger health complications; *e.g*., hyperlipidemia, tumors, and diabetes. Umaya and Manpal [104] reported that eating fatty food is the major reason for increasing obesity and animal metabolic diseases, and they found that carvacrol reduced the accumulation of intercellular fat and fat cell differentiation in 3T3 -L1 mouse embryo cells. The results also showed that a carbohydrate-rich fat diet reduced plasma total cholesterol and total visceral fat in mice. Besides, carvacrol reduced the gene expression responsible for forming lipids in visceral adipose tissue. Stevanovic *et al*. [100] stated that carvacrol reduced levels of free fatty acids and RNA levels.

CONCLUDING REMARKS

Many studies explored the usage and nature of essential oils in poultry nutrition. The active compounds in EOs exhibited antioxidant, antimicrobial, anticancer, and anti-inflammatory effects. Antioxidant properties of EOs increased body weight and other growth and productive performance traits. The biological activity of a mixture of EOs needs more experiments because the effect of these compounds on poultry nutrition is still insufficient to reach the optimum level of the extract.

CONSENT FOR PUBLICATION

Not applicable.

CONFLICT OF INTEREST

The author declares no conflict of interest, financial or otherwise.

ACKNOWLEDGEMENTS

Declared none.

REFERENCES

[1]   Brenes A, Roura E. Essential oils in poultry nutrition: Main effects and modes of action. Anim Feed Sci Technol 2010; 158(1-2): 1-4.
[http://dx.doi.org/10.1016/j.anifeedsci.2010.03.007]

[2]   Zhai H, Liu H, Wang S, Wu J, Kluenter AM. Potential of essential oils for poultry and pigs. Anim Nutr 2018; 4(2): 179-86.
[http://dx.doi.org/10.1016/j.aninu.2018.01.005] [PMID: 30140757]

[3]   Sadhasivam S, Shapiro OH, Ziv C, Barda O, Zakin V, Sionov E. Synergistic Inhibition of Mycotoxigenic Fungi and Mycotoxin Production by Combination of Pomegranate Peel Extract and Azole Fungicide. Front Microbiol 2019; 10: 1919.
[http://dx.doi.org/10.3389/fmicb.2019.01919] [PMID: 31481948]

[4]   Loi M, Paciolla C, Logrieco AF, Mulè G. Plant Bioactive Compounds in Pre- and Postharvest Management for Aflatoxins Reduction. Front Microbiol 2020; 11: 243.
[http://dx.doi.org/10.3389/fmicb.2020.00243] [PMID: 32226415]

[5]   Abd El-Hack ME, Mahgoub SA, Alagawany M, Dhama K. Influences of dietary supplementation of antimicrobial cold pressed oils mixture on growth performance and intestinal microflora of growing Japanese quails. Int J Pharmacol 2015; 11: 689-96.
[http://dx.doi.org/10.3923/ijp.2015.689.696]

[6]   Mathlouthi N, Bouzaienne T, Oueslati I, *et al.* Use of rosemary, oregano, and a commercial blend of essential oils in broiler chickens: *in vitro* antimicrobial activities and effects on growth performance. J Anim Sci 2012; 90(3): 813-23.
[http://dx.doi.org/10.2527/jas.2010-3646] [PMID: 22064737]

[7]   Alp M, Midilli M, Kocaba NL, *et al.* The effects of dietary oregano essential oil on live performance, carcass yield, serum immunoglobulin G level, and oocyst count in broilers. J Appl Poult Res 2012; 21: 630-6.
[http://dx.doi.org/10.3382/japr.2012-00551]

[8]   Chaves Lobón N, Ferrer de la Cruz I, Alías Gallego JC. Autotoxicity of diterpenes present in leaves of *Cistus ladanifer* L. Plants (Basel) 2019; 8(2): 27.
[http://dx.doi.org/10.3390/plants8020027] [PMID: 30678267]

[9]   Jang IS, Ko HY, Kang SY, Lee CY. Effect of commercial essential oils on growth performance, digestive enzyme activity and intestinal microflora population in broiler chickens. Anim Feed Sci Technol 2007; 134: 305-15.
[http://dx.doi.org/10.1016/j.anifeedsci.2006.06.009]

[10]   Basmacioğlu-Malayoğlu H, Özdemir P, Bağriyanik HA. Influence of an organic acid blend and essential oil blend, individually or in combination, on growth performance, carcass parameters, apparent digestibility, intestinal microflora and intestinal morphology of broilers. Br Poult Sci 2016; 57(2): 227-34.
[http://dx.doi.org/10.1080/00071668.2016.1141171] [PMID: 26785140]

[11]   Negera M, Washe AP. Use of natural dietary spices for reclamation of food quality impairment by aflatoxin. J Food Qual 2019; 4371206.
[http://dx.doi.org/10.1155/2019/4371206]

[12]   Oviedo-Rondón EO, Hume ME, Hernández C, Clemente-Hernández S. Intestinal microbial ecology of broilers vaccinated and challenged with mixed *Eimeria* species, and supplemented with essential oil

blends. Poult Sci 2006; 85(5): 854-60.
[http://dx.doi.org/10.1093/ps/85.5.854] [PMID: 16673762]

[13] Evans JW, Plunkett MS, Bandfield MJ. Effect of an essential oil blend on coccidiosis in broiler chicks. Poult Sci 2001; 80: 258. [abstract].

[14] Lee SJ, Umano K, Shibamoto T, Lee K. Identification of volatile components in basil (*Ocimum basilicum* L.) and thyme leaves (Thymus vulgaris L.) and their antioxidant properties. Food Chem 2005; 91(1): 131-7.
[http://dx.doi.org/10.1016/j.foodchem.2004.05.056]

[15] Tilford L. Gregory Edible and Medicinal Plants of the West. Missoula, MT: Mountain Press Publishing 1997.

[16] Norwitz G, Nataro N, Keliher PN. Study of the steam distillation of phenolic compounds using ultraviolent spectrometry. Anal Chem 1986; 58: 639-41.
[http://dx.doi.org/10.1021/ac00294a034]

[17] Nostro A, Blanco AR, Cannatelli MA, *et al.* Susceptibility of methicillin-resistant staphylococci to oregano essential oil, carvacrol and thymol. FEMS Microbiol Lett 2004; 230(2): 191-5.
[http://dx.doi.org/10.1016/S0378-1097(03)00890-5] [PMID: 14757239]

[18] Akyurek H, Yel A. Influence of dietary thymol and carvacrol preparation and/or an organic acid blend on growth performance, digestive organs and intestinal microbiota of broiler chickens. Afr J Microbiol Res 2011; 5: 979-84.
[http://dx.doi.org/10.5897/AJMR10.203]

[19] Farag MR, Alagawany MM, Dhama K. Antidotal effect of Turmeric (*Curcuma longa*) against endosulfan-induced cytogenotoxicity and immunotoxicity in broiler chicks. Int J Pharmacol 2014; 10: 429-39.
[http://dx.doi.org/10.3923/ijp.2014.429.439]

[20] Palaniappan K, Holley RA. Use of natural antimicrobials to increase antibiotic susceptibility of drug resistant bacteria. Int J Food Microbiol 2010; 140(2-3): 164-8.
[http://dx.doi.org/10.1016/j.ijfoodmicro.2010.04.001] [PMID: 20457472]

[21] Ahmad A, Khan A, Yousuf S, Khan LA, Manzoor N. Proton translocating ATPase mediated fungicidal activity of eugenol and thymol. Fitoterapia 2010; 81(8): 1157-62.
[http://dx.doi.org/10.1016/j.fitote.2010.07.020] [PMID: 20659536]

[22] Guo N, Liu J, Wu X, *et al.* Antifungal activity of thymol against clinical isolates of fluconazole-sensitive and -resistant *Candida albicans*. J Med Microbiol 2009; 58(Pt 8): 1074-9.
[http://dx.doi.org/10.1099/jmm.0.008052-0] [PMID: 19528168]

[23] Mezzoug N, Elhadri A, Dallouh A, *et al.* Investigation of the mutagenic and antimutagenic effects of Origanum compactum essential oil and some of its constituents. Mutat Res 2007; 629(2): 100-10.
[http://dx.doi.org/10.1016/j.mrgentox.2007.01.011] [PMID: 17383930]

[24] Andersen A. Final report on the safety assessment of sodium p-chloro-m-cresol, p-chloro-m-cresol, chlorothymol, mixed cresols, m-cresol, o-cresol, p-cresol, isopropyl cresols, thymol, o-cymen-5-ol, and carvacrol. Int J Toxicol 2006; 25(1) (Suppl. 1): 29-127.
[PMID: 16835130]

[25] Platel K, Srinivasan K. Digestive stimulant action of spices: a myth or reality? Indian J Med Res 2004; 119(5): 167-79.
[PMID: 15218978]

[26] Lee KW, Everts H, Kappert HJ, Frehner M, Losa R, Beynen AC. Effects of dietary essential oil components on growth performance, digestive enzymes and lipid metabolism in female broiler chickens. Br Poult Sci 2003; 44(3): 450-7. a
[http://dx.doi.org/10.1080/0007166031000085508] [PMID: 12964629]

[27] Cross DE, McDevitt RM, Hillman K, Acamovic T. The effect of herbs and their associated essential

oils on performance, dietary digestibility and gut microflora in chickens from 7 to 28 days of age. Br Poult Sci 2007; 48(4): 496-506.
[http://dx.doi.org/10.1080/00071660701463221] [PMID: 17701503]

[28]   Botsoglou NA, Florou-Paneri P, Christaki E, Fletouris DJ, Spais AB. Effect of dietary oregano essential oil on performance of chickens and on iron-induced lipid oxidation of breast, thigh and abdominal fat tissues. Br Poult Sci 2002; 43(2): 223-30.
[http://dx.doi.org/10.1080/00071660120121436] [PMID: 12047086]

[29]   Hashemipour H, Kermanshahi H, Golian A, Veldkamp T. Effect of thymol and carvacrol feed supplementation on performance, antioxidant enzyme activities, fatty acid composition, digestive enzyme activities, and immune response in broiler chickens. Poult Sci 2013; 92(8): 2059-69.
[http://dx.doi.org/10.3382/ps.2012-02685] [PMID: 23873553]

[30]   Ashour EA, Alagawany M, Reda FM, Abd El-Hack ME. Effect of supplementation of yucca schidigera extract to growing rabbit diets on growth performance, carcass characteristics, serum biochemistry and liver oxidative status. Asian J Anim Vet Adv 2014; 9: 732-42.
[http://dx.doi.org/10.3923/ajava.2014.732.742]

[31]   Alagawany MM, Farag MR, Dhama K. Nutritional and biological effects of turmeric (*Curcuma longa*) supplementation on performance, serum biochemical parameters and oxidative status of broiler chicks exposed to endosulfan in the diets. Asian J Anim Vet Adv 2015; 10: 86-96. b
[http://dx.doi.org/10.3923/ajava.2015.86.96]

[32]   Acamovic T, Brooker JD. Biochemistry of plant secondary metabolites and their effects in animals. Proc Nutr Soc 2005; 64(3): 403-12.
[http://dx.doi.org/10.1079/PNS2005449] [PMID: 16048675]

[33]   Influence of two plant extracts derived from thyme and cinnamon on broiler performance. Pak Vet J 2009; 29(4): 169-73.

[34]   Yanishlieva NV, Marinova EM, Gordon MH, Raneva VG. Antioxidant activity and mechanism of action of thymol and carvacrol in two lipid systems. Food Chem 1999; 64: 59-66.
[http://dx.doi.org/10.1016/S0308-8146(98)00086-7]

[35]   Youdim KA, Deans SG. Effect of thyme oil and thymol dietary supplementation on the antioxidant status and fatty acid composition of the ageing rat brain. Br J Nutr 2000; 83(1): 87-93.
[http://dx.doi.org/10.1017/S000711450000012X] [PMID: 10703468]

[36]   Lin CC, Wu SJ, Chang CH, Ng LT. Antioxidant activity of Cinnamomum cassia. Phytother Res 2003; 17(7): 726-30.
[http://dx.doi.org/10.1002/ptr.1190] [PMID: 12916067]

[37]   Luna A, Lábaque MC, Zygadlo JA, Marin RH. Effects of thymol and carvacrol feed supplementation on lipid oxidation in broiler meat. Poult Sci 2010; 89(2): 366-70.
[http://dx.doi.org/10.3382/ps.2009-00130] [PMID: 20075292]

[38]   Deb DD, Parimala G, Saravana Devi S, Chakraborty T. Effect of thymol on peripheral blood mononuclear cell PBMC and acute promyelotic cancer cell line HL-60. Chem Biol Interact 2011; 193(1): 97-106.
[http://dx.doi.org/10.1016/j.cbi.2011.05.009] [PMID: 21640085]

[39]   Alagawany MM, Farag MR, Dhama K, Abd El-Hack ME, Tiwari R, Alam GM. Mechanisms and beneficial applications of resveratrol as feed additive in animal and poultry nutrition: a review. Int J Pharmacol 2015; 11: 213-21. a
[http://dx.doi.org/10.3923/ijp.2015.213.221]

[40]   Burt S. Essential oils: their antibacterial properties and potential applications in foods--a review. Int J Food Microbiol 2004; 94(3): 223-53.
[http://dx.doi.org/10.1016/j.ijfoodmicro.2004.03.022] [PMID: 15246235]

[41]   Simitzis PE. Enrichment of animal diets with essential oils-a great perspective on improving animal

performance and quality characteristics of the derived products. Medicines (Basel) 2017; 4(2): 35.
[http://dx.doi.org/10.3390/medicines4020035] [PMID: 28930250]

[42]   Nieddu M, Rassu G, Boatto G, *et al.* Improvement of thymol properties by complexation with cyclodextrins: *in vitro* and *in vivo* studies. Carbohydr Polym 2014; 102(15): 393-9.
[http://dx.doi.org/10.1016/j.carbpol.2013.10.084] [PMID: 24507296]

[43]   Oskuee RK, Behravan J, Ramezani M. Chemical composition, antimicrobial activity and antiviral activity of essential oil of Carum copticum from Iran. Avicenna J Phytomed 2011; 1(2): 83-90.

[44]   Sánchez ME, Turina AV, García DA, Nolan MV, Perillo MA. Surface activity of thymol: implications for an eventual pharmacological activity. Colloids Surf B Biointerfaces 2004; 34(2): 77-86.
[http://dx.doi.org/10.1016/j.colsurfb.2003.11.007] [PMID: 15261077]

[45]   Nevas M, Korhonen AR, Lindström M, Turkki P, Korkeala H. Antibacterial efficiency of Finnish spice essential oils against pathogenic and spoilage bacteria. J Food Prot 2004; 67(1): 199-202.
[http://dx.doi.org/10.4315/0362-028X-67.1.199] [PMID: 14717375]

[46]   Dwivedy AK, Singh VK, Prakash B, Dubey NK. Nanoencapsulated Illicium verum Hook.f. essential oil as an effective novel plant-based preservative against aflatoxin B_1 production and free radical generation. Food Chem Toxicol 2018; 111: 102-13.
[http://dx.doi.org/10.1016/j.fct.2017.11.007] [PMID: 29126800]

[47]   Johny AK, Darre MJ, Donoghue AM, Donoghue DJ, Venkitanarayanan K. Antibacterial effect of trans-cinnamaldehyde, eugenol, carvacrol, and thymol on *Salmonella Enteritidis* and *Campylobacter jejuni* in chicken cecal contents *in vitro*. J Appl Poult Res 2010; 19(3): 237-44.
[http://dx.doi.org/10.3382/japr.2010-00181]

[48]   Arsi K, Donoghue AM, Venkitanarayanan K, *et al.* The efficacy of the natural plant extracts, thymol and carvacrol against campylobacter colonization in broiler chickens. J Food Saf 2014; 34(4): 321-5.
[http://dx.doi.org/10.1111/jfs.12129]

[49]   Soković M, Glamočlija J, Marin PD, Brkić D, van Griensven LJ. Antibacterial effects of the essential oils of commonly consumed medicinal herbs using an *in vitro* model. Molecules 2010; 15(11): 7532-46.
[http://dx.doi.org/10.3390/molecules15117532] [PMID: 21030907]

[50]   Soković M, Tzakou O, Pitarokili D, Couladis M. Antifungal activities of selected aromatic plants growing wild in Greece. Nahrung 2002; 46(5): 317-20.
[http://dx.doi.org/10.1002/1521-3803(20020901)46:5<317::AID-FOOD317>3.0.CO;2-B]   [PMID: 12428445]

[51]   Lu Y, Wu C. Reduction of *Salmonella enterica* contamination on grape tomatoes by washing with thyme oil, thymol, and carvacrol as compared with chlorine treatment. J Food Prot 2010; 73(12): 2270-5.
[http://dx.doi.org/10.4315/0362-028X-73.12.2270] [PMID: 21219747]

[52]   Pinto E, Pina-Vaz C, Salgueiro L, *et al.* Antifungal activity of the essential oil of *Thymus pulegioides* on Candida, Aspergillus and dermatophyte species. J Med Microbiol 2006; 55(Pt 10): 1367-73.
[http://dx.doi.org/10.1099/jmm.0.46443-0] [PMID: 17005785]

[53]   Astani A, Schnitzler P. Antiviral activity of monoterpenes beta-pinene and limonene against herpes simplex virus *in vitro*. Iran J Microbiol 2014; 6(3): 149-55.
[PMID: 25870747]

[54]   Sheu SJ, Liu NC, Ou CC, *et al.* Resveratrol stimulates mitochondrial bioenergetics to protect retinal pigment epithelial cells from oxidative damage. Physiol Pharmacol 2013; 54(9): 6426-37.
[http://dx.doi.org/10.1167/iovs.13-12024]

[55]   Yao CS, Lin M, Liu X, Wang YH. Stilbene derivatives from Gnetum cleistostachyum. J Asian Nat Prod Res 2005; 7(2): 131-7.
[http://dx.doi.org/10.1080/10286020310001625102] [PMID: 15621615]

[56] Farina A, Ferranti C, Marra C. An improved synthesis of resveratrol. Nat Prod Res 2006; 20(3): 247-52.
[http://dx.doi.org/10.1080/14786410500059532] [PMID: 16401555]

[57] Trantas E, Panopoulos N, Ververidis F. Metabolic engineering of the complete pathway leading to heterologous biosynthesis of various flavonoids and stilbenoids in *Saccharomyces cerevisiae*. Metab Eng 2009; 11(6): 355-66.
[http://dx.doi.org/10.1016/j.ymben.2009.07.004] [PMID: 19631278]

[58] Vuong TV, Franco C, Zhang W. Treatment strategies for high resveratrol induction in *Vitis vinifera* L. cell suspension culture. Biotechnol Rep (Amst) 2014; 1-2(2): 15-21.
[http://dx.doi.org/10.1016/j.btre.2014.04.002] [PMID: 28435798]

[59] Murcia MA, Martínez-Tomé M. Antioxidant activity of resveratrol compared with common food additives. J Food Prot 2001; 64(3): 379-84.
[http://dx.doi.org/10.4315/0362-028X-64.3.379] [PMID: 11252483]

[60] Alcaín FJ, Villalba JM. Sirtuin activators. Expert Opin Ther Pat 2009; 19(4): 403-14.
[http://dx.doi.org/10.1517/13543770902762893] [PMID: 19441923]

[61] Macmillan-Crow LA, Cruthirds DL. Invited review: manganese superoxide dismutase in disease. Free Radic Res 2001; 34(4): 325-36.
[http://dx.doi.org/10.1080/10715760100300281] [PMID: 11328670]

[62] Hu D, Cao P, Thiels E, *et al.* Hippocampal long-term potentiation, memory, and longevity in mice that overexpress mitochondrial superoxide dismutase. Neurobiol Learn Mem 2007; 87(3): 372-84.
[http://dx.doi.org/10.1016/j.nlm.2006.10.003] [PMID: 17129739]

[63] Leiro J, Arranz JA, Fraiz N, Sanmartín ML, Quezada E, Orallo F. Effect of cis-resveratrol on genes involved in nuclear factor kappa B signaling. Int Immunopharmacol 2005; 5(2): 393-406.
[http://dx.doi.org/10.1016/j.intimp.2004.10.006] [PMID: 15652768]

[64] Benitez DA, Pozo-Guisado E, Alvarez-Barrientos A, Fernandez-Salguero PM, Castellón EA. Mechanisms involved in resveratrol-induced apoptosis and cell cycle arrest in prostate cancer-derived cell lines. J Androl 2007; 28(2): 282-93.
[http://dx.doi.org/10.2164/jandrol.106.000968] [PMID: 17050787]

[65] Olson ER, Naugle JE, Zhang X, Bomser JA, Meszaros JG. Inhibition of cardiac fibroblast proliferation and myofibroblast differentiation by resveratrol. Am J Physiol Heart Circ Physiol 2005; 288(3): H1131-8.
[http://dx.doi.org/10.1152/ajpheart.00763.2004] [PMID: 15498824]

[66] Bhat KP, Lantvit D, Christov K, Mehta RG, Moon RC, Pezzuto JM. Estrogenic and antiestrogenic properties of resveratrol in mammary tumor models. Cancer Res 2001; 61(20): 7456-63.
[PMID: 11606380]

[67] Wang Y, Lee KW, Chan FL, Chen S, Leung LK. The red wine polyphenol resveratrol displays bilevel inhibition on aromatase in breast cancer cells. Toxicol Sci 2006; 92(1): 71-7.
[http://dx.doi.org/10.1093/toxsci/kfj190] [PMID: 16611627]

[68] Pisoschi AM, Pop A, Cimpeanu C, Predoi G. Antioxidant capacity determination in plants and plant-derived products: a review. Oxid Med Cell Longev 2016; 2016: 9130976.
[http://dx.doi.org/10.1155/2016/9130976] [PMID: 28044094]

[69] Olas B, Wachowicz B. Resveratrol, a phenolic antioxidant with effects on blood platelet functions. Platelets 2005; 16(5): 251-60.
[http://dx.doi.org/10.1080/09537100400020591] [PMID: 16011975]

[70] Stojanović S, Sprinz H, Brede O. Efficiency and mechanism of the antioxidant action of trans-resveratrol and its analogues in the radical liposome oxidation. Arch Biochem Biophys 2001; 391(1): 79-89.
[http://dx.doi.org/10.1006/abbi.2001.2388] [PMID: 11414688]

[71]   Dixon RA. Natural products and plant disease resistance. Nature 2001; 411(6839): 843-7.
[http://dx.doi.org/10.1038/35081178] [PMID: 11459067]

[72]   Sharan S, Nagar S. Pulmonary metabolism of resveratrol: *in vitro* and *in vivo* evidence. Drug Metab Dispos 2013; 41(5): 1163-9.
[http://dx.doi.org/10.1124/dmd.113.051326] [PMID: 23474649]

[73]   Wenzel E, Somoza V. Metabolism and bioavailability of trans-resveratrol. Mol Nutr Food Res 2005; 49(5): 472-81.
[http://dx.doi.org/10.1002/mnfr.200500010] [PMID: 15779070]

[74]   Das A. Heat stress-induced hepatotoxicity and its prevention by resveratrol in rats. Toxicol Mech Methods 2011; 21(5): 393-9.
[http://dx.doi.org/10.3109/15376516.2010.550016] [PMID: 21426263]

[75]   Liu ZP, Li WX, Yu B, *et al.* Effects of trans-resveratrol from Polygonum cuspidatum on bone loss using the ovariectomized rat model. J Med Food 2005; 8(1): 14-9.
[http://dx.doi.org/10.1089/jmf.2005.8.14] [PMID: 15857203]

[76]   Hao Ren, Yu Fei, Zhao Yue1, *et al.* Effects of resveratrol on lipid peroxidation in mice with high fat and high cholesterol diet. Chin Med J 2011; 40(1): 17-25.

[77]   Dal-Pan A, Blanc S, Aujard F. Resveratrol suppresses body mass gain in a seasonal non-human primate model of obesity. BMC Physiol 2010; 10: 11.
[http://dx.doi.org/10.1186/1472-6793-10-11] [PMID: 20569453]

[78]   Moon YS, Lee HS, Lee SE. Inhibitory effects of three monoterpenes from ginger essential oil on growth and aflatoxin production of *Aspergillus flavus* and their gene regulation in aflatoxin biosynthesis. Appl Biol Chem 2018; 61: 243-50.
[http://dx.doi.org/10.1007/s13765-018-0352-x]

[79]   Viveros A, Chamorro S, Pizarro M, Arija I, Centeno C, Brenes A. Effects of dietary polyphenol-rich grape products on intestinal microflora and gut morphology in broiler chicks. Poult Sci 2011; 90(3): 566-78.
[http://dx.doi.org/10.3382/ps.2010-00889] [PMID: 21325227]

[80]   Sahin K, Akdemir F, Orhan C, Tuzcu M, Hayirli A, Sahin N. Effects of dietary resveratrol supplementation on egg production and antioxidant status. Poult Sci 2010; 89(6): 1190-8.
[http://dx.doi.org/10.3382/ps.2010-00635] [PMID: 20460666]

[81]   Guo Y, Tang Q, Yuan J, Jiang Z. Effects of supplementation with vitamin E on the performance and the tissue peroxidation of broiler chicks and the stability of thigh meat against oxidative deterioration. Anim Feed Sci Technol 2001; 89: 165-73.
[http://dx.doi.org/10.1016/S0377-8401(00)00228-5]

[82]   Sahin N, Akdemir F, Orhan C, Kucuk O, Hayirli A, Sahin K. Lycopene enriched quail egg as functional food for humans. Food Res Int 2008; 41: 295-300.
[http://dx.doi.org/10.1016/j.foodres.2007.12.006]

[83]   Liu LL, He JH, Xie HB, Yang YS, Li JC, Zou Y. Resveratrol induces antioxidant and heat shock protein mRNA expression in response to heat stress in black-boned chickens. Poult Sci 2014; 93(1): 54-62.
[http://dx.doi.org/10.3382/ps.2013-03423] [PMID: 24570423]

[84]   Sgambato A, Ardito R, Faraglia B, Boninsegna A, Wolf FI, Cittadini A. Resveratrol, a natural phenolic compound, inhibits cell proliferation and prevents oxidative DNA damage. Mutat Res 2001; 496(1-2): 171-80.
[http://dx.doi.org/10.1016/S1383-5718(01)00232-7] [PMID: 11551493]

[85]   López-Vélez M, Martínez-Martínez F, Del Valle-Ribes C. The study of phenolic compounds as natural antioxidants in wine. Crit Rev Food Sci Nutr 2003; 43(3): 233-44.
[http://dx.doi.org/10.1080/727072831] [PMID: 12822671]

[86]   Rubiolo JA, Mithieux G, Vega FV. Resveratrol protects primary rat hepatocytes against oxidative stress damage: activation of the Nrf2 transcription factor and augmented activities of antioxidant enzymes. Eur J Pharmacol 2008; 591(1-3): 66-72.
[http://dx.doi.org/10.1016/j.ejphar.2008.06.067] [PMID: 18616940]

[87]   Sahin K, Orhan C, Akdemir F, Tuzcu M, Iben C, Sahin N. Resveratrol protects quail hepatocytes against heat stress: modulation of the Nrf2 transcription factor and heat shock proteins. J Anim Physiol Anim Nutr (Berl) 2012; 96(1): 66-74.
[http://dx.doi.org/10.1111/j.1439-0396.2010.01123.x] [PMID: 21244525]

[88]   Kalli V, Kollia E, Roidaki A, Proestos C, Markaki P. Cistus incanus L. extract inhibits aflatoxin B1 production by *Aspergillus parasiticus* in macadamia nuts. Ind Crops Prod 2018; 111: 63-8.
[http://dx.doi.org/10.1016/j.indcrop.2017.10.003]

[89]   Sridhar M, Suganthi RU, Thammiaha V. Effect of dietary resveratrol in ameliorating aflatoxin B1-induced changes in broiler birds. J Anim Physiol Anim Nutr (Berl) 2015; 99(6): 1094-104.
[http://dx.doi.org/10.1111/jpn.12260] [PMID: 25319220]

[90]   Momchilova A, Petkova D, Staneva G, *et al.* Resveratrol alters the lipid composition, metabolism and peroxide level in senescent rat hepatocytes. Chem Biol Interact 2014; 207(207): 74-80.
[http://dx.doi.org/10.1016/j.cbi.2013.10.016] [PMID: 24183824]

[91]   Kucinska M, Piotrowska H, Luczak MW, *et al.* Effects of hydroxylated resveratrol analogs on oxidative stress and cancer cells death in human acute T cell leukemia cell line: prooxidative potential of hydroxylated resveratrol analogs. Chem Biol Interact 2014; 209(25): 96-110.
[http://dx.doi.org/10.1016/j.cbi.2013.12.009] [PMID: 24398169]

[92]   Aburjai TA. Anti-platelet stilbenes from aerial parts of Rheum palaestinum. Phytochemistry 2000; 55(5): 407-10.
[http://dx.doi.org/10.1016/S0031-9422(00)00341-1] [PMID: 11140601]

[93]   Santos AC, Veiga F, Ribeiro AJ. New delivery systems to improve the bioavailability of resveratrol. Expert Opin Drug Deliv 2011; 8(8): 973-90.
[http://dx.doi.org/10.1517/17425247.2011.581655] [PMID: 21668403]

[94]   De Vincenzi M, Stammati A, De Vincenzi A, Silano M. Constituents of aromatic plants: carvacrol. Fitoterapia 2004; 75(7-8): 801-4.
[http://dx.doi.org/10.1016/j.fitote.2004.05.002] [PMID: 15567271]

[95]   Hu Y, Zhang J, Kong W, Zhao G, Yang M. Mechanisms of antifungal and anti-aflatoxigenic properties of essential oil derived from turmeric (*Curcuma longa* L.) on *Aspergillus flavus*. Food Chem 2017; 220: 1-8.
[http://dx.doi.org/10.1016/j.foodchem.2016.09.179] [PMID: 27855875]

[96]   More UB, Narkhede HP, Dalal DS, Mahulikar PP. Synthesis of biologically active Carvacrol compounds using different solvents and supports. Synth Commun 2007; 37(12): 1957-64.
[http://dx.doi.org/10.1080/00397910701354608]

[97]   Ultee A, Slump RA, Steging G, Smid EJ. Antimicrobial activity of carvacrol toward *Bacillus cereus* on rice. J Food Prot 2000; 63(5): 620-4.
[http://dx.doi.org/10.4315/0362-028X-63.5.620] [PMID: 10826719]

[98]   Basmacioğlu Malayoğlu H, Baysal S, Misirlioğlu Z, Polat M, Yilmaz H, Turan N. Effects of oregano essential oil with or without feed enzymes on growth performance, digestive enzyme, nutrient digestibility, lipid metabolism and immune response of broilers fed on wheat-soybean meal diets. Br Poult Sci 2010; 51(1): 67-80.
[http://dx.doi.org/10.1080/00071660903573702] [PMID: 20390571]

[99]   Austgulen LT, Solheim E, Scheline RR. Metabolism in rats of p-cymene derivatives: carvacrol and thymol. Pharmacol Toxicol 1987; 61(2): 98-102.
[http://dx.doi.org/10.1111/j.1600-0773.1987.tb01783.x] [PMID: 2959918]

[100] Zora Dajić Stevanović, Jasna Bošnjak-Neumüller, Ivana Pajić-Lijaković, Jog Raj, Marko Vasiljević. Essential oils as feed additives - future perspectives. Molecules 2018; 23(7): 1717. [http://dx.doi.org/10.3390/molecules23071717]

[101] Jamroz D, Kamel C. Plant extracts enhance broiler performance. J Anim Sci 2002; 80: 4. [Abstr.].

[102] Jaafari A, Tilaou M, Mouse HA, *et al.* Comparative study of the antitumor effect of natural monoterpenes: relationship to cell cycle analysis. Braz J Pharmacog 2012; 22: 534-40. [http://dx.doi.org/10.1590/S0102-695X2012005000021]

[103] Lee KW, Everts H, Kappert HJ, Yeom KH, Beynen AC. Dietary Carvacrol Lowers Body Weight Gain but Improves Feed Conversion in Female Broiler Chickens. J Appl Poult Res 2003; 12: 394-9. b [http://dx.doi.org/10.1093/japr/12.4.394]

[104] Umaya RS, Manpal S. Biological and pharmacological of actions carvacrol and its effects on poultry: an updated review. World J Pharm Pharm Sci 2013; 2(5): 3581-95.

[105] Veldhuizen EJ, Tjeerdsma-van Bokhoven JL, Zweijtzer C, Burt SA, Haagsman HP. Structural requirements for the antimicrobial activity of carvacrol. J Agric Food Chem 2006; 54(5): 1874-9. [http://dx.doi.org/10.1021/jf052564y] [PMID: 16506847]

[106] Baser KHC. Biological and pharmacological activities of carvacrol and carvacrol bearing essential oils. Curr Pharm Des 2008; 14(29): 3106-19. [http://dx.doi.org/10.2174/138161208786404227] [PMID: 19075694]

[107] Burt SA, Vlielander R, Haagsman HP, Veldhuizen EJ. Increase in activity of essential oil components carvacrol and thymol against *Escherichia coli* O157:H7 by addition of food stabilizers. J Food Prot 2005; 68(5): 919-26. [http://dx.doi.org/10.4315/0362-028X-68.5.919] [PMID: 15895722]

[108] Burt SA, Fledderman MJ, Haagsman HP, van Knapen F, Veldhuizen EJ. Inhibition of *Salmonella enterica* serotype Enteritidis on agar and raw chicken by carvacrol vapour. Int J Food Microbiol 2007; 119(3): 46-350. 3

[109] Azirak S, Rencuzogullari E. The *in vivo* genotoxic effects of carvacrol and thymol in rat bone marrow cells. Environ Toxicol 2008; 23(6): 728-35. [http://dx.doi.org/10.1002/tox.20380] [PMID: 18361405]

[110] Aristatile B, Numair AKS, Assaf AHA, Veeramani C, Pugalendi KV. Protective effect of carvacrol on oxidative stress and cellular DNA damage induced by UVB irradiation in human peripheral lymphocytes. J Biochem Mol Toxicol 2015; 29(11): 497-507. [http://dx.doi.org/10.1002/jbt.20355] [PMID: 26768646]

[111] Ipeka E, Zeytinoglua H, Okaya S, Tuylua BA, Kurkcuoglub M, Can Baserb KH. Genotoxicity and antigenotoxicity of Origanum oil and carvacrol evaluated by Ames Salmonella/microsomal test. Food Chem 2005; 93(3): 551-6. [http://dx.doi.org/10.1016/j.foodchem.2004.12.034]

[112] Karkabounas S, Kostoula OK, Daskalou T, *et al.* Anticarcinogenic and antiplatelet effects of carvacrol. Exp Oncol 2006; 28(2): 121-5. [PMID: 16837902]

[113] Yin QH, Yan FX, Zu XY, *et al.* Anti-proliferative and pro-apoptotic effect of carvacrol on human hepatocellular carcinoma cell line HepG-2. Cytotechnology 2012; 64(1): 43-51. [http://dx.doi.org/10.1007/s10616-011-9389-y] [PMID: 21938469]

[114] Aristatile B, Al-Numair KS, Veeramani C, Pugalendi KV. Antihyperlipidemic effect of carvacrol on D-galactosamine-induced hepatotoxic rats. J Basic Clin Physiol Pharmacol 2009; 20(1): 15-27. a [http://dx.doi.org/10.1515/JBCPP.2009.20.1.15] [PMID: 19601392]

[115] Aristatile B, Al-Numair KS, Veeramani C, Pugalendi KV. Effect of carvacrol on hepatic marker enzymes and antioxidant status in D-galactosamine-induced hepatotoxicity in rats. Fundam Clin

Pharmacol 2009; 23(6): 757-65. b
[http://dx.doi.org/10.1111/j.1472-8206.2009.00721.x] [PMID: 19650854]

[116] Trabace L, Zotti M, Morgese MG, *et al.* Estrous cycle affects the neurochemical and neurobehavioral profile of carvacrol-treated female rats. Toxicol Appl Pharmacol 2011; 255(2): 169-75.
[http://dx.doi.org/10.1016/j.taap.2011.06.011] [PMID: 21723308]

[117] Marchand F, Perretti M, McMahon SB. Role of the immune system in chronic pain. Nat Rev Neurosci 2005; 6(7): 521-32.
[http://dx.doi.org/10.1038/nrn1700] [PMID: 15995723]

[118] Guimaraes AG, Xavier MA, Santana MT. Carvacrol attenuates mechanical hypernociception and inflammatory response. N- S Arch Pharmacol 2012; 385: 253-63.

CHAPTER 14

Organic Acids as Eco-Friendly Growth Promoters in Poultry Feed

Mohamed E. Abd El-Hack[1,*], **Elwy A. Ashour**[1], **Muhammad Arif**[2], **Maria Tabassum Chaudhry**[3], **Mohamed Emam**[4], **Asmaa F. Khafaga**[5], **Ayman E. Taha**[6], **Dairon Más**[7], **Kuldeep Dhama**[8], **Mayada R. Farag**[9] and **Mahmoud Alagawany**[1,*]

[1] *Departmentof Poultry, Faculty of Agriculture, Zagazig University, Zagazig 44511, Egypt*

[2] *Department of Animal Sciences, College of Agriculture, University of Sargodha 40100, Pakistan*

[3] *Institute of Animal Nutrition, Northeast Agricultural University, Harbin 150030, China*

[4] *Department of Nutrition and Clinical Nutrition, Faculty of Veterinary Medicine, Damanhour University, Damanhour 22516, Egypt*

[5] *Department of Pathology, Faculty of Veterinary Medicine, Alexandria University, Edfina 22758, Egypt*

[6] *Department of Animal Husbandry and Animal Wealth Development, Faculty of Veterinary Medicine, Alexandria University, Edfina 22578, Egypt*

[7] *Laboratory of Animal Nutrition, Faculty of Natural Sciences, Autonomous University of Queretaro, Queretaro 76230, Mexico*

[8] *Division of Pathology, ICAR-Indian Veterinary Research Institute, Izatnagar, Bareilly, Uttar Pradesh - 243122, India*

[9] *Forensic Medicine and Toxicology Department, Veterinary Medicine Faculty, Zagazig University, Zagazig 44511, Egypt*

Abstract: Organic acids (OAs) have been used as natural preservatives for food products and as hygiene promoters to inhibit microbial growth, thereby improving the freshness and shelf-life of food items. The impact of OAs on microbial growth makes it an alternative to antibiotic growth promoters. The characteristic of inhibiting microbial growth is a useful feature that has been recently used in poultry production. Organic acids are chemically weak, and they modulate the beneficial competitive exclusion in the gastrointestinal tract (GIT) and diminish the production of metabolites harmful to the body by decreasing the proliferation and colonization of pathogenic bacteria in the GIT. Further, they improve the ability of the intestinal wall to absorb nutrients by improving the structure of the villi and the digestive secretions that lead to enhanced absorption of proteins, carbohydrates, and minerals.

* **Corresponding authors Mahmoud Alagawany and Mohamed E. Abd El-Hack:** Poultry Department, Faculty of Agriculture, Zagazig University, Zagazig, Egypt; E-mails: mmalagwany@zu.edu.eg and m.ezzat@zu.edu.eg

The use of 15g/kg of citric acid in broiler diets reduced the cecal total bacterial count and *Enterobacteriaceae* by 62.26% and 80%, respectively, in comparison with control. However, the same level of fumaric acid reduced the cecal total bacterial count and *Enterobacteriaceae* by 88.63 and 78.57%, respectively. Similarly, the inclusion of 30g/kg of fumaric acid reduced the cecal total bacterial count and *Enterobacteriaceae* by 95.84 and 88.57%, respectively. The immunity of broilers can thus be improved as a normal consequence of all previously mentioned advantages. The use of 0.30 g/kg blends of sorbic acid, fumaric acid, and thymol improved the spleen size of broiler chickens by 50% when compared to control. Dietary inclusion of formic acid up to 5 and 10 g/kg significantly improved feed conversion ratio by 9.37 and 16.66% and improved ileal digestibility of crude protein by 19.85 and 21.08%, respectively. This chapter summarizes the possible modes of action of dietary OAs and their effects on the growth and health of poultry.

Keywords: Antimicrobial activity, Nutrition, Organic acid types, Performance, Poultry.

INTRODUCTION

Antibiotic growth promoters (AGPs) are either banned or under control as they lead to antibiotic resistance in both humans and animals [1 - 4]. In January 2006, the European Union, as a step in minimizing and eliminating the use of AGPs in the poultry industry, started with the prevention of the use of sub-therapeutic antibiotics (European Parliament and Council Regulation (EC) No 1831/2003) in food production. However, the removal of AGPs resulted in delayed performance effects, therefore, researchers developed several alternatives to AGPs such as prebiotics, probiotics, organic minerals, bacteriophages, plant additives, and organic acids (OAs) [5 - 11].

Dietary acids used in poultry nutrition are divided into organic and inorganic acids [12, 13]. OAs are defined as carboxylic acids that have R-COOH group in their chemical structure such as fatty acids and among them only OAs with excellent physical and chemical characteristics are used in the poultry industry. The commonly used acids are the short-chain OAs such as formic, acetic, propionic, and butyric acids, in addition to other OAs such as lactic, malic, tartaric, fumaric, and citric acids [14]. Dietary OA supplementation gained considerable attention as an alternative to AGPs owing to its effect on pathogenic bacteria; it reduces the pH in the gastrointestinal tract (GIT), thus improving the absorption of different nutrients in poultry [15, 16]. Further, OAs improve growth performance, feed utilisation, and disease resistance [14, 17, 18]. The main objective of this chapter is to describe the workable mode of action of dietary OAs for poultry and its effects on the growth rate and health aspects.

DEFINITION AND CHEMICAL STRUCTURE OF ORGANIC ACIDS [OAS]

R-COOH group is the main component of the OA structure that gives it acidic properties; such as fatty and amino acids. In general, OAs are weak acids that cannot completely dissociate in water. The most important property for measuring the strength and activity of an OA is the measure of its dissociation, which is determined using pKa; the pKa value which is lower in a healthier and more dissociable acid. To have an antimicrobial effect, the pKa value of the OA should be between 3–5 [14]; although all OAs exhibit partial dissociation, all of them do not have the same antimicrobial effect. Short-chain acids between C1 and C7 with one carboxylic group are formic, propionic, butyric acids tartaric, lactic, malic, and citric acids, which have antimicrobial properties. Furthermore, fumaric and sorbic acids have an extra advantage of an anti-fungal effect. OAs and their salts have not only an antimicrobial effect on both the feed and the GIT but also a performance enhancement effect [19].

Action Mechanisms of Dietary OAs

As OAs are not clearly described in previous articles, their application in broiler diets is limited. Several modes of actions have been proposed, and they focus on [a] the decrease in the pH in the feed and the GIT; [b] the increase in nutrient retention, which increases nutrient utilization; and [c] antimicrobial effects [9, 20, 21]. The dietary butyric acid and its salt could act asglycolysis intermediates accumulate in the cell, which confirms that butyrate is a preferred energy substrate over glucose. Further, dietary butyrate spares the oxidation of some amino acids, increasing their digestion and absorption. Al-Kassi and Mohssen [19] indicated that enzyme activity plays a role in the enhanced performance resulting from different doses of some OAs. This improved performance is partially attributed to the increase in pepsin activity, pancreatic enzyme activities [trypsin and lipase], and intestinal enzyme activities [leucine-aminopeptidase and phosphatases].

Antimicrobial Activity of OAs

Organic acids are economically viable and biologically active alternatives to AGPs. For several years, OAs have been added effectively in the feed of birds to reduce the presence of pathogens, especially *Salmonella* spp. and mycotoxins produced by fungi [22]. Attia *et al.* [23] reported that OAs modulate the intestinal pH, inhibit the growth of pathogenic microorganisms, and maintain the microbial balance in the GIT. Further, Saki *et al.* [24] and Nair and Johny [25] showed that

OAs reduce *Salmonella* spp. and bacteria of the family *Enterobacteriaceae* in broiler chicken. Besides, several other studies showed that formic acid and propionic acid have a bactericidal effect against *Salmonella* spp., *coliforms*, and *Escherichia coli* in bird GITs [17, 26, 27]. Nair and Johny [25] also indicated that OAs in the diet decreased the vertical transmission of *Salmonella* in chickens. Regassa and Nyachoti [28] reported that the addition of butyric acid in the diet of birds could reduce a *Salmonella Enteritidis* infection in the GIT.

The inclusion of up to 30 g/kg of citric acid and fumaric acid in the diet for broilers minimizes the total number of bacteria and the *Enterobacteriaceae* in the caecum; however, the addition of 15 g/kg is recommended considering economic viability [23]. Palamidi and Mountzouris [29] found that the addition of OAs positively affected the microbial ratio in the caecum and increased the activity of glycolytic enzymes produced by beneficial bacteria in the ileum. They also observed that the subgroups of *C. leptum* and *C. coccoides* in the broiler caecum increased significantly with OAs compared with avilamycin [29]. This demonstrates the ability of using OAs as alternatives to AGPs. The bactericidal and bacteriostatic effects of OAs are dependent on the pH of the GIT; in particular, lactic, fumaric, and citric acids whch culd eliminate the pathogenic bacteria sensitive to pH changes in the stomach, while formic, acetic, butyric, propionic, and sorbic acids act directly on the cell wall of gram-negative bacteria [22, 30].

Acetic, propionic, butyric, fumaric, and lactic acids are weak fatty acids that can lower the pH of the bacterial cytoplasm because, in an undissociated form, they can cross the cell wall of bacteria without lowering the intestinal pH and modify the beneficial microbiota [22]. Ricke [17] reported that OAs decreased nutrient transport and energy metabolism due to their effect on the bacterial membrane. Yadav and Jha [31] stated that, hydrophobicity, the value of pKa, and the ability to change from the non-dissociated to the dissociated form, are fundamental elements for OAs to exhibit excellent antibacterial activity. Papatsiros *et al.* [30] reported that a pKa value between 3 and 5 is optimal for using weak OAs as antibacterials in diets for poultry. Organic acids also improved the digestive physiology of birds; the activity of proteolytic enzymes, and the digestibility of nutrients, increase pancreatic secretions, and balance the intestinal microbiota of birds [22]. In Broiler chickens, birds fed diets enriched with OAs and medium chain fatty acids (MCFAs) showed a linear decrease [P = 0.002] in *E. coli* count and increase [P = 0.042] in Lactobacillus count [32]. Tartaric acid, acetic acid, and citric acid inhibited *S. typhimurium* by 0.312%, 0.512% and 0.625% for the three levels of the strain: 10, 100, and 103 CFU/ml, respectively [33]. Use of 0.2

g/kg organic acids or 0.2 g/kg probiotics or their combination enhanced gut microflora by increasing the *Lactobacillus spp.* to *E. coli* ratio and decreasing the count of *E. coli* [34].

Impact of OAs on The pH of The GIT

Organic acids decrease the pH of the diet and, consequently, the digesta, which influenced the pKa values and the pH of the GIT [35]. The dietary addition of OAs considerably decreased the pH in the upper part of the intestine compared to that in the lower part. Paul *et al.* [36] and Samanta *et al.* [37] showed that OAs decreased the pH of the crop, and the reduction in the pH of the crop depended on the dose of the OA. In several experiments, OAs decreased the pH of the proventriculus with an average of 0.12, which is lower than the pH of the crop [38, 39]. Further, the pH of the duodenum was reduced by the inclusion of OAs in the diets for birds; however, there is a contradiction in the results for the intestinal portion [37, 40, 41]. Further, a similar pH reduction was recorded for the jejunum, ileum, and caecum. A small amount of OAs was not absorbed in the upper part, and they continued to be in the lower part of the GIT [42]. This may be another reason that explains why the pH of the lower part of the GIT is not affected by the addition of OAs. As described previously, we can conclude that dietary OAs reduce pH primarily in the upper portion of the GIT in broiler chickens.

Impact of OAs on Immunity

The immune system of a bird plays an essential role in maintaining and regulating its health [43]. According to Sharma [44], environmental, nutritional, physiological, and genetic factors affect the immune mechanisms of birds. However, avian defense mechanisms are very similar to that of mammals, in birds, a protective immune response is achieved *via* the complex integration of several cells and soluble factors. In birds, unlike mammals, the primary lymphoid organs [bursa of Fabricius and thymus] involute and immune cells migrate to the secondary lymphoid organs [spleen, lymphoid tissues associated with the intestine, Harder's gland, and bone marrow]; the bone and the lymphoid tissues then be associated with the bronchi [44]. According to Dibner and Buttin [14], the use of OAs in the diet considerably affected the immunological state of birds. The increase in beneficial bacteria in the intestine and the decrease in subclinical infectious diseases improve the digestibility of nutrients. Chowdhury *et al.* [45] indicated an improvement in the immunological status of broiler chickens fed 0.5% citric acid; Rahmani and Speer [46] and Abdel-Fattah *et al.* [47] showed a similar increase in the immune response of broiler chickens due to OAs supplementation.

The action of OAs modifies lymphoid organs; Yang *et al.* [43] found an increase in the size of the spleen in birds that consumed 0.30 g/kg of OAs [sorbic acid, fumaric acid, and thymol] during the grower or the finisher periods, and also, on day 42. In the duodenal and ileal mucosa, higher concentrations of immunoglobulin A were found. Also, there were significant improvements [linear, P = 0.011] in the concentration of IgG associated with the supplementation of the blend of OAs and MCFAslevels in the broiler diets. But, bursa of Fabricius weight was reduced [linear, P = 0.052] by OAs and MCFAs supplementation [32].

Impact of Different Sources of OAs on Poultry Performance

The supplementation of 2.25 g/kg of humic acid in the diets of broiler chickens improved weight gain and the feed conversion ratio (FCR) and decreased the levels of cholesterol and low-density lipoproteins (LDL) in the blood [48]. Disetlhe *et al.* [49] found that the inclusion of humic acid in diets based on canola meal had beneficial effects on the quality of meat and the proportion of polyunsaturated fatty acids (PUFAs), n-6 and n-3 fatty acids, and the PUFA/saturated fatty acid ratio. On the other hand, feeding with commercial feed containing humic acid did not modify the productive behavior of broiler chickens of both sexes; however, it transformed the intestinal morphometry and the expression of mucin 2 [MUC2] and tumor necrosis factor alpha [TNF-α] without affecting interleukin-1 beta and interleukin-10 [50]. Further, formic acid was supplemented in the water and feed of broilers to improve production indicators, microbiota, and digestibility; however, Açıkgöz *et al.* [51] found that acidification of water up to pH 4.5 in male chickens more than five days old did not improve growth performance, microflora, and contamination of the carcass.

The growth performance parameters of broilers improved by the inclusion of up to 10,000 ppm of formic acid in addition to a change in the intestinal morphology was also observed (increased depth of the crypts without modifying the surface of the villi); besides, the apparent ileal digestibility of all nutrients were improved [52]. Hernández *et al.* [53] reported that the ileal digestibility of dry matter enhanced by the addition of 10 g/kg of formic acid in the feed for broiler chickens; however, the pH of the jejunum and the histo-morphology of the intestine did not change with this addition. Paul *et al.* [36] reported a decrease in the feed intake of broilers when 3 g/kg of ammonium formate was added to the feed [ammonium salt of formic acid]; however, this addition improved the body weight and FCR.

In broilers, the growth rate was improved when up to 30 g/kg of acetic acid was included in the diet; further, the pH of the proventriculus and ventriculus was significantly reduced compared to a diet without OAs [54]. The live weight, FCR, and weight gain were improved with the supplementation of 1.5 and 3% acetic or citric acids in the diet, respectively; the pH also reduced in the gizzard and portions of the small intestine [47]. Similarly, in laying hens, a 600-ppm dose of acetic acid in the diet improved egg production, egg weight, and external and internal quality parameters [55].

Paul *et al.* [36] included a salt of propionic acid [calcium propionate] in the diet of broilers and found an increase in the body weight and FCR, despite a lower feed intake. Some butyric acid derivatives such as partially protected sodium butyrate(PSB) and sodium butyrate (sodium salt) were included in chicken diets as growth promoters [56, 57]. According to Chamba *et al.* [57], a greater weight gain and FCR was noted in the growth and finishing phase of broiler chickens fed 700 ppm of PSB. Besides, the relative weight of the digestive organs was not modified at any productive period. However, at 14 days, the length of the small intestine increased post-treatment with PSB; similarly, the villi of the jejunum increased with an experimental treatment in correspondence to the control diet, at 42 days of age [57]. Adil *et al.* [56] reported an increase in the body weight gain and a better FCR in broiler chickens post supplementation of 2% and 3% sodium butyrate in the diet; however this supplementation did not affect voluntary food intake.

The addition of 0.5% and 1.0% fumaric acid to the diet of broilers increased body weight without affecting feed efficiency [58]. However, body weight and nutritional efficiency are not affected by the substitution of 0.5%, 1.0%, or 1.5% wheat with fumaric acid [59]. On the other hand, the inclusion of 2% citric acid in diets for broiler chickens increased the digestion of dry matter, crude protein, and neutral detergent fiber; however, it decreased the daily weight gain and feed consumption [60]. Bozkurt *et al.* [61] indicated that, with a dose of 1.0 g/kg of citric acid, the FCR of broilers at 21 days of age was improved. Esmaeilipour *et al.* [62] indicated an increase in FCR with 20 and 40 g/kg of citric acid in the diet of chickens; however, it caused a decrease in feed intake and weight gain. The inclusion of citric acid up to 50 g/kg of dry matter for broilers improved live weight and FCR [39]. Chowdhury *et al.* [45] reported an increase in growth, feed intake, feed efficiency, and carcass yield of broiler chickens that were fed on a diet containing 0.5% citric acid. Not all OAs have a beneficial effect on the performance and digestive physiology of broilers. Józefiak *et al.* [63] reported a decrease in the body growth and cecal pH of chickens fed 0.2% benzoic acid; however, there was no change in pH of other portions of the GIT. The impact of different sources of OAs on various poultry species is summarized in Table **1**.

Table 1. Impacts of different sources of organic acids on poultry.

Type of OAs	Doses	Bird Species	Results	Reference
Humic acid	0, 0.75, 1.5, 2.25 and 3 g/kg diet.	Broiler chickens	The level of 2.25 g/kg caused improved weight gain and feed conversion ratio (FCR) in addition to reducing blood cholesterol and low-density lipoprotein [LDL].	[48]
Acetic acid	0, 10, 20, 30 g/kg diet.	Broiler chickens	The results showed that AA supplementation improved weight gain (WG) and FCR . A significant reduction in pH of proventriculus and ventriculus was observed within a dose-related manner.	[54]
Formic acid	Acidified drinking water [pH 4.5] after 5 d of age.	Male broilers	The acidification of the drinking water didn't show beneficial effects on performance, microflora, or carcass contamination.	[51]
Fumaric acid	3% in the diet.	Broiler chickens	The best improvement in body weight gain (BWG) and FCR was obtained at 3% fumaric acid in the diet.	[64]
Formic acid	5,000 ppm of formic acid; 10,000 ppm of formic acid.	Broiler chickens	Both doses showed improvement in growth performance parameters. The group fed the 10,000 ppm had the most significant crypt depth, but the villus surface area was not influenced.	[52]
Formic acid	5 and 10 g/kg diet	Broiler chickens	10 g/kg slightly improved ileal dry matter (DM) digestibility compared to the other treatment groups. Jejunum pH was not affected when 5 or 10 g/kg formic acid was added, and the results do not clearly show a positive effect of formic acid on the intestinal histomorphology.	[53]
Ammonium formate	3gm/kg diet	Broiler chickens	Ammonium formate in the diet had decreased feed intake, but BWG was comparable to control birds, the FCR had been improved.	[36]
Calcium propionate	3gm/kg diet	Broiler chickens	Calcium propionate in the diet lowered feed intake, but BWG was comparable to control birds, and thus improved FCR.	[36]
Lactic acid	3% in the diet.	Broiler chickens	Significantly improved BWG and FCR. No effect on cumulative feed consumption.	[56]
Na-butyrate	2% and 3% in the diet.	Broiler chickens	Significant improvement in body weight gains and feed conversion ratio. No effect on cumulative feed consumption.	[56]

(Table 1) cont.....

Type of OAs	Doses	Bird Species	Results	Reference
Butyric acid	partially protected sodium butyrate (PSB) at 700 ppm	Broiler chickens	Chicks fed PSB in grower and finisher phases had the highest BWG and the best FCR. Relative digestive organs' weights were not affected by treatment in any period. The jejunum and small intestine relative lengths of birds fed PSB at 14 days were longer than those of birds fed the control diet. Jejunal villi of birds fed PSB at 42 days were higher than those in birds fed the control diet.	[57]
Citric acid	2% of the diet	Broiler chickens	Significantly increased the retention of DM, crude proten (CP), and neutral detergent fiber (NDF), but decreased feed intake and BWG.	[60]
	1. of the diet	Broiler chickens	Decreased FCR.	[60]
	1.0 g /kg diet	Broiler chickens	Significantly improved the FCR at day 21.	[61]
	1.5 and 3% of the diet	Broiler chickens	Improved LBW, BWG, FCR.	[47]
	0, 20 and 40 mg/kg of diet	Broiler chickens	The addition of citric acid [40 g/kg of dry diet matter] decreased feed consumption and BWG. However, significant improvement in the FCR was observed by the supplementation of citric acid (20 and 40 g/kg of diet).	[62]
	6.25, 12.5, 25 and 50 g/kg of diet dry matter	Broiler chickens	Significant improvement in LBW and FCR were observed with the supplementation of a higher levels compared with other levels of citric acid.	[39]
Acetic acid	1.5 and 3% of the diet	Broiler chickens	Higher life body weight (LBW) Higher BWG Better FCR.	[47]
Acetic acid	600, 400 and 200 ppm	Laying hens during the hot season	The drinking acetic acid significantly improved egg production, external and internal egg quality parameters. An increase in the supplemental acetic acid produced a linear increase in external egg qualities such as egg weight The most marked results were obtained with 600 ppm acetic acid supplementation.	[55]
Fumaric acid	2% and 3% in the diet	Broiler chickens	Improved BWG and FCR. No effect on cumulative feed consumption was observed.	[56]

(Table 1) cont.....

Type of OAs	Doses	Bird Species	Results	Reference
Fumaric acid	Replacing 0.5%, 1.0% or 1.5% of the wheat.	Broiler chickens	No significant effect on BWG or feed efficiency. lower numbers of *Lactic acid bacteria* and *Coliforms* in the ileum and caeca. lower levels of endogenous losses compared to control fed birds.	[59]
Fumaric acid	Fumaric acid was added at 0, 0.5, 1.0 and 1.5%	Broiler chickens	The addition of 0.5 or 1.0% fumaric acid significantly [P<0.05] improved the body weights of broilers but did not influence feed utilization.	[58]
Benzoic acid	0.2%	Broiler chickens	Depressed the growth of broiler chickens . - Increased the DM of the digesta in the crop and caeca . The pH of the caecal contents decreased . No differences were found in the pH of the crop, ileal, gizzard digesta, and rectum content. Lactic acid bacteria populations were lowered Coliform bacteria decreased in the caeca.	[63]

CONCLUSION

The published data from the available reports showed that OAs improved growth performance and the health status of birds; thus, they could be considered potential alternatives for AGPs. Organic acids have the following advantages: 1] reducing the pH in the diet and increase nutrient absorption in the GIT; 2] having an antimicrobial effect on pathogenic bacteria, targeting zoonotic bacteria; for example, *Campylobacter, E. coli*, and *Salmonella*, both in the diet and in the GIT of poultry; 3] minimizing the microbial load in poultry meat products; 4] improving the growth of the mucosa, width, height, and depth of the villi, and decrease the pH of the intestines; and 5] improving the immune system and the digestibility of proteins, carbohydrates, and minerals.

CONSENT FOR PUBLICATION

Not applicable.

CONFLICT OF INTEREST

The author declares no conflict of interest, financial or otherwise.

ACKNOWLEDGEMENTS

Declared none.

REFERENCES

[1] Shewita RS, Taha AE. Influence of dietary supplementation of ginger powder at different levels on growth performance, haematological profiles, slaughter traits and gut morphometry of broiler chickens. S Afr J Anim Sci 2018; 48(6): 997-1008.

[2] Arif M, Hayat Z, Abd El-Hack ME, *et al.* Impacts of supplementing broiler diets with a powder mixture of black cumin, Moringa and chicory seeds. S Afr J Anim Sci 2019; 49(3): 564-72.
[http://dx.doi.org/10.4314/sajas.v49i3.17]

[3] Taha AE, Hassan SS, Shewita RS, *et al.* Effects of supplementing broiler diets with coriander seed powder on growth performance, blood haematology, ileum microflora and economic efficiency. J Anim Physiol Anim Nutr (Berl) 2019; 103(5): 1474-83.
[http://dx.doi.org/10.1111/jpn.13165] [PMID: 31368211]

[4] Ashour EA, El-Kholy MS, Alagawany M, *et al.* Effect of dietary supplementation with *Moringa oleifera* leaves and/or seeds powder on production, egg characteristics, hatchability and blood chemistry of laying japanese quails. Sustainability 2020; 12(6): 2463.
[http://dx.doi.org/10.3390/su12062463]

[5] Yan L, Hong SM, Kim IH. Effect of bacteriophage supplementation on the growth performance, nutrient digestibility, blood characteristics, and fecal microbial shedding in growing pigs. Asian-Australas J Anim Sci 2012; 25(10): 1451-6.
[http://dx.doi.org/10.5713/ajas.2012.12253] [PMID: 25049502]

[6] Ashour EA, Alagawany M, Reda FM, Abd El-Hack ME. Effect of supplementation of *Yucca schidigera* extract to growing rabbit diets on growth performance, carcass characteristics, serum biochemistry and liver oxidative status. Asian J Anim Vet Adv 2014; 9(11): 732-42.
[http://dx.doi.org/10.3923/ajava.2014.732.742]

[7] Abd El-Hack ME, Alagawany M. Performance, egg quality, blood profile, immune function, and antioxidant enzyme activities in laying hens fed diets with thyme powder. J Anim Feed Sci 2015; 24(2): 127-33.
[http://dx.doi.org/10.22358/jafs/65638/2015]

[8] Ni H, Martínez Y, Guan G, *et al.* Analysis of the impact of isoquinoline alkaloids, derived from *Macleaya cordata* extract, on the development and innate immune response in swine and poultry. BioMed Res Int 2016; 2016: 1352146.
[http://dx.doi.org/10.1155/2016/1352146] [PMID: 28042566]

[9] Yadav AS, Kolluri G, Gopi M, Karthik K, Singh Y. Exploring alternatives to antibiotics as health promoting agents in poultry-A review. J Exp Biol 2016; 4(10): 3.

[10] Abd El-Hack ME, Alagawany M, Ragab Farag M, *et al.* Beneficial impacts of thymol essential oil on health and production of animals, fish and poultry: a review. J Essent Oil Res 2016; 28(5): 365-82.
[http://dx.doi.org/10.1080/10412905.2016.1153002]

[11] Abd El-Hack ME, Abdelnour SA, Abd El-Moneim AEE, *et al.* Putative impacts of phytogenic additives to ameliorate lead toxicity in animal feed. Environ Sci Pollut Res Int 2019; 26(23): 23209-18.
[http://dx.doi.org/10.1007/s11356-019-05805-8] [PMID: 31243654]

[12] Polycarpo GV, Andretta I, Kipper M, *et al.* Meta-analytic study of organic acids as an alternative performance-enhancing feed additive to antibiotics for broiler chickens. Poult Sci 2017; 96(10): 3645-53.
[http://dx.doi.org/10.3382/ps/pex178] [PMID: 28938776]

[13] Salah AS, Ahmed-Farid OA, El-Tarabany MS. Carcass yields, muscle amino acid and fatty acid profiles, and antioxidant indices of broilers supplemented with synbiotic and/or organic acids. J Anim Physiol Anim Nutr (Berl) 2019; 103(1): 41-52.
[http://dx.doi.org/10.1111/jpn.12994] [PMID: 30280428]

[14] Dibner JJ, Buttin P. Use of organic acids as a model to study the impact of gut microflora on nutrition and metabolism. J Appl Poult Res 2002; 11(4): 453-63.
[http://dx.doi.org/10.1093/japr/11.4.453]

[15] Partanen K. Organic acids-their efficacy and modes of action in pigs Gut environment in pigs/A Piva, KE Bach Knudsen. JE Lindberg 2001.

[16] Kil DY, Kwon WB, Kim BG. Dietary acidifiers in weanling pig diets: a review. Rev Colomb Cienc Pecu 2011; 24(3): 231-47.

[17] Ricke SC. Perspectives on the use of organic acids and short chain fatty acids as antimicrobials. Poult Sci 2003; 82(4): 632-9.
[http://dx.doi.org/10.1093/ps/82.4.632] [PMID: 12710485]

[18] Islam KM. Use of citric acid in broiler diets. Worlds Poult Sci J 2012; 68(1): 104-18.
[http://dx.doi.org/10.1017/S0043933912000116]

[19] Al-Kassi AG, Mohssen MA. Comparative study between single organic acid effect and synergistic organic acid effect on broiler performance. Pak J Nutr 2009; 8(6): 896-9.
[http://dx.doi.org/10.3923/pjn.2009.896.899]

[20] Afsharmanesh M, Pourreza J. Effects of calcium, citric acid, ascorbic acid, vitamin D3 on the efficacy of microbial phytase in broiler starters fed wheat-based diets I. Performance, bone mineralization and ileal digestibility. Int J Poult Sci 2005; 4: 418-24.
[http://dx.doi.org/10.3923/ijps.2005.418.424]

[21] Mroz Z, Jongbloed AW, Partanen K, et al. Ileal digestibility of amino acids in pigs feddiets of different buffering capacity and with supplementaryorganic acids. J Anim Feed Sci 1998; (Suppl. 1): 191-7.

[22] Dittoe DK, Ricke SC, Kiess AS. Organic acids and potential for modifying the avian gastrointestinal tract and reducing pathogens and disease. Front Vet Sci 2018; 5: 216.
[http://dx.doi.org/10.3389/fvets.2018.00216] [PMID: 30238011]

[23] Attia FM. Effect of organic acids supplementation on nutrients digestibility, gut microbiota and immune response of broiler chicks. Egyptian Poult Sci J 2018; 38(1): 223-39.

[24] Saki AA, Harcini RN, Rahmatnejad E, Salary J. Herbal additives and organic acids as antibiotic alternatives in broiler chickens' diet for organic production. Afr J Biotechnol 2012; 11(8): 2139-45.

[25] Nair DV, Johny AK. *Salmonella* in Poultry Meat Production. Food Safety in Poultry Meat Production. Cham: Springer 2019; pp. 1-24.
[http://dx.doi.org/10.1007/978-3-030-05011-5_1]

[26] Ruhnke I, Röhe I, Goodarzi Boroojeni F, et al. Feed supplemented with organic acids does not affect starch digestibility, nor intestinal absorptive or secretory function in broiler chickens. J Anim Physiol Anim Nutr (Berl) 2015; 99 (Suppl. S1): 29-35.
[http://dx.doi.org/10.1111/jpn.12313] [PMID: 25865420]

[27] Gowda V, Shivakumar S. Novel Biocontrol Agents: Short Chain Fatty Acids and More Recently, Polyhydroxyalkanoates. Biotechnological Applications of Polyhydroxyalkanoates. Singapore: Springer 2019; pp. 323-45.
[http://dx.doi.org/10.1007/978-981-13-3759-8_12]

[28] Regassa A, Nyachoti CM. Application of resistant starch in swine and poultry diets with particular reference to gut health and function. Anim Nutr 2018; 4(3): 305-10.
[http://dx.doi.org/10.1016/j.aninu.2018.04.001] [PMID: 30175259]

[29] Palamidi I, Mountzouris KC. Diet supplementation with an organic acids-based formulation affects gut microbiota and expression of gut barrier genes in broilers. Anim Nutr 2018; 4(4): 367-77.
[http://dx.doi.org/10.1016/j.aninu.2018.03.007] [PMID: 30564756]

[30] Papatsiros VG, Katsoulos PD, Koutoulis KC, Karatzia M, Dedousi A, Christodoulopoulos G.

Alternatives to antibiotics for farm animals. Perspect Agric Vet Sci Nutr Nat Resour 2013; 8: 1-5.
[http://dx.doi.org/10.1079/PAVSNNR20138032]

[31]   Yadav S, Jha R. Strategies to modulate the intestinal microbiota and their effects on nutrient utilization, performance, and health of poultry. J Anim Sci Biotechnol 2019; 10(1): 2.
[http://dx.doi.org/10.1186/s40104-018-0310-9] [PMID: 30651986]

[32]   Nguyen DH, Lee KY, Mohammadigheisar M, Kim IH. Evaluation of the blend of organic acids and medium-chain fatty acids in matrix coating as antibiotic growth promoter alternative on growth performance, nutrient digestibility, blood profiles, excreta microflora, and carcass quality in broilers. Poult Sci 2018; 97(12): 4351-8.
[http://dx.doi.org/10.3382/ps/pey339] [PMID: 30165535]

[33]   El Baaboua A, El Maadoudi M, Bouyahya A, *et al.* Evaluation of antimicrobial activity of four organic acids used in chicks feed to control *Salmonella* typhimurium: suggestion of amendment in the search standard. Int J Microbiol 2018; 2018: 7352593.
[http://dx.doi.org/10.1155/2018/7352593] [PMID: 30364137]

[34]   Rodjan P, Soisuwan K, Thongprajukaew K, *et al.* Effect of organic acids or probiotics alone or in combination on growth performance, nutrient digestibility, enzyme activities, intestinal morphology and gut microflora in broiler chickens. J Anim Physiol Anim Nutr (Berl) 2018; 102(2): e931-40.
[http://dx.doi.org/10.1111/jpn.12858] [PMID: 29250860]

[35]   Kim D, Kim J, Kim S, *et al.* A study on the efficacy of dietary supplementation of organic acid mixture in broiler chicks. J Anim Sci Technol 2009; 51(3): 207-16.
[http://dx.doi.org/10.5187/JAST.2009.51.3.207]

[36]   Paul SK, Halder G, Mondal MK, Samanta G. Effect of organic acid salt on the performance and gut health of broiler chicken. J Poult Sci 2007; 44(4): 389-95.
[http://dx.doi.org/10.2141/jpsa.44.389]

[37]   Samanta S, Haldar S, Ghosh TK. Production and carcase traits in broiler chickens given diets supplemented with inorganic trivalent chromium and an organic acid blend. Br Poult Sci 2008; 49(2): 155-63.
[http://dx.doi.org/10.1080/00071660801946950] [PMID: 18409089]

[38]   Panda AK, Rao SV, Raju MV, Sunder GS. Effect of butyric acid on performance, gastrointestinal tract health and carcass characteristics in broiler chickens. Asian-Aust J Anim Sci 2009; 22(7): 31-1026.
[http://dx.doi.org/10.5713/ajas.2009.80298]

[39]   Salgado-Tránsito L, Del Río-García JC, Arjona-Román JL, Moreno-Martínez E, Méndez-Albores A. Effect of citric acid supplemented diets on aflatoxin degradation, growth performance and serum parameters in broiler chickens. Arch Med Vet 2011; 43(3): 215-22.
[http://dx.doi.org/10.4067/S0301-732X2011000300003]

[40]   Panda AK, Raju MV, Rao SR, Sunder GS, Reddy MR. Effect of graded levels of formic acid on gut microflora count, serum biochemical parameters, performance and carcass yield of broiler chickens. Indian J Anim Sci 2009; 79(11): 1165-8. b

[41]   Nourmohammadi R, Hosseini SM, Saraee H, Arab A. Plasma thyroid hormone concentrations and pH values of some GI-tract segments of broilers fed on different dietary citric acid and microbial phytase levels. Am J Anim Vet Sci 2011; 6: 1-6.
[http://dx.doi.org/10.3844/ajavsp.2011.1.6]

[42]   Hume ME, Corrier DE, Ivie GW, Deloach JR. Metabolism of [14C]propionic acid in broiler chicks. Poult Sci 1993; 72(5): 786-93.
[http://dx.doi.org/10.3382/ps.0720786] [PMID: 8502603]

[43]   Yang X, Xin H, Yang C, Yang X. Impact of essential oils and organic acids on the growth performance, digestive functions and immunity of broiler chickens. Anim Nutr 2018; 4(4): 388-93.
[http://dx.doi.org/10.1016/j.aninu.2018.04.005] [PMID: 30564758]

[44] Sharma JM. The avian immune system. Dis Poult 2003; 11: 5-16.

[45] Chowdhury R, Islam KM, Khan MJ, *et al.* Effect of citric acid, avilamycin, and their combination on the performance, tibia ash, and immune status of broilers. Poult Sci 2009; 88(8): 1616-22.
[http://dx.doi.org/10.3382/ps.2009-00119] [PMID: 19590076]

[46] Rahmani HR, Speer W. Natural additives influence the performance and humoral immunity of broilers. Int J Poult Sci 2005; 4(9): 713-7.
[http://dx.doi.org/10.3923/ijps.2005.713.717]

[47] Abdel-Fattah SA, El-Sanhoury MH, El-Mednay NM, Abdel-Azeem F. Thyroid activity, some blood constituents, organs morphology and performance of broiler chicks fed supplemental organic acids. Int J Poult Sci 2008; 7(3): 215-22.
[http://dx.doi.org/10.3923/ijps.2008.215.222]

[48] Arif M, Rehman A, Saeed M, *et al.* Impacts of dietary humic acid supplementation on growth performance, some blood metabolites and carcass traits of broiler chicks. Indian J Anim Sci 2016; 86: 1073-8.

[49] Disetlhe ARP, Marume U, Mlambo V, Hugo A. Effects of dietary humic acid and enzymes on meat quality and fatty acid profiles of broiler chickens fed canola-based diets. Asian-Australas J Anim Sci 2019; 32(5): 711-20.
[http://dx.doi.org/10.5713/ajas.18.0408] [PMID: 30208685]

[50] Aristimunha PC, Mallheiros RD, Ferket PR, *et al.* Effect of dietary organic acids and humic substance supplementation on performance, immune response and gut morphology of broiler chickens. J Appl Poult Res 2020; 29(1): 85-94.
[http://dx.doi.org/10.3382/japr/pfz031]

[51] Açıkgöz Z, Bayraktar H, Altan ÖZ. Effects of formic acid administration in the drinking water on performance, intestinal microflora and carcass contamination in male broilers under high ambient temperature. Asian-Australas J Anim Sci 2010; 24(1): 96-102.
[http://dx.doi.org/10.5713/ajas.2011.10195]

[52] García V, Catala-Gregori P, Hernandez F, Megias MD, Madrid J. Effect of formic acid and plant extracts on growth, nutrient digestibility, intestine mucosa morphology, and meat yield of broilers. J Appl Poult Res 2007; 16(4): 555-62.
[http://dx.doi.org/10.3382/japr.2006-00116]

[53] Hernández F, García V, Madrid J, Orengo J, Catalá P, Megías MD. Effect of formic acid on performance, digestibility, intestinal histomorphology and plasma metabolite levels of broiler chickens. Br Poult Sci 2006; 47(1): 50-6.
[http://dx.doi.org/10.1080/00071660500475574] [PMID: 16546797]

[54] Ur Rehman Z, Ul Haq A, Akram N, *et al.* Growth performance, intestinal histomorphology, blood hematology and serum metabolites of broilers chickens fed diet supplemented with graded levels of acetic acid. Int J Pharmacol 2016; 12(8): 874-83.
[http://dx.doi.org/10.3923/ijp.2016.874.883]

[55] Kadim IT, Al-Marzooqi W, Mahgoub O, Al-Jabri A, Al-Waheebi SK. Effect of acetic acid supplementation on egg quality characteristics of commercial laying hens during hot season. Int J Poult Sci 2008; 7(10): 1015-21.

[56] Adil S, Banday T, Bhat GA, Mir MS, Rehman M. Effect of dietary supplementation of organic acids on performance, intestinal histomorphology, and serum biochemistry of broiler chicken 2010; 2010: 479485.
[http://dx.doi.org/10.4061/2010/479485]

[57] Chamba F, Puyalto M, Ortiz A, Torrealba H, Mallo JJ, Riboty R. Effect of partially protected sodium butyrate on performance, digestive organs, intestinal villi and *E. coli* development in broilers chickens. Int J Poult Sci 2014; 13(7): 390-6.

[http://dx.doi.org/10.3923/ijps.2014.390.396]

[58]   Patten JD, Waldroup PW. Use of organic acids in broiler diets. Poult Sci 1988; 67(8): 1178-82.
[http://dx.doi.org/10.3382/ps.0671178] [PMID: 3217307]

[59]   Pirgozliev V, Murphy TC, Owens B, George J, McCann ME. Fumaric and sorbic acid as additives in broiler feed. Res Vet Sci 2008; 84(3): 387-94.
[http://dx.doi.org/10.1016/j.rvsc.2007.06.010] [PMID: 17765939]

[60]   Ao T, Cantor AH, Pescatore AJ, Ford MJ, Pierce JL, Dawson KA. Effect of enzyme supplementation and acidification of diets on nutrient digestibility and growth performance of broiler chicks. Poult Sci 2009; 88(1): 111-7.
[http://dx.doi.org/10.3382/ps.2008-00191] [PMID: 19096065]

[61]   Bozkurt M, Küçükyılmaz K, Çatlı AU, Çınar M. Effect of dietary mannan oligosaccharide with or without oregano essential oil and hop extract supplementation on the performance and slaughter characteristics of male broilers. S Afr J Anim Sci 2009; 39: 3.
[http://dx.doi.org/10.4314/sajas.v39i3.49157]

[62]   Esmaeilipour O, Shivazad M, Moravej H, Aminzadeh S, Rezaian M, van Krimpen MM. Effects of xylanase and citric acid on the performance, nutrient retention, and characteristics of gastrointestinal tract of broilers fed low-phosphorus wheat-based diets. Poult Sci 2011; 90(9): 1975-82.
[http://dx.doi.org/10.3382/ps.2010-01264] [PMID: 21844263]

[63]   Józefiak D, Kaczmarek S, Rutkowski A. The effects of benzoic acid supplementation on the performance of broiler chickens. J Anim Physiol Anim Nutr (Berl) 2010; 94(1): 29-34.
[http://dx.doi.org/10.1111/j.1439-0396.2008.00875.x] [PMID: 19138347]

[64]   Adil S, Banday T, Ahmad Bhat G, Salahuddin M, Raquib M, Shanaz S. Response of broiler chicken to dietary supplementation of organic acids. J Cent Eur Agric 2011; 12: 3.
[http://dx.doi.org/10.5513/JCEA01/12.3.947]

CHAPTER 15

Beneficial Impacts of Probiotics on Poultry Nutrition

Mohamed E. Abd El-Hack[1,*], Mohammed A. E. Naiel[2], Samar S. Negm[3], Asmaa F. Khafaga[4], Mayada R. Farag[5], Shaaban S. Elnesr[6] and Mahmoud Alagawany[1,*]

[1] *Department of Poultry, Faculty of Agriculture, Zagazig University, Zagazig 44511, Egypt*

[2] *Department of Animal Production, Faculty of Agriculture, Zagazig University, Zagazig 44511, Egypt*

[3] *Fish Biology and Ecology Department, Central Lab for Aquaculture Research Abassa, Agriculture Research Centre, Giza, Egypt*

[4] *Department of Pathology, Faculty of Veterinary Medicine, Alexandria University, Edfina 22758, Egypt*

[5] *Forensic Medicine and Toxicology Department, Veterinary Medicine Faculty, Zagazig University, Zagazig 44519, Egypt*

[6] *Poultry Production Department, Faculty of Agriculture, Fayoum University, Fayoum 63514, Egypt*

Abstract: Antibiotics have been commonly used as growth enhancers to promote performance and feed efficiency in poultry production. It is essential to find new and safe alternative compounds to antibiotics due to their numerous harmful effects, such as antibiotic resistance, destruction of the gastrointestinal microbiota community, and dysbacteriosis. Improving poultry production using probiotics as feed additives is one of the decent alternative options to antibiotics. Probiotics are described as "living microorganisms that confer a benefit on the host health when applied in adequate quantities". Probiotics as feed additives help in feed digestion by creating the nutrients in an available form to grow faster. Also, poultry diets supplemented with probiotics improve immunity status. Besides, fortified poultry diets with probiotics enhance meat characterization and egg quality traits. Additionally, the use of probiotics in poultry feed could prevent various infectious diseases. Thus, obtaining optimum results requires a good selection of probiotic strains. This chapter focuses on the probiotics' mode of action and their relevance in poultry diet supplementation to improve production and preserve poultry health.

Keywords: Health, Mechanisms, Performance, Poultry, Probiotics.

---

* **Corresponding authors Mahmoud Alagawany and Mohamed E. Abd El-Hack:** Poultry Department, Faculty of Agriculture, Zagazig University, Zagazig, Egypt; E-mails: mmalagwany@zu.edu.eg and m.ezzat@zu.edu.eg

INTRODUCTION

Since the 1940s, antibiotics have been used as feed additives or growth promoters. It was found that using chlortetracycline supplemented diets with *Streptomyces aureofaciens* enhanced the bird's growth performance [1]. Since 2006, the European Union (EU) has restricted antibiotics use as growth promoter agents or for food supplementation; the ban to the antibiotics use was due to induction of bacterial resistance strains against antibiotics used for a long time to prevent poultry diseases. Also, antibiotics induce several other problems, such as the destruction of various gastrointestinal beneficial microbiota. Furthermore, the EU observed that using antibiotics may lead to growth reduction, which might lead to a growing prevalence of subclinical dysbacteriosis and necrotic enteritis [2].

The demand from customers and their fears about the adverse effects of antibiotic usage in poultry diets and the EU's restriction encouraged researchers to consider antibiotics [3]. These alternatives are aimed to induce a high survival rate against infectious diseases, being a safe animal product while protecting the consumer's health and environment. Many research papers have accomplished to search for natural substances with similar positive effects as traditional growth promoters [4]. However, there are a variety of non-therapeutic compounds that could be alternative antibiotics. Amongst these, the common are prebiotics, probiotics, natural organic acids, synthetic enzymes, immunostimulant agents, bacterial proteinaceous, phages, phenolic compounds, nanoparticles, and volatile oils [5]. Probiotics' beneficial and protective effects are evident in numerous features. These could be recommended as a valuable strategy for preventing pathogenic bacteria and enhancing performance, egg quality, nutrients absorption, thereby improving poultry health [6 - 8]. Hence, probiotics play a vital role as the profit alternative to antibiotics due to their several useful impacts on animals' growth, involving fish and poultry [9].

FAO/WHO [10] defined probiotics as a live microorganism. When fortified into suitable quantities, itconfers a profit on the host health. Additionally, Hill, Guarner [11] recommended this definition of a probiotic. Likewise, Abd El-Hack, Mahgoub [12] have defined probiotics as live microorganisms used as feed supplements which positively enhanc the gastrointestinal tract *via* improving the gut microbiota community and improving nutrient absorption, performance, feed efficiency and economic aspects of poultry. This enhancement is supported by decreasing intestinal pH, microbiota and increasing the digestive enzymes [13, 14]. The probiotics' mode of action depends on the endogenous enzymes' stimulation, reduction of toxic substances, metabolism [15], and produced antibacterial compounds or vitamins [16]. Probiotic bacteria produce antibacterial proteins such as bacteriocins, which prevent toxins and promote the development of pathogenic bacterial strains [17]. Therefore, Probiotics enhance the immune status and improve resistance to pathogenic bacterial colonization [16]. For example, supplementation of chicken feed with *Enterococcus faecium*in showed an antimicrobial effect on the small intestine microflora [18]. Similar results were described by Latha, Vinothini [19] using *Streptomyces* sp. The study by Zhang, Cho [20] revealed that supplementing broiler diets with 10^5 cfu of *Bacillus subtilis* prevents necrotic enteritis, increases body weight and the thymus relative weight percentage. Furthermore, treating chicken with probiotic reduced the NH_3 and H_2S production levels in excretions, consequently leading to smaller odor emissions. Selecting suitable probiotic strains could reduce the harmful effects of antibiotic usage and have many useful outcomes due to its capability to prevent the pathogen's development.

Probiotics include numerous species, for example, beneficial intestinal microbiota, yeast or fungi, and the mainly recommended probiotics strains are *Bacillus subtilis, Bifidobacterium, Lactobacillus,* and *Streptococcus*, which inhibit the development of several pathogenic bacteria such as *Clostridium perfringens, Staphylococcus aureus, Salmonella typhimurium, Escherichia coli, etc.* [13 - 15, 21]. Besides, probiotics show several affirmative effects on the characterization of poultry meat [8, 16]. They enhance pH values, meat color, the profile of fatty acid, body chemical composition, the capacity of water retention and oxidative status [8, 12]. The probiotics also increase the meat contents from protein and fat and, therefore, the quality of meat. Abdurrahman, Pramono [22] stated a strong correlation between the oxidation of lipids and the feed quality deterioration. Other research may support this hypothesis by showing that the presence of *Aspergillus awamori* and *Saccharomyces cerevisiae* in chicken diets deprives the blood content of saturated fatty acids and increases polyunsaturated fatty acids [23]. Another related study carried out by Liu, Yan [24] found that supplementing broiler chicken diets with *Bacillus licheniformis* enhanced color, flavor and juiciness of produced meat, and increased the protein percentage and the respective aromatic and indispensable amino acids. Probiotics might prevent the incidence of the coccoidal diseases. Also, Giannenas, Papadopoulos [25] showed that treating chicken with probiotics in the absence of anticoccidial infections decreases the influence of parasite infection. Besides, using probiotics exerted coccidio static influence against *Eimeria tenella*. This could reduce the high risk and spread of coccidiosis and preserve gastrointestinal health [3].

This chapter highlights the probiotics sources, mode of action and healthy profits. Besides, the probiotics application in poultry diets, effects on the production and immune status have been defined here, which could be beneficial for researchers, veterinarians, nutritionists, and poultry producers.

THE PROBIOTIC APPROACH IN POULTRY NUTRITION

Fig. (**1**) shows the modes of action and beneficial activities of probiotics in poultry. At the beginning of the 20th century, the use of antibiotics collaborated with poultry production. Antibiotics are well known for high feed efficiency, improved animal production, and reduced mortality rates due to lower clinical and subclinical disease occurrences [26]. Since 1951, the National Research Council of Food and Drug Administration permits further use of specific antibiotics on livestock feeds [27]. Recently, the European Union restricted antibiotics use as growth promoter agents to minimize the risk of developing antibiotic-resistant organisms, which could pose a risk to human health [28] and cause an increased prevalence of poultry disease, an imbalance between pathogenic and beneficial microbiota, and the development of tolerant bacterial strains to antibiotics [3]. Thus, there is a massive interest in discovering antibiotic alternatives for poultry production. Probiotics have been identified as effective alternatives to growth promoters or antibiotics and safe feed additives that can prevent inflammatory gastrointestinal diseases and produce healthy poultry products [29 - 32].

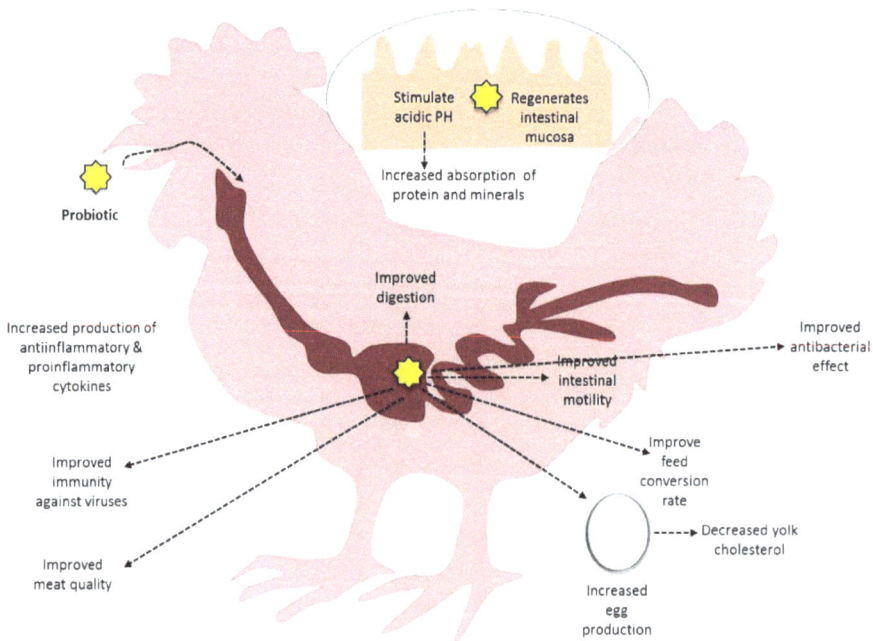

Fig. (1). Modes of action and beneficial activities of probiotics in poultry.

Probiotics are described as a live microbial feed supplement that benefits the host by improving the intestinal microbiota balance and maintaining the gut's optimum pH level, thus improving the bird's health immune status [33]. A more recent national Food Ingredient Association [NFA] definition that a probiotic [direct-fed microbial, DFM] is a resource of live, natural microorganisms, including bacteria, fungi and yeast [34]. The broiler performance is also enhanced and of probiotic, which supports producing high meat quality without any drug contaminants [35]. The concepts and developments discussed regarding the implementation of probiotic would be useful to researchers, poultry farmers, feed manufactures, and veterinarians and will improve economic benefits and profits by enhancing the safety and development of poultry sector through feed alteration.

There are numerous natural resources from probiotics, for example, bacterial strains [*Bacillus subtilis, Lactobacillus, Bifidobacterium* and *Streptococcus*], fungi [*Aspergillus*] and yeast [*Saccharomyces cerevisiae, Saccharomyces boulardii* and *Candida*]. Two main groups of microbiota may live in the gastrointestinal tract [36]. The first type arises in near contact with the intestinal epithelium and the second is free in the lumen of the gut [37].

The Active Probiotic Strains Used Within Poultry Feeds

Therefore, the adhesion capability of the microorganism would not be essential, and probiotic organisms can be formulated for poultry either to create beneficial microbiota absent from the gastrointestinal tract or even provide certain beneficial bacteria [38]. The bacterial species of *Lactobacillus* and *S. Fecium* are commonly found in the gastrointestinal tract, while *Bacillus* spp. and yeasts are discovered only sporadically in the gut microflora [39]. Besides, *lactobacillus* preparations are among the first group: they develop on the small intestine and exert antibacterial compounds effects against defined pathogenic bacterium [40]. Additionally, these can generate large quantities of carbohydrate lactate and tolerate a high acidity that is usually lethal to other bacterial strains [41]. A beneficial lactic acid microflora was formed in the gastrointestinal tract 24 hours after chicks were supplemented with live *lactobacillus bacteria* [35]. Groups of direct-fed probiotic microorganisms such as lactic acid bacteria are remarkably fragile. They must be technologically covered to protect them from the heat and pressure during the processing of feed [without protection, *lactobacilli*, yeasts and *streptococci* tolerate only up to 52, 63 and 71°C, respectively] [42]. However, spore *Bacillus* species are more tolerant and easily survive pelleting during feed manufacture [43].

Many probiotic strains are uncommon, like *Leuconostoc mesenteroides* and *Lactobacillus plantarum,* which could be isolated from fresh plants [44]. In bird's diets, the probiotic used may consist of a single bacterial strain or a mixture of two or more species [45]. Furthermore, various types of probiotics such as oil, powder, gel, paste, and granules are commonly found in pellets, tablets, bags, *etc.*

[21]. Dry dosage type of probiotics has a longer shelf life and a greater tolerance to the gastrointestinal condition. The usage of hydroxypropyl methylcellulose phthalate 55 by oral delivery has good probiotic efficacy in the poultry [46].

Mechanisms of Beneficial Probiotic in Poultry

Probiotic action mechanisms function in two ways: the prior enhances growth efficiency, whereas the latter improves immune status. The function or mechanism of different bacterial strains in a probiotic community can differentiate [47]. For example, isolating bacteria may be unique within the same species and might have different adherence areas, similar immune responses, and other physiological behavior [48]. Therefore, probiotics containing related bacterial species can differ in their effectiveness [33].

The stimulating growth performance mechanism of probiotic could occur either in a direct or indirect way. Regulatory growth efficiency in poultry occurs directly by maintaining epithelial barriers that increase nutrient absorption and promote growth [49]. It can also promote digestive enzyme production, increasing the availability of nutrients in the gastrointestinal tract [50]. The *Lactobacillus spp.* and *Bacillus spp.* could induce indirect enhancement in the poultry gastrointestinal tract *via* regulation of the production of volatile fatty acids [VFA] by encouragement of nutrient availability [51, 52]. The VFA can also support gastrointestinal health by direct stimulation of epithelial cell proliferation [53]. Such fatty acids, mainly acetate, propionate, and butyrate, are ingested immediately in the hindgut and used as energy sources in tissues [54]. Mechanistically, butyrate can affect this by regulating antioxidant gene expression such as peroxisome proliferator-activated receptor-gamma 1-alpha [PGC-1α], peroxisome proliferator-activated receptor alpha [PPARα], carnitine palmitoyl transferase 1 [CPT1a], and acyl CoA oxidase [ACO] and deceased fatty acid synthase [FAS] in adipocytes [55, 56]. Butyrate can also control chicken growth by selectively partitioning nutrients away from the liver and adipose tissue into the muscle by selectively controlling the expression of the muscle insulin receptor β subunit [IRβ] [57]. Therefore, probiotics can stimulate growth by increased production of VFA in poultry and by active regulation of insulin signaling in various tissues [58]. However, they can act as direct moderators of gene expression and phenotype by functioning as epigenetic promoters of multiple gene expression that can have significant implications for poultry's health and growth [59, 60].

The second mechanism was the control of the immune response by the probiotics. Activation of the immune response results in synthetic nutrients being redirected from successful pathways such as tissue accretion or egg production *via* the immune regulation process [26, 61 - 63]. Probiotic was blocked for all pathogens by generating organic acid compounds and antibacterial molecules such as hydrogen peroxide, bacteriocins and defensins, preventing pathogenic bacterial permeability to intestinal receptors using competitive inhibitors [64]. Also, it can modulate the innate immune response by affecting regulatory T-cells, cell-presenting antigen, T- and B-cells and enterocytes, and intestinal mucosal regeneration [65, 66].

However, Roselli, Finamore [67] and Tiwari, Tiwari [64] reported that probiotics might also regulate the development of anti- and pro-inflammatory cytokine and help stimulate antibody mass production [sIgA], actually enhance the behavior of lymphocytes and macrophages [NK] cells, transmit the function and phenotype of dendritic cells, accentuate the AP-1 and NF-kB pathways, modulate apoptosis, and generate nitric oxide. It may also enhance epithelial layer function, regulate mucous development and gastric motility, and promote acid pH, which stimulates the absorption of proteins and minerals such as copper, calcium, iron, manganese, and magnesium [68]. The immunostimulant role of probiotic species is demonstrated in a strain-specific manner *via* its influence on T-helper cells, as well as, the fact that it can activate specific cytokines [69]. It can also alleviate cardiovascular diseases because of its capability to decrease cholesterol levels [70]. Rather, Choi [71] study showed that probiotic bacteria [*Lactobacillus plantarum* YML009] does have an anti-viral capacity against the H1N1 influenza virus; however, its mechanisms still need to be discovered.

The Applications of Probiotics in Poultry Feeds

In the diet of broiler chicks, the probiotics substantially develop an immune response [35]. Probiotics feeding has also been confirmed to increase antibodies titers against viral diseases such as Newcastle Disease (ND) and Infectious Bursal Disease (IBD) [72]. It improves the bird's resistance to defend off microbial pathogens and the adverse effects on its growth [73]. The probiotic decreases the pathogenic bacterial load of the intestine and reduces pathogenic bacteria spreading in the poultry housing farm through contamination of fecal. Probiotic multiple strains must be used correctly and periodically in feed to avoid various pathogens, including bacterial, fungal, protozoan and viral agents [33]. At the same trend, using probiotics as feed additives can decrease the flock mortality rate caused by immunosuppressive diseases such as IBD, anemia, Marek's disease, mycotoxins, *etc.* [74].

In recent years, the emphasis seems to be on probiotics as an alternative feed supplement to antibiotics due to its critical demand in the poultry industry [75]. Studies have reported probiotics' ability to regulate the gastrointestinal tract's bacterial alance and, subsequently, the animal natural defense mechanism against pathogenic bacteria [76 - 78]. Such species have been aided by the normal adaptation of numerous lactic acid bacteria to the gastrointestinal environment and its antibacterial compounds [peptidic toxins and organic acids] with a suitable benefit compared to other microorganisms to be used as a probiotic supplementation [79]. Numerous studies have indicated that supplemented feed diets with probiotics have good effects on feed efficiency and utilization, performance, and the survival rate [31, 80, 81]. The efficacy of probiotics mainly depends on applying more productive strains, gene modulation, the relationship among several strains, and the mixture of probiotics and therapeutically acting compounds [33]. The use of multi-strain probiotics is an excellent way to potentiate the useful effects of probiotics by enhancing beneficial bacteria's development against pathogenic bacterium antagonism in the gut tract of birds [35].

Probiotics exert numerous advantages on the host, such as promoting the mucosal immune status and enhancing the intestinal lumen environment, epithelial and mucosal barrier functions [82]. These feed additives can increase the appetite and treat the maldigestion by depressing gastrointestinal disturbance. These could also be used as immune promoters by stimulating the immune properties and improving the specific humoral vaccine effects and cell-mediated immunity reactions in the host [83]. The valuable probiotics applications are their role as anti-oxidant, anti-inflammatory, anti-allergic, anti-cancerous, strong anti-mutagenic, anti-diabetic, and antiviral against many poultry viruses [84]. Furthermore, probiotic additives have been used efficiently in examining the pathogenic bacterial load of meat and meat products throughout packaging and processing [35]. Additionally, supplemented broiler diets with *Bacillus subtilis* spore [GalliPro®] at 0.2 g kg^{-1} could reduce the amino acid requirements, and as a result, decrease the feeding cost [85]. Apata [86] reported that supplemented broiler diets with probiotics [*Lactobacillus bulgaricus* at 20, 40 and 60 mg kg^{-1}] significantly enhanced the apparent digestion coefficients of some nutrients such as crude protein and amino acids.

Enhancing Growth Performance and Production

Probiotics have also been used to enhance the digestion and absorption of the nutrients; assistance in the metabolism of minerals and vitamins synthesis process [Biotin, Vitamin-B1, B2, B12 and K] are liable for promoting growth and metabolism functions. These can also deactivate toxins exerted by pathogenic bacteria *via* producing anti-enterotoxin compounds [acidolin, acidophilin and lactin] and have also been verified to bind feed mycotoxins [87]. This has been useful in alleviating the litter ammonia production by their reversal effects against ammonifying bacteria and decreased urease activity, thus inhibiting kerato conjunctivitis development [74]. Supplemented poultry diets with *L. acidophilus* and *L. casei* alone or combined throughout the feed or even the water significantly reduced the serum triglycerides levels [33]. This decrease in the lipid content may be due to the modification in fat digestion and gallbladder acids [88]. Besides, broiler chickens fed with dietary *Bacillus subtilis* supplemented diets exhibited decreased serum liver and carcass triglyceride levels because of their efficiency in restricting the rate of fatty acids synthesis *via* diminishing the acetyl coenzyme A carboxylase activities [89].

Supplementing laying hen diets with a commercial probiotic product [Protexin®; a mixture of beneficial bacterial strains] improved the growth performance and egg quality traits [90]. Besides, feeding ISA-Brown and Leghorn laying hens diets supplemented with probiotics [mixture from *Lactobacillus*, *Bifidobacterium*, *Streptococcus* and *Enterococcus* spp.] at 0.1% and 0.2% enhanced the egg mass [91]. In contrast, Ramasamy, Abdullah [92] revealed that using probiotics as feed additives had no significant effect on egg yield and production. Whereas *Lactobacillus* supplemented diets promoted egg weight and size during the laying period of hens. Also, Probiotic *(Bacillus subtilis)* at rate 1×10^8 cfu kg^{-1} in diets had a valuable influence on layer performance, egg quality traits and cholesterol levels of yolk lipids [93]. Likewise, supplementation of *Bacillus subtilis* at 8×10^5 cfu g^{-1} and multi-strain probiotics [MP] at 0.4% levels in layer diets enhanced egg quality, improved egg production, and decreased the feed costs [94]. Thus, probiotics as natural products could be a good strategy alternative for using antibiotics in poultry diets, probably to increase the productive performance, egg quality traits, and feed efficiency [95].

Using *Bacillus amyloliquefaciens* probiotic [BAP] as a direct broiler chickens feed additive [20 g kg^{-1}] for 35 days significantly enhanced the growth performance. This is suitable for improving gastrointestinal health by enhancing the digestion and absorption of the gut [15]. As well, it may cause improved digestibility or increae the all nutrients availability [96]. Also, broilers diets supplemented with *Bacillus coagulans* NJ0516 revealed a significant increase in amylase and protease activities and enhanced starch and protein digestibility, consequently improving the broilers' performance [50]. Another study, using fermented Ginkgo biloba and Camelia sinensis based probiotics as feed additives in Ross broilers at 0.1% or 0.2%, significantly displayed promoted growth and feed efficiency. Also, the pathogenic *E. coli* bacterial load was lowered in their caecal flora [97]. Conversely, Afsari, Mohebbifar [98] found that supplementing laying hens' feed diets with probiotic has no significant impact on egg production and size. *In ovo* supplementation [embryonic age of 18d] with PrimaLac®

[*Lactobacillus acidophilus, Lactobacillus casei, Enterococcus faecium* and *Bifidobacterium bifidium*] at 1×10^6 cfu improved the growth performance first-week post-hatch without any adverse effects on the hatchability rate [99].

Health and Immunity

The use of probiotics in freshly hatched chicks is recommended to develop gut microbial equilibrium and prevent early chick mortality and stressful environmental effects during rearing management. Probiotics are now approved for use during antibiotic treatment to preserve the necessary microflora intestinal balance and minimize diarrhea without influencinging antibiotics' effectiveness. Probiotics are also seen as decent alternatives to antibiotics for growth promotion that benefits from reducing antibiotic residues in poultry products and eliminating drug-resistant microbes [32].

Probiotics products may be a useful alternative to antibiotics in poultry nutrition and are expected to improve bird health and immunity status [95]. A study [100] results revealed that using *Clostridium butyricum* at concentration 2×10^7 cfu or 3×10^7 cfu kg^{-1} in broilers' feed diets promoted the intestinal microbiota balance and enhanced the immune status. By the way, Bai, Wu [101] found that supplementing broilers feed diets with 1×10^7 cfu g^{-1} *Lactobacillus fermentum* and 2×10^7 cfu g^{-1}*Saccharomyces cerevisiae* at 0.1% or 0.2% in combined form might improve the T-cell production in the intestine without inducing any harmful effects on growth. Furthermore, Lee, Lillehoj [102] stated that supplementing chicken diets with *Bacillus* [5×10^6 cfu per 0.5 ml sterile distilled water] significantly decreased the gastrointestinal lesions score induced by *Eimeria maxima* infection. It may be attributed to enhanced immunity, as shown by increased serum nitric oxide levels in birds fed with probiotic enriched diets.

Likewise, Liao, Ma [103] investigated that feeding broilers with 2.5×10^8 or 5×10^8 or 1×10^9 cfu *Clostridium butyricum* kg^{-1} diet enhanced immune response and antioxidant status. Fortified feed diets with probiotic products [contain *Bacillus subtilis, Clostridium butyricum and Lactobacillus acidophilus*] promoted humoral immunity and amino acid digestion in broilers [104]. Besides, Al-Fataftah and Abdelqader [105] confirmed that supplemented broiler diets with 1 g *B. subtilis* kg^{-1} under heat stress conditions were efficient in alleviating the adverse effects on performance through enhancing the beneficial gastrointestinal microbiota colonization and developing the impaired villus-crypt construct. The use of probiotics in poultry diets also increases the effectiveness of vaccines in them. Treated drinking water with Probiotic at 200g kg^{-1} promoted the humoral immune status during the Lasota Newcastle disease vaccine in broiler chickens. This was due to their influence resulting in increased expression of IL-7 mRNA in Harder's gland, caecal tonsils, duodenum and patch of ileal Peyer [106]. Also, using gel probiotics [Poultry Star®] with coccidia vaccine was realized to enhance defense mechanisms against *Eimeria* infection disease [6]. This may be due to the ability of *Saccharomyces boulardii* and *Bacillus subtilis* B10 to improve mRNA expression [cloudin2 and cloudin3], consequently modifying the intestinal ultrastructure [107]. Ramasamy, Abdullah [108] showed that supplemented laying hens with probiotic [*Lactobacillus* culture] reduced the contents of the egg from cholesterol by 10.4% at 28 weeks of age. In addition, Tang, Sieo [109] showed a significant decrease in the egg yolk cholesterol and total saturated fatty acids after supplementing layer diets with probiotic [0.1% PrimaLac®] at 28 weeks of age and improved total unsaturated fatty acids content during 28, 32 and 36 weeks of age.

Countering Infectious Pathogens

In poultry, probiotic bacterial colonization, as determined by colony-forming units [CFU], increases the amount from the beak to the colon [110]. The feed ingredients, proventriculus, and gizzard have a minimum load of anaerobic bacteria due to the oxygen absorbed in the feed and the small luminal pH, mainly associated with hydrochloric acid in the proventriculus [111]. The small intestine has large amounts of facultative anaerobe bacteria such as *Lactobacilli* spp., *Streptococci* and *Enterobacteria*, *Bifidobacterium spp.*, *Bacteroides spp.* and *Clostridia* spp., with rates between 10^4 and 10^8 CFU ml^{-1} [112]. The most heavily colonized gastrointestinal [GI] tract regions are the colon and cecum with the colonization of 10^{10} to 10^{13} CFU ml^{-1} [113].

Using probiotics as feed additives plays a vital role in protecting against enteric bacterial infections induced by certain pathogenic bacteria. *Lactobacillus*'s specific strain*s* have beneficial effects on raw chicken meat induced *Listeria monocytogenes* and *Salmonella* enteridite infection [114]. Supplementing feed diets with *L. johnsonii* FI9785 strain reduced the necrotic enteritis lesion score induced by *Clostridium perfringens* infection [13, 100, 103]. *Bacillus longum* can survive in chicken's gastrointestinal tract and has significant antimicrobial activity against *Campylobacter* infection, thereby minimizing the contamination load of the intestinal pathogens in the farm and chicken meat [115]. Besides, *Bacillus licheniformis* was effective in improving productivity and the quality of meat of the broiler [24]. Also, Giannenas, Papadopoulos [25] found that dietary probiotics have been valuable in promoting the growth of broiler chickens challenged with *E. tenella*.

Supplemented feed and water with probiotics have been found to enhance performance, feed efficiency, and poultry birds' health against *Eimeria* species infections, causing coccidiosis [6]. *In ovo* injection of probiotic bacteria [Prima Lac®] at level 1×10⁶ cfu in 18d embryonic age showed hatched chicks protection against mixed *Eimeria* spp. challenge at 3d post-hatch [116]. This may be because of their activating effect on caecal and ileum immune system response genes [99]. The use of probiotics may also help prevent *Listeria monocytogenes* in poultry [29]. Administration of probiotic Prima Lac® in poultry diets has been proven to increase antibody titers to mitigate viral diseases such as Newcastle disease [ND] and infectious bursal disease [IBD] [117]. Also, Hasanzadeh and Far [118] reported that supplemented feed diets with *Echinacea purpurea* and protexin® probiotic enhanced mucosal immunity against NDV and ND diseases in turkey.

Several studies have shown the effect of dietary supplementation of probiotics on reducing numerous types of gut pathogens such as *Salmonella enteritidis, Salmonella gallinarum, Salmonella typhimurium* and *Campylobacter jejuni* [14, 119 - 122]. Besides, probiotic supplementation decreased *Escherichia coli* and total coliform counts and increased *lactobacilli* in the broiler chickens' intestines [80]. The probiotic mixture [*Lactobacillus pentosus* ITA23 and *Lactobacillus acidophilus* ITA44] increased the bacterial count of cecal by lowering the number of *Escherichia coli* and growing beneficial bacteria [123]. The latter action could be due to several modes of actions by direct-fed microorganisms, depending on the strains or species in different products used in such experiments. For example, Prima Lac® prevents infection of *Campylobacter jejuni* in broilers due to its ability to release organic acid and protein molecules from probiotic bacteria that destroy pathogenic bacteria and that are hypersensitive to low pH conditions [124]. At the same trend, fortified birds fed diets with *Bacillus subtilis* C-3102 possibly could decrease *Campylobacter* growing in poultry [125]. *Lactobacillus gasseri* SBT2055 inhibited the adhesion, invasion, and colonization of *C. jejuni* [126]. An *in vivo* experiment was performed with various isolates *Bacillus sp.* in chickens to prevent the *Campylobacter sp.* infection [115]. Supplementing poultry diet with *Lactobacillus salivarius* 59 and *Enterococcus faecium* PXN33 combination instigated a decrease in *Salmonella Enteritidis* S1400 colonization [120]. A probiotic strain of *E. coli* Nissle 1917 was restructured at the genetic level to secrete Microcin J25, an antimicrobial peptide. Forkus, Ritter [127] showed that the utilization of developed *E. coli* might diminish gastrointestinal *Salmonella* enterica in turkeys. Researchers examined various bacteria as a probiotic source based on their function. Examination of the ability of three *B. subtilis* on reducing *C. jejuni* colonization showed that the good isolate motility had increased capability to reduce colonization due to its capability to reach the *C. jejuni* site faster [128]. Schematic representation for the antimicrobial activities of probiotics on intestinal mucosa is illustrated in Fig. (**2**).

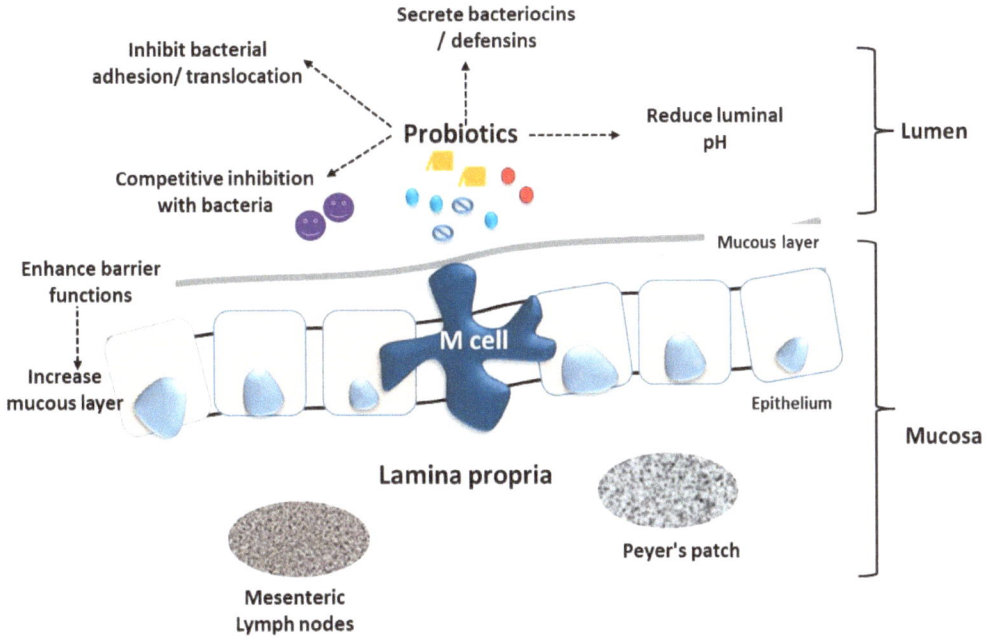

Fig. (2). Schematic representation for the antimicrobial activities of probiotics on the intestinal mucosa.

CONCLUDING REMARKS

The probiotics practically in poultry diets lead to numerous health and production profits. Indeed, they will act as the proper alternative strategy for using antibiotics in poultry diets. Immunomodulatory effects are additional benefits for producing healthy meat and eggs besides reducing feed cost and the inhibition of bird loss or drug expenditure. We also realize differences in the researcher's findings with no additional advantages of the probiotic application. The vital issue to address in this pathway is to achieve the ideal dose and suitable strain of probiotic for particular required action. Enhancement in their form and transport methods will also support in realizing a high potential of probiotics. A further area of profit can also be discovered, which could be attained throughout their possible use with more experimental trials and encouraging research. Additionally, their mode of action will be useful in obtaining more advantages from them. Even though a significant amount of work exists, the positive effects of using probiotics in poultry feed on production still require additional investigation to derive out some specific protocol for their application.

CONSENT FOR PUBLICATION

Not applicable.

CONFLICT OF INTEREST

The author declares no conflict of interest, financial or otherwise.

ACKNOWLEDGEMENTS

All the authors acknowledge and thank their respective Institutes and Universities.

REFERENCES

[1]　Eckert N, Lee J, Hyatt D, *et al.* Influence of probiotic administration by feed or water on growth parameters of broilers reared on medicated and nonmedicated diets. J Appl Poult Res 2010; 19(1): 59-67.
[http://dx.doi.org/10.3382/japr.2009-00084]

[2]　M'Sadeq SA, Wu S, Swick RA, Choct M. Towards the control of necrotic enteritis in broiler chickens with in-feed antibiotics phasing-out worldwide. Anim Nutr 2015; 1(1): 1-11.
[http://dx.doi.org/10.1016/j.aninu.2015.02.004] [PMID: 29766984]

[3]　Mehdi Y, Létourneau-Montminy M-P, Gaucher M-L, *et al.* Use of antibiotics in broiler production: Global impacts and alternatives. Animal nutrition 2018; 4(2): 8-170.

[4]　Yadav AS, Kolluri G, Gopi M, Karthik K, Singh Y. Exploring alternatives to antibiotics as health promoting agents in poultry-a review. J Exp Biol 2016; 4(3S-10.18006): 3S.

[5]　Tiwari R, Chakraborty S, Dhama K, Wani MY, Kumar A, Kapoor S. Wonder world of phages: potential biocontrol agents safeguarding biosphere and health of animals and humans- current scenario and perspectives. Pak J Biol Sci 2014; 17(3): 316-28.
[http://dx.doi.org/10.3923/pjbs.2014.316.328] [PMID: 24897785]

[6]　Ritzi MM, Abdelrahman W, Mohnl M, Dalloul RA. Effects of probiotics and application methods on performance and response of broiler chickens to an *Eimeria* challenge. Poult Sci 2014; 93(11): 2772-8.
[http://dx.doi.org/10.3382/ps.2014-04207] [PMID: 25214558]

[7]　Alagawany M, Abd El-Hack ME, Farag MR, Sachan S, Karthik K, Dhama K. The use of probiotics as eco-friendly alternatives for antibiotics in poultry nutrition. Environ Sci Pollut Res Int 2018; 25(11): 10611-8.
[http://dx.doi.org/10.1007/s11356-018-1687-x] [PMID: 29532377]

[8]　Popova T. Effect of probiotics in poultry for improving meat quality. Curr Opin Food Sci 2017; 14: 72-7.
[http://dx.doi.org/10.1016/j.cofs.2017.01.008]

[9]　Zorriehzahra MJ, Delshad ST, Adel M, *et al.* Probiotics as beneficial microbes in aquaculture: an update on their multiple modes of action: a review. Vet Q 2016; 36(4): 228-41.
[http://dx.doi.org/10.1080/01652176.2016.1172132] [PMID: 27075688]

[10]　FAO/WHO. Guidelines for the Evaluation of Probiotics in Food. London, ON: FAO/WHO 2002.

[11]　Hill C, Guarner F, Reid G, *et al.* Expert consensus document. The International Scientific Association for Probiotics and Prebiotics consensus statement on the scope and appropriate use of the term probiotic. Nat Rev Gastroenterol Hepatol 2014; 11(8): 506-14.
[http://dx.doi.org/10.1038/nrgastro.2014.66] [PMID: 24912386]

[12]　Abd El-Hack ME, Mahgoub SA, Alagawany M, Ashour EA. Improving productive performance and mitigating harmful emissions from laying hen excreta *via* feeding on graded levels of corn DDGS with or without *Bacillus subtilis* probiotic. J Anim Physiol Anim Nutr (Berl) 2017; 101(5): 904-13.
[http://dx.doi.org/10.1111/jpn.12522] [PMID: 27184423]

[13] Hussein EOS, Ahmed SH, Abudabos AM, *et al.* Effect of Antibiotic, Phytobiotic and Probiotic Supplementation on Growth, Blood Indices and Intestine Health in Broiler Chicks Challenged with *Clostridium perfringens.* Animals (Basel) 2020; 10(3): 507.
[http://dx.doi.org/10.3390/ani10030507] [PMID: 32197455]

[14] El-Shall NA, Awad AM, El-Hack MEA, *et al.* The Simultaneous Administration of a Probiotic or Prebiotic with Live *Salmonella* Vaccine Improves Growth Performance and Reduces Fecal Shedding of the Bacterium in *Salmonella*-Challenged Broilers. Animals (Basel) 2019; 10(1): 70.
[http://dx.doi.org/10.3390/ani10010070] [PMID: 31906020]

[15] Arif M, Iram A, Bhutta MAK, *et al.* The Biodegradation Role of *Saccharomyces cerevisiae* against Harmful Effects of Mycotoxin Contaminated Diets on Broiler Performance, Immunity Status, and Carcass characteristics. Animals (Basel) 2020; 10(2): 238.
[http://dx.doi.org/10.3390/ani10020238] [PMID: 32028628]

[16] Hassanein SM, Soliman NK. Effect of probiotic [Saccharomyces cerevisiae] adding to diets on intestinal microflora and performance of Hy-Line layers hens. J Am Sci 2010; 6(11): 159-69.

[17] Pan D, Yu Z. Intestinal microbiome of poultry and its interaction with host and diet. Gut Microbes 2014; 5(1): 108-19.
[http://dx.doi.org/10.4161/gmic.26945] [PMID: 24256702]

[18] Levkut M, Revajová V, Lauková A, *et al.* Leukocytic responses and intestinal mucin dynamics of broilers protected with *Enterococcus faecium* EF55 and challenged with *Salmonella Enteritidis.* Res Vet Sci 2012; 93(1): 195-201.
[http://dx.doi.org/10.1016/j.rvsc.2011.06.021] [PMID: 21767856]

[19] Latha S, Vinothini G, John Dickson Calvin D, Dhanasekaran D. *In vitro* probiotic profile based selection of indigenous actinobacterial probiont *Streptomyces sp.* JD9 for enhanced broiler production. J Biosci Bioeng 2016; 121(1): 124-31.
[http://dx.doi.org/10.1016/j.jbiosc.2015.04.019] [PMID: 26111601]

[20] Zhang Z, Cho J, Kim I. Effects of *Bacillus subtilis* UDT-MO2 on growth performance, relative immune organ weight, gas concentration in excreta, and intestinal microbial shedding in broiler chickens. Livest Sci 2013; 155(2-3): 343-7.
[http://dx.doi.org/10.1016/j.livsci.2013.05.021]

[21] Iannitti T, Palmieri B. Therapeutical use of probiotic formulations in clinical practice. Clin Nutr 2010; 29(6): 701-25.
[http://dx.doi.org/10.1016/j.clnu.2010.05.004] [PMID: 20576332]

[22] Abdurrahman Z, Pramono Y, Suthama N. Meat Characteristic of Crossbred Local Chicken Fed Inulin of Dahlia Tuber and *Lactobacillus sp.* Media Peternakan 2016; 39. [2].
[http://dx.doi.org/10.5398/medpet.2016.39.2.112]

[23] Saleh AA, Eid YZ, Ebeid TA, *et al.* The modification of the muscle fatty acid profile by dietary supplementation with Aspergillus awamori in broiler chickens. Br J Nutr 2012; 108(9): 1596-602.
[http://dx.doi.org/10.1017/S0007114511007069] [PMID: 22289635]

[24] Liu X, Yan H, Lv L, *et al.* Growth performance and meat quality of broiler chickens supplemented with Bacillus licheniformis in drinking water. Asian-Australas J Anim Sci 2012; 25(5): 682-9.
[http://dx.doi.org/10.5713/ajas.2011.11334] [PMID: 25049614]

[25] Giannenas I, Papadopoulos E, Tsalie E, *et al.* Assessment of dietary supplementation with probiotics on performance, intestinal morphology and microflora of chickens infected with *Eimeria tenella.* Vet Parasitol 2012; 188(1-2): 31-40.
[http://dx.doi.org/10.1016/j.vetpar.2012.02.017] [PMID: 22459110]

[26] Ajuwon KM. Chronic immune stimulation in adipose tissue and its consequences for health and performance in the pig. Vet Immunol Immunopathol 2014; 159(3-4): 166-70.
[http://dx.doi.org/10.1016/j.vetimm.2014.02.013] [PMID: 24646651]

[27]   NRC tNRC Issues specific to antibiotics The Use of Drugs in Food Animals: Benefits and Risks:. [US]: National Academies Press 1999.

[28]   Ronquillo MG, Hernandez JCA. Antibiotic and synthetic growth promoters in animal diets: review of impact and analytical methods. Food Control 2017; 72: 255-67.
[http://dx.doi.org/10.1016/j.foodcont.2016.03.001]

[29]   Dhama K, Karthik K, Tiwari R, *et al.* Listeriosis in animals, its public health significance (food-borne zoonosis) and advances in diagnosis and control: a comprehensive review. Vet Q 2015; 35(4): 211-35.
[http://dx.doi.org/10.1080/01652176.2015.1063023] [PMID: 26073265]

[30]   Edens F. An alternative for antibiotic se in poultry: probiotics. Braz J Poult Sci 2003; 5(2): 75-97.
[http://dx.doi.org/10.1590/S1516-635X2003000200001]

[31]   Park YH, Hamidon F, Rajangan C, *et al.* Application of probiotics for the production of safe and high-quality poultry meat. Han-gug Chugsan Sigpum Hag-hoeji 2016; 36(5): 567-76.
[http://dx.doi.org/10.5851/kosfa.2016.36.5.567] [PMID: 27857531]

[32]   Dhama K, Verma V, Sawant P, Tiwari R, Vaid R, Chauhan R. Applications of probiotics in poultry: Enhancing immunity and beneficial effects on production performances and health-A review. J Clin Immunol 2011; 13(1): 1-19.

[33]   Markowiak P, Śliżewska K. The role of probiotics, prebiotics and synbiotics in animal nutrition. Gut Pathog 2018; 10(1): 21.
[http://dx.doi.org/10.1186/s13099-018-0250-0] [PMID: 29930711]

[34]   Khan RU, Naz S, Dhama K, *et al.* Direct-fed microbial: beneficial applications, modes of action and prospects as a safe tool for enhancing ruminant production and safeguarding health. Int J Pharmacol 2016; 12(3): 220-31.
[http://dx.doi.org/10.3923/ijp.2016.220.231]

[35]   Lutful Kabir SM. The role of probiotics in the poultry industry. Int J Mol Sci 2009; 10(8): 3531-46.
[http://dx.doi.org/10.3390/ijms10083531] [PMID: 20111681]

[36]   Rouger A, Tresse O, Zagorec M. Bacterial contaminants of poultry meat: sources, species, and dynamics. Microorganisms 2017; 5(3): 50.
[http://dx.doi.org/10.3390/microorganisms5030050] [PMID: 28841156]

[37]   Vancamelbeke M, Vermeire S. The intestinal barrier: a fundamental role in health and disease. Expert Rev Gastroenterol Hepatol 2017; 11(9): 821-34.
[http://dx.doi.org/10.1080/17474124.2017.1343143] [PMID: 28650209]

[38]   Roto SM, Rubinelli PM, Ricke SC. An introduction to the avian gut microbiota and the effects of yeast-based prebiotic-type compounds as potential feed additives. Front Vet Sci 2015; 2: 28.
[http://dx.doi.org/10.3389/fvets.2015.00028] [PMID: 26664957]

[39]   Fijan S. Microorganisms with claimed probiotic properties: an overview of recent literature. Int J Environ Res Public Health 2014; 11(5): 4745-67.
[http://dx.doi.org/10.3390/ijerph110504745] [PMID: 24859749]

[40]   Liévin-Le Moal V, Servin AL. Anti-infective activities of *lactobacillus strains* in the human intestinal microbiota: from probiotics to gastrointestinal anti-infectious biotherapeutic agents. Clin Microbiol Rev 2014; 27(2): 167-99.
[http://dx.doi.org/10.1128/CMR.00080-13] [PMID: 24696432]

[41]   Corcoran BM, Stanton C, Fitzgerald GF, Ross RP. Survival of probiotic lactobacilli in acidic environments is enhanced in the presence of metabolizable sugars. Appl Environ Microbiol 2005; 71(6): 3060-7.
[http://dx.doi.org/10.1128/AEM.71.6.3060-3067.2005] [PMID: 15933002]

[42]   Invernizzi G, Bontempo V, Savoini G. The beneficial role of probiotics in monogastric animal nutrition and health. J Dairy Vet Anim Res 2015; 2: 116-32.

[43] Maciorowski K, Herrera P, Jones F, Pillai S, Ricke S. Effects on poultry and livestock of feed contamination with bacteria and fungi. Anim Feed Sci Technol 2007; 133(1-2): 109-36.
[http://dx.doi.org/10.1016/j.anifeedsci.2006.08.006]

[44] Sornplang P, Piyadeatsoontorn S. Probiotic isolates from unconventional sources: a review. J Anim Sci Technol 2016; 58(1): 26.
[http://dx.doi.org/10.1186/s40781-016-0108-2] [PMID: 27437119]

[45] Collins MD, Gibson GR. Probiotics, prebiotics, and synbiotics: approaches for modulating the microbial ecology of the gut. Am J Clin Nutr 1999; 69(5): 1052S-7S.
[http://dx.doi.org/10.1093/ajcn/69.5.1052s] [PMID: 10232648]

[46] Jiang T, Li H-S, Han GG, et al. Oral delivery of probiotics in poultry using pH-sensitive tablets. J Microbiol Biotechnol 2017; 27(4): 739-46.
[http://dx.doi.org/10.4014/jmb.1606.06071] [PMID: 28081355]

[47] Hemarajata P, Versalovic J. Effects of probiotics on gut microbiota: mechanisms of intestinal immunomodulation and neuromodulation. Therap Adv Gastroenterol 2013; 6(1): 39-51.
[http://dx.doi.org/10.1177/1756283X12459294] [PMID: 23320049]

[48] Hibbing ME, Fuqua C, Parsek MR, Peterson SB. Bacterial competition: surviving and thriving in the microbial jungle. Nat Rev Microbiol 2010; 8(1): 15-25.
[http://dx.doi.org/10.1038/nrmicro2259] [PMID: 19946288]

[49] Awad WA, Ghareeb K, Böhm J. Effect of addition of a probiotic micro-organism to broiler diet on intestinal mucosal architecture and electrophysiological parameters. J Anim Physiol Anim Nutr (Berl) 2010; 94(4): 486-94.
[http://dx.doi.org/10.1111/j.1439-0396.2009.00933.x] [PMID: 19906141]

[50] Wang Y, Gu Q. Effect of probiotic on growth performance and digestive enzyme activity of Arbor Acres broilers. Res Vet Sci 2010; 89(2): 163-7.
[http://dx.doi.org/10.1016/j.rvsc.2010.03.009] [PMID: 20350733]

[51] Wu L, Fang Y, Tan R, Shi K. A comparison of cecal microflora and volatile fatty acid concentration in goslings fed diets supplemented with or without a dried *Bacillus subtilis* culture. J Appl Anim Res 2009; 36(2): 231-4.
[http://dx.doi.org/10.1080/09712119.2009.9707066]

[52] Meimandipour A, Shuhaimi M, Soleimani AF, et al. Selected microbial groups and short-chain fatty acids profile in a simulated chicken cecum supplemented with two strains of *Lactobacillus*. Poult Sci 2010; 89(3): 470-6.
[http://dx.doi.org/10.3382/ps.2009-00495] [PMID: 20181862]

[53] Ichikawa H, Shineha R, Satomi S, Sakata T. Gastric or rectal instillation of short-chain fatty acids stimulates epithelial cell proliferation of small and large intestine in rats. Dig Dis Sci 2002; 47(5): 1141-6.
[http://dx.doi.org/10.1023/A:1015014829605] [PMID: 12018914]

[54] Chapman MA, Grahn MF, Boyle MA, Hutton M, Rogers J, Williams NS. Butyrate oxidation is impaired in the colonic mucosa of sufferers of quiescent ulcerative colitis. Gut 1994; 35(1): 73-6.
[http://dx.doi.org/10.1136/gut.35.1.73] [PMID: 8307454]

[55] Lu H, Su S, Ajuwon K. Butyrate supplementation to gestating sows and piglets induces muscle and adipose tissue oxidative genes and improves growth performance. Anim Sci J 2012; 90(4): 2-430.
[http://dx.doi.org/10.2527/jas.53817]

[56] Gao Z, Yin J, Zhang J, et al. Butyrate improves insulin sensitivity and increases energy expenditure in mice. Diabetes 2009; 58(7): 1509-17.
[http://dx.doi.org/10.2337/db08-1637] [PMID: 19366864]

[57] Mátis G, Neogrády Z, Csikó G, et al. Epigenetic effects of dietary butyrate on hepatic histone acetylation and enzymes of biotransformation in chicken. Acta Vet Hung 2013; 61(4): 477-90.

[http://dx.doi.org/10.1556/avet.2013.033] [PMID: 23974937]

[58] Ajuwon K. Toward a better understanding of mechanisms of probiotics and prebiotics action in poultry species. J Appl Poult Res 2016; 25(2): 277-83.
[http://dx.doi.org/10.3382/japr/pfv074]

[59] Canani RB, Nocerino R, Terrin G, *et al.* Effect of *Lactobacillus* GG on tolerance acquisition in infants with cow's milk allergy: a randomized trial. J Allergy Clin Immunol 2012; 129(2): 2-580.

[60] Kang S-J, Park Y-I, So B, Kang H-G. Sodium butyrate efficiently converts fully reprogrammed induced pluripotent stem cells from mouse partially reprogrammed cells. Cell Reprog [Formerly" Cloning and Stem Cells"] 2014; 16(5): 54-345.
[http://dx.doi.org/10.1089/cell.2013.0087]

[61] Gabler N, Spurlock M. Integrating the immune system with the regulation of growth and efficiency. J Anim Sci 2008; 86(14): 64-74.
[http://dx.doi.org/10.2527/jas.2007-0466]

[62] Cao GT, Zeng XF, Chen AG, *et al.* Effects of a probiotic, *Enterococcus faecium*, on growth performance, intestinal morphology, immune response, and cecal microflora in broiler chickens challenged with *Escherichia coli* K88. Poult Sci 2013; 92(11): 2949-55.
[http://dx.doi.org/10.3382/ps.2013-03366] [PMID: 24135599]

[63] Kim JS, Ingale SL, Kim YW, *et al.* Effect of supplementation of multi-microbe probiotic product on growth performance, apparent digestibility, cecal microbiota and small intestinal morphology of broilers. J Anim Physiol Anim Nutr (Berl) 2012; 96(4): 618-26.
[http://dx.doi.org/10.1111/j.1439-0396.2011.01187.x] [PMID: 21699585]

[64] Tiwari G, Tiwari R, Pandey S, Pandey P. Promising future of probiotics for human health: Current scenario. Chron Young Sci 2012; 3(1): 17.
[http://dx.doi.org/10.4103/2229-5186.94308]

[65] Oelschlaeger TA. Mechanisms of probiotic actions - A review. Int J Med Microbiol 2010; 300(1): 57-62.
[http://dx.doi.org/10.1016/j.ijmm.2009.08.005] [PMID: 19783474]

[66] Perdigon G, Alvarez S, Rachid M, Agüero G, Gobbato N. Immune system stimulation by probiotics. J Dairy Sci 1995; 78(7): 1597-606.
[http://dx.doi.org/10.3168/jds.S0022-0302(95)76784-4] [PMID: 7593855]

[67] Roselli M, Finamore A, Britti MS, Bosi P, Oswald I, Mengheri E. Alternatives to in-feed antibiotics in pigs: Evaluation of probiotics, zinc or organic acids as protective agents for the intestinal mucosa. A comparison of *in vitro* and *in vivo* results. Anim Res 2005; 54(3): 203-18.
[http://dx.doi.org/10.1051/animres:2005012]

[68] Kiela PR, Ghishan FK. Physiology of intestinal absorption and secretion. Best Pract Res Clin Gastroenterol 2016; 30(2): 145-59.
[http://dx.doi.org/10.1016/j.bpg.2016.02.007] [PMID: 27086882]

[69] Fong FLY, Shah NP, Kirjavainen P, El-Nezami H. Mechanism of action of probiotic bacteria on intestinal and systemic immunities and antigen-presenting cells. Int Rev Immunol 2016; 35(3): 179-88.
[http://dx.doi.org/10.3109/08830185.2015.1096937] [PMID: 26606641]

[70] Jones ML, Tomaro-Duchesneau C, Martoni CJ, Prakash S. Cholesterol lowering with bile salt hydrolase-active probiotic bacteria, mechanism of action, clinical evidence, and future direction for heart health applications. Expert Opin Biol Ther 2013; 13(5): 631-42.
[http://dx.doi.org/10.1517/14712598.2013.758706] [PMID: 23350815]

[71] Rather IA, Choi K-H, Bajpai VK, Park Y-H. Antiviral mode of action of *Lactobacillus plantarum* YML009 on Influenza virus H1N1. Bangladesh J Pharmacol 2015; 10(2): 475-82.
[http://dx.doi.org/10.3329/bjp.v10i2.23068]

[72] Talebi A, Amani A, Pourmahmod M, Saghaei P, Rezaie R, Eds. Synbiotic enhances immune responses

against infectious bronchitis, infectious bursal disease, Newcastle disease and avian influenza in broiler chickens Veterinary Research Forum. Urmia, Iran: Faculty of Veterinary Medicine, Urmia University 2015.

[73]   Lillehoj H, Liu Y, Calsamiglia S, *et al.* Phytochemicals as antibiotic alternatives to promote growth and enhance host health. Vet Res (Faisalabad) 2018; 49(1): 76.
[http://dx.doi.org/10.1186/s13567-018-0562-6] [PMID: 30060764]

[74]   Dhama K, Tiwari R, Khan RU, *et al.* Growth promoters and novel feed additives improving poultry production and health, bioactive principles and beneficial applications: the trends and advances-a review. Int J Pharmacol 2014; 10(3): 129-59.
[http://dx.doi.org/10.3923/ijp.2014.129.159]

[75]   Kesarcodi-Watson A, Kaspar H, Lategan MJ, Gibson L. Probiotics in aquaculture: the need, principles and mechanisms of action and screening processes. Aquaculture 2008; 274(1): 1-14.
[http://dx.doi.org/10.1016/j.aquaculture.2007.11.019]

[76]   Mathipa MG, Thantsha MS. Probiotic engineering: towards development of robust probiotic strains with enhanced functional properties and for targeted control of enteric pathogens. Gut Pathog 2017; 9(1): 28.
[http://dx.doi.org/10.1186/s13099-017-0178-9] [PMID: 28491143]

[77]   La Fata G, Weber P, Mohajeri MH. Probiotics and the gut immune system: indirect regulation. Probiotics Antimicrob Proteins 2018; 10(1): 11-21.
[http://dx.doi.org/10.1007/s12602-017-9322-6] [PMID: 28861741]

[78]   Lee K, Lillehoj HS, Siragusa GR. Direct-fed microbials and their impact on the intestinal microflora and immune system of chickens. J Poult Sci 2010; 1001160039.
[http://dx.doi.org/10.2141/jpsa.009096]

[79]   Vieco-Saiz N, Belguesmia Y, Raspoet R, *et al.* Benefits and inputs from lactic acid bacteria and their bacteriocins as alternatives to antibiotic growth promoters during food-animal production. Front Microbiol 2019; 10: 57.
[http://dx.doi.org/10.3389/fmicb.2019.00057] [PMID: 30804896]

[80]   Dibaji SM, Seidavi A, Asadpour L, Moreira da Silva F. Effect of a synbiotic on the intestinal microflora of chickens. J Appl Poult Res 2014; 23(1): 1-6.
[http://dx.doi.org/10.3382/japr.2012-00709]

[81]   Vinderola G, Ouwehand A, Salminen S, von Wright A. Lactic acid bacteria: microbiological and functional aspects. Crc Press 2019.
[http://dx.doi.org/10.1201/9780429057465]

[82]   D'Angelo C, Reale M, Costantini E. Microbiota and probiotics in health and HIV infection. Nutrients 2017; 9(6): 615.
[http://dx.doi.org/10.3390/nu9060615] [PMID: 28621726]

[83]   Watarai S, Iwase T, Tajima T, Yuba E, Kono K, Sekiya Y. Application of pH-sensitive fusogenic polymer-modified liposomes for development of mucosal vaccines. Vet Immunol Immunopathol 2014; 158(1-2): 62-72.
[http://dx.doi.org/10.1016/j.vetimm.2013.05.005] [PMID: 23790647]

[84]   Nazir Y, Hussain SA, Abdul Hamid A, Song Y. Probiotics and their potential preventive and therapeutic role for cancer, high serum cholesterol, and allergic and HIV diseases. Res Intern 2018; 2018: 3428437.
[http://dx.doi.org/10.1155/2018/3428437]

[85]   Zaghari M, Zahroojian N, Riahi M, Parhizkar S. Effect of *Bacillus subtilis* spore [GalliPro®] nutrients equivalency value on broiler chicken performance. Ital J Anim Sci 2015; 14(1): 3555.
[http://dx.doi.org/10.4081/ijas.2015.3555]

[86]   Apata D. Growth performance, nutrient digestibility and immune response of broiler chicks fed diets

supplemented with a culture of *Lactobacillus bulgaricus*. J Sci Food Agric 2008; 88(7): 1253-8.
[http://dx.doi.org/10.1002/jsfa.3214]

[87]   Yoshii K, Hosomi K, Sawane K, Kunisawa J. Metabolism of dietary and microbial vitamin B family in the regulation of host immunity. Front Nutr 2019; 6: 48.
[http://dx.doi.org/10.3389/fnut.2019.00048] [PMID: 31058161]

[88]   Carey MC, Hernell O. Digestion and absorption of fat. Semin Gastrointest Dis 1992; 3: 189-208.

[89]   Santoso U, Tanaka K, Ohtani S. Effect of dried *Bacillus subtilis* culture on growth, body composition and hepatic lipogenic enzyme activity in female broiler chicks. Br J Nutr 1995; 74(4): 523-9.
[http://dx.doi.org/10.1079/BJN19950155] [PMID: 7577890]

[90]   Youssef AW, Hassan H, Ali H, Mohamed M. Effect of probiotics, prebiotics and organic acids on layer performance and egg quality. Asian J Polit Sci 2013; 7(2): 65-74.

[91]   Yörük MA, Gül M, Hayirli A, Macit M. The effects of supplementation of humate and probiotic on egg production and quality parameters during the late laying period in hens. Poult Sci 2004; 83(1): 84-8.
[http://dx.doi.org/10.1093/ps/83.1.84] [PMID: 14761088]

[92]   Ramasamy K, Abdullah N, Jalaludin S, Wong M, Ho YW. Effects of *Lactobacillus cultures* on performance of laying hens, and total cholesterol, lipid and fatty acid composition of egg yolk. J Sci Food Agric 2009; 89(3): 482-6.
[http://dx.doi.org/10.1002/jsfa.3477]

[93]   Sobczak A, Kozłowski K. The effect of a probiotic preparation containing *Bacillus subtilis* ATCC PTA-6737 on egg production and physiological parameters of laying hens. Ann Anim Sci 2015; 15(3): 711-23.
[http://dx.doi.org/10.1515/aoas-2015-0040]

[94]   Ribeiro V Jr, Albino L, Rostagno H, *et al.* Effects of the dietary supplementation of *Bacillus subtilis* levels on performance, egg quality and excreta moisture of layers. Anim Feed Sci Technol 2014; 195: 142-6.
[http://dx.doi.org/10.1016/j.anifeedsci.2014.06.001]

[95]   Cox CM, Dalloul RA. Immunomodulatory role of probiotics in poultry and potential *in ovo* application. Benef Microbes 2015; 6(1): 45-52.
[http://dx.doi.org/10.3920/BM2014.0062] [PMID: 25213028]

[96]   Hrnčár C, Gašparovič M, Weis J, *et al.* Effect of three-strain probiotic on productive performance and carcass characteristics of broiler chickens. Lucr Stiint Zooteh Biotehnol 2016; 49: 149-54.

[97]   Kim Y-J, Bostami A, Islam M, Mun HS, Ko S, Yang C-J. Effect of fermented ginkgo biloba and camelia sinensis-based probiotics on growth performance, immunity and caecal microbiology in broilers. Int J Poult Sci 2016; 15(2): 62-71.
[http://dx.doi.org/10.3923/ijps.2016.62.71]

[98]   Afsari M, Mohebbifar A, Torki M. Effects of dietary inclusion of olive pulp supplemented with probiotics on productive performance, egg quality and blood parameters of laying hens. Annu Res Rev Biol 2014; 198-211.
[http://dx.doi.org/10.9734/ARRB/2014/5212]

[99]   Pender CM, Kim S, Potter TD, Ritzi MM, Young M, Dalloul RA. *In ovo* supplementation of probiotics and its effects on performance and immune-related gene expression in broiler chicks. Poult Sci 2017; 96(5): 1052-62.
[http://dx.doi.org/10.3382/ps/pew381] [PMID: 28158826]

[100]   Yang CM, Cao GT, Ferket PR, *et al.* Effects of probiotic, *Clostridium butyricum*, on growth performance, immune function, and cecal microflora in broiler chickens. Poult Sci 2012; 91(9): 2121-9.

[http://dx.doi.org/10.3382/ps.2011-02131] [PMID: 22912445]

[101]   Bai SP, Wu AM, Ding XM, *et al.* Effects of probiotic-supplemented diets on growth performance and intestinal immune characteristics of broiler chickens. Poult Sci 2013; 92(3): 663-70.
[http://dx.doi.org/10.3382/ps.2012-02813] [PMID: 23436517]

[102]   Lee K-W, Lillehoj HS, Jang SI, *et al.* Effect of Bacillus-based direct-fed microbials on *Eimeria maxima* infection in broiler chickens. Comp Immunol Microbiol Infect Dis 2010; 33(6): e105-10.
[http://dx.doi.org/10.1016/j.cimid.2010.06.001] [PMID: 20621358]

[103]   Liao XD, Ma G, Cai J, *et al.* Effects of *Clostridium butyricum* on growth performance, antioxidation, and immune function of broilers. Poult Sci 2015; 94(4): 662-7.
[http://dx.doi.org/10.3382/ps/pev038] [PMID: 25717087]

[104]   Zhang ZF, Kim IH. Effects of multistrain probiotics on growth performance, apparent ileal nutrient digestibility, blood characteristics, cecal microbial shedding, and excreta odor contents in broilers. Poult Sci 2014; 93(2): 364-70.
[http://dx.doi.org/10.3382/ps.2013-03314] [PMID: 24570458]

[105]   Al-Fataftah A-R, Abdelqader A. Effects of dietary *Bacillus subtilis* on heat-stressed broilers performance, intestinal morphology and microflora composition. Anim Feed Sci Technol 2014; 198: 279-85.
[http://dx.doi.org/10.1016/j.anifeedsci.2014.10.012]

[106]   Hu L, Shao Y, Jiang N, *et al.* Effects of probiotic on the expression of IL-7 gene and immune response to Newcastle disease vaccine in broilers. Int J Health Sci Res 2016; 4: 140-8.

[107]   Rajput IR, Li LY, Xin X, *et al.* Effect of *Saccharomyces boulardii* and *Bacillus subtilis* B10 on intestinal ultrastructure modulation and mucosal immunity development mechanism in broiler chickens. Poult Sci 2013; 92(4): 956-65.
[http://dx.doi.org/10.3382/ps.2012-02845] [PMID: 23472019]

[108]   Ramasamy K, Abdullah N, Wong MC, Karuthan C, Ho YW. Bile salt deconjugation and cholesterol removal from media by *Lactobacillus strains* used as probiotics in chickens. J Sci Food Agric 2010; 90(1): 65-9.
[http://dx.doi.org/10.1002/jsfa.3780] [PMID: 20355013]

[109]   Tang SGH, Sieo CC, Kalavathy R, *et al.* Chemical compositions of egg yolks and egg quality of laying hens fed prebiotic, probiotic, and synbiotic diets. J Food Sci 2015; 80(8): C1686-95.
[http://dx.doi.org/10.1111/1750-3841.12947] [PMID: 26174350]

[110]   Liao SF, Nyachoti M. Using probiotics to improve swine gut health and nutrient utilization. Anim Nutr 2017; 3(4): 331-43.
[http://dx.doi.org/10.1016/j.aninu.2017.06.007] [PMID: 29767089]

[111]   Kiarie EG, Mills A. Role of feed processing on gut health and function in pigs and poultry: conundrum of optimal particle size and hydrothermal regimens. Front Vet Sci 2019; 6: 19.
[http://dx.doi.org/10.3389/fvets.2019.00019] [PMID: 30838217]

[112]   Abenavoli L, Scarpellini E, Colica C, *et al.* Gut microbiota and obesity: a role for probiotics. Nutrients 2019; 11(11): 2690.
[http://dx.doi.org/10.3390/nu11112690] [PMID: 31703257]

[113]   Hillman ET, Lu H, Yao T, Nakatsu CH. Microbial ecology along the gastrointestinal tract. Microbes Environ 2017; 32(4): 300-13.
[http://dx.doi.org/10.1264/jsme2.ME17017] [PMID: 29129876]

[114]   Maragkoudakis PA, Mountzouris KC, Psyrras D, *et al.* Functional properties of novel protective lactic acid bacteria and application in raw chicken meat against *Listeria monocytogenes* and *Salmonella* enteritidis. Int J Food Microbiol 2009; 130(3): 219-26.
[http://dx.doi.org/10.1016/j.ijfoodmicro.2009.01.027] [PMID: 19249112]

[115]   Saint-Cyr MJ, Guyard-Nicodème M, Messaoudi S, *et al.* Recent advances in screening of anti-

Campylobacter activity in probiotics for use in poultry. Front Microbiol 2016; 7: 553.
[http://dx.doi.org/10.3389/fmicb.2016.00553] [PMID: 27303366]

[116] Pender CM, Kim S, Potter TD, Ritzi MM, Young M, Dalloul RA. Effects of *in ovo* supplementation of probiotics on performance and immunocompetence of broiler chicks to an *Eimeria* challenge. Benef Microbes 2016; 7(5): 699-705.
[http://dx.doi.org/10.3920/BM2016.0080] [PMID: 27726419]

[117] Murarolli VDA, Burbarelli MFdC, Polycarpo GV, Ribeiro PdAP, Moro MEG, Albuquerque Rd. Prebiotic, probiotic and symbiotic as alternative to antibiotics on the performance and immune response of broiler chickens. Braz J Poult Sci 2014; 16(3): 279-84.
[http://dx.doi.org/10.1590/1516-635x1603279-284]

[118] Hasanzadeh M, Far R. Efficacy of *Echinacea purpurea* and protexin on systemic and mucosal immune response to Newcastle diseases virus vaccination [VG/GA strain] in commercial turkey poults. Iran J Vet Med 2017; 11(1): 85-95.

[119] Swaggerty CL, Callaway TR, Kogut MH, Piva A, Grilli E. Modulation of the immune response to improve health and reduce foodborne pathogens in poultry. Microorganisms 2019; 7(3): 65.
[http://dx.doi.org/10.3390/microorganisms7030065] [PMID: 30823445]

[120] Carter A, Adams M, La Ragione RM, Woodward MJ. Colonisation of poultry by *Salmonella Enteritidis* S1400 is reduced by combined administration of *Lactobacillus salivarius* 59 and *Enterococcus faecium* PXN-33. Vet Microbiol 2017; 199: 100-7.
[http://dx.doi.org/10.1016/j.vetmic.2016.12.029] [PMID: 28110775]

[121] Oh JK, Pajarillo EAB, Chae JP, Kim IH, Yang DS, Kang D-K. Effects of *Bacillus subtilis* CSL2 on the composition and functional diversity of the faecal microbiota of broiler chickens challenged with *Salmonella Gallinarum*. J Anim Sci Biotechnol 2017; 8(1): 1.
[http://dx.doi.org/10.1186/s40104-016-0130-8] [PMID: 28070331]

[122] Park JH, Kim IH. The effects of the supplementation of *Bacillus subtilis* RX7 and B2A strains on the performance, blood profiles, intestinal *Salmonella* concentration, noxious gas emission, organ weight and breast meat quality of broiler challenged with *Salmonella typhimurium*. J Anim Physiol Anim Nutr (Berl) 2015; 99(2): 326-34.
[http://dx.doi.org/10.1111/jpn.12248] [PMID: 25244020]

[123] Faseleh Jahromi M, Wesam Altaher Y, Shokryazdan P, *et al.* Dietary supplementation of a mixture of *Lactobacillus strains* enhances performance of broiler chickens raised under heat stress conditions. Int J Biometeorol 2016; 60(7): 1099-110.
[http://dx.doi.org/10.1007/s00484-015-1103-x] [PMID: 26593972]

[124] Ebrahimi H, Rahimi S, Khaki P, Grimes JL, Kathariou S. The effects of probiotics, organic acid, and a medicinal plant on the immune systemand gastrointestinal microflora in broilers challenged with *Campylobacter jejuni*. Turk J Vet Anim Sci 2016; 40(3): 329-36.
[http://dx.doi.org/10.3906/vet-1502-68]

[125] Fritts C, Kersey J, Motl M, *et al. Bacillus subtilis* C-3102 [Calsporin] improves live performance and microbiological status of broiler chickens. J Appl Poult Res 2000; 9(2): 149-55.
[http://dx.doi.org/10.1093/japr/9.2.149]

[126] Nishiyama K, Seto Y, Yoshioka K, *et al. Lactobacillus gasseri* SBT2055 reduces infection by and colonization of *Campylobacter jejuni*. PLoS One 2014; 9(9): e108827. [9].
[http://dx.doi.org/10.1371/journal.pone.0108827] [PMID: 25264604]

[127] Forkus B, Ritter S, Vlysidis M, Geldart K, Kaznessis YN. Antimicrobial probiotics reduce *Salmonella* enterica in turkey gastrointestinal tracts. Sci Rep 2017; 7(1): 40695.
[http://dx.doi.org/10.1038/srep40695] [PMID: 28094807]

[128] Aguiar VF, Donoghue AM, Arsi K, *et al.* Targeting motility properties of bacteria in the development of probiotic cultures against *Campylobacter jejuni* in broiler chickens. Foodborne Pathog Dis 2013; 10(5): 435-41.

CHAPTER 16

Nutritional Applications of Nanotechnology in Poultry with Special References to Minerals

Mahmoud Alagawany[1,*], **Sameh A. Abdelnour**[2], **Mayada R. Farag**[3], **Shaaban S. Elnesr**[4], **Mohamed S. El-Kholy**[1] and **Mohamed E. Abd El-Hack**[1]

[1] *Department of Poultry, Faculty of Agriculture, Zagazig University, Zagazig, 44511, Egypt*

[2] *Animal Production Department, Faculty of Agriculture, Zagazig University, Zagazig, 44511, Egypt*

[3] *Forensic Medicine and Toxicology Department, Faculty of Veterinary Medicine, Zagazig University, Zagazig 44511, Egypt*

[4] *Poultry Production Department, Faculty of Agriculture, Fayoum University, Fayoum, 63514, Egypt*

Abstract: The prefix "Nano" comes from the Latin word "nanus", which means "dwarf". Nanotechnology can be defined as the manipulation of materials at the nanoscale as it deals with particles sized between 1-100 nm. Nanotechnology, can open up opportunities for improving feed particles' utilization to the benefit of livestock production. Nanotechnology can also act as new vehicle for nutrient delivery to improve the digestion and absorption pathway for better nutrient metabolism. Minerals administered in the nanoparticle form as feed additives can pass through the wall of intestinal cells and other body cells more speedily than ordinary minerals, thus boosting their bioavailability. Therefore, nanotechnology can be used in animal feed to improve production performance, nutrient bioavailability, and livestock's immune response after considering nanotechnology's social, economic, legal and ethical implications. In conclusion, nanotechnology applications can provide solutions for poultry and livestock production systems to enhance the final product quality.

Keywords: Immunity, Nanotechnology, Nutrient bioavailability, Poultry, Production performance.

INTRODUCTION

The nanoparticles produced by various methods have been indicated as a novel industrial revolution as they have been utilized in numerous biological and industrial applications [1].

---

* **Corresponding author Mahmoud Alagawany:** Department of Poultry, Faculty of Agriculture, Zagazig University, Zagazig - 44511, Egypt; E-mail: mmalagwany@zu.edu.eg

Mahmoud Alagawany & Mohamed E. Abd El-Hack (Eds.)

The material at the nanometer dimension exhibits some novel properties (higher surface activity, greater specific surface area, stronger adsorbing ability, high catalytic efficiency) that are different from its normal-sized particles [2, 3]. In the last decades, in agricultural industry, the execution of nanotech-based tools has gained momentum. The implementation of nano-fertilizers and nano-pesticides as the nanotechnology intervention in the agriculture has enhanced the efficacy of nutrients and production level, and relieved the soil and water from pollutants. Concerning the animal production sector, the application of nanotechnology in this field facilitates the improvement of animal productivity, reduces the efforts and time, decreases the amounts of feed additives in diet, and lowers the cost of high prices of feed additives, thus leading to the sustainability of the livestock sector. Nanotechnology is important because it increases the trace mineral absorption by decreasing the antagonistic influence among the bi-valent cations. This novel approach can be exploited in poultry and livestock nutrition for better utilization of feedstuffs through an efficient uptake of nutrients and other supplements [4]. The use of nanoscale metal instead of inorganic mineral allows animals to absorb feed minerals, hence noticeably lessening environmental contamination risks [5, 6]. Although this technology is very promising for better poultry production, studies are very limited. There is still concern regarding the impact of nanoparticles on health and the environment. Thus, it is important to overview the applications of this technologyas a significant tool in promoting the poultry sector. This chapter covers different aspects of nanotechnology, including the role of nano Se, Zn and Cu particles in poultry nutrition and their up-coming prospectives.

EFFECTS OF NANO-SELENIUM ON POULTRY PERFORMANCE

Nano Se revealed strong nutritional and biological effects on improving poultry's productive and physiological performance (Fig. 1). Table 1 shows different effects of nano-Se on various parameters of some poultry types during the last five years.

Table 1. Effects of nano-Se on poultry (available literature during the last five years).

Dose	Size of Nanoparticles	Poultry Type and Age	Effects	Reference
Nano Se (0.075, 0.15, 0.225 and 0.3 µg/egg)	< 100 nm	Broiler chicken *in ovo* (18th day incubation)	No harmful effects on the developing embryo and hatchability	[7]
0.3 mg nano-Se/kg diet	100 to 500 nm	15-30 days old	Enhanced growth performance by improving antioxidative or immune properties	[8]

(Table 1) cont.....

Dose	Size of Nanoparticles	Poultry Type and Age	Effects	Reference
nano-Se (0.3mg/kg diet)	50-100 nm	Laying hen 9-20 weeks	Increased CBH response after immunization, antibody titers against SRBC, SOD and GSHPx activity	[9]
Se nanoparticles (0.075, 0.1125. 0.1875 and 0.225 mg/kg)	30 – 60 nm	Broiler chicken 1-35 days old	Improved oxidation resistance Increased serum SOD activity and GSHPx activity Decreased malondialdehyde level	[10]
Nano-Se(0.075, 0.1125, 0.1875 and 0.225 mg/kg)	30 – 60 nm	Broiler chicken 1-35 days old	Increased expression of liver GSHP×1 mRNA gene Improved oxidation resistance	[11]
0.5 mg/kg Nano-Se	20–80 nm	Broiler chicken 1-42 days old	Improvement of function, immunity and total antioxidant activity of blood serum	[12]
0.15 and 0.30 ppm Nano Se	80 nm	Broiler chicken 1-40 days old	Better growth performance and quality of broiler meat	[13]
nano-Se (0.1, 0.2, 0.3, 0.4, 0.5 mg/kg)	N/A	Broiler Chicken 1-42 days old	Improved growth performance, carcass parts and immune function Increased anti-ND hemagglutination inhibition titer No effect on glucose and total protein concentrations	[14]
50, 150 and 300 ppb nano Se	N/A	Giriraja chicken1-56 days old	Improved water holding capacity of meat No effect on production parameters and carcass characteristics	[15]

N/A = not available; CBH = cutaneous basophil hypersensitivity SRBC = sheep red blood cell; GSHPx = gluthatione peroxidase; SOD = superoxidase dismutase; ND = Newcastle disease.

Results showed that supplementing the diet with nano-Se improved the feed efficiency, body weight gain (BWG) and final body weight of Guangxi Yellow chicken [16]. This improvement may be attributed to small particle size and high specific surface area of nano-Se. Thus, good intestinal absorption could be obtained because of the creation of nanoemulsion droplets [17]. Enriching heat-stressed hens diets with nano-Se (0.3 ppm) provided the greatest value in both egg mass and egg production percentage (8.56%, 19.60%, respectively), also improving feed conversion ratio (FCR) by 4.05% compared to the organic selenium group [8]. Additionally, Ahmadi *et al.* [14] recently demonstrated that nano-Se dietary supplementation significantly enhanced feed efficiency and daily body gain in growing broilers. Also, they concluded that the addition of nano-Se enhanced the protein and energy utilization than the untreated group by 0.397 and 5.9 *vs*. 0.414 and 6.2, respectively. Actually, selenium has certain functions in protein and energy metabolism [18], so this may allow better efficiency of protein and energy metabolism in growing broiler [14]. Also, feeding broiler with nano-Se (0.3%) combined with *AspergillusAwamori* (0.5%) increased significantly the BWG, protein and energy digestibility, reduced feed intake and enhanced feed efficiency [19].

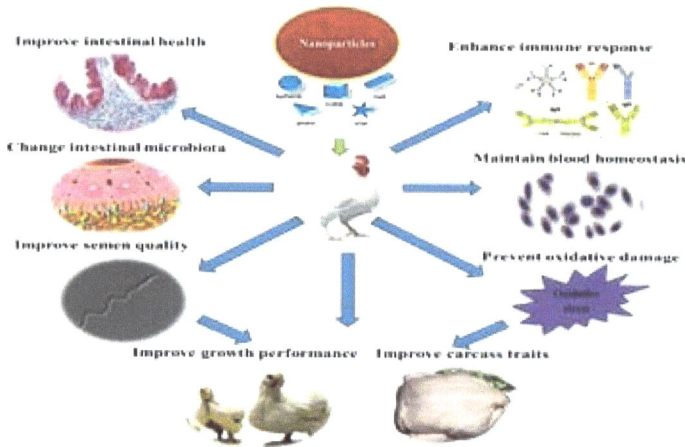

Fig. (1). Applications of Nanotechnology in Poultry.

In contrast, Payne and Southern [20] and Ryu *et al.* [21] presented that feed competence and body weight were not influenced by enrichment of feeds with selenium . No opposing effect on the growth was detected during the study period. It has also been illustrated that the supplementation of 0.3mg nano-Se/kg diet showed no differences in the feed consumption, feed conversion and daily weight gain [22] in comparison with the control group. Moreover, Boostani *et al.* [23] demonstrated that nano-Se enriched diets in broiler fed did not enhance growth performance. Similarly, in laying hens, it was indicated that feed intake, egg weight and body weight were not significantly influenced by nano-Se supplementation to diet under heat stress conditions [8]. Gangadoo *et al.* [24] showed that nano-Se inclusion in broilers' diet did not significantly affect bird weight.

EFFECTS OF NANO-SELENIUM ON BLOOD CONSTITUENTS

Broiler receiving selenium nanoparticles (SeNPs) (0.3 mg/kg of diet) had a higher muscular level of Se and GPX activity in the liver and plasma [25]. Nano selenium supplemented to the stressed broiler diet increased the cholesterol level, heterophil to lymphocyte (H:L) ratio and improved the glucose amount compared with control groups [25]. Circulatory corticoids could play an effective role in diminishing the number of lymphocytes [25]. Besides, the increase of H:L in nano-Se groups improved immune competence in the birds. It has been indicated that dietary supplementation of nano-Se (0.3mg/kg diet) exhibited a significant reduction in plasma total lipid and serum AST, while improved total proteins and globulins levels in laying hens under Egyptian summer conditions [8] and albumin in broiler [14]. Se may be effective in depressing cholesterol by regulating the activity of GSH-Px that plays an important role as antioxidant enzyme [26]. Saleh [19] observed that growing broiler fed with a mixture of *Aspergillus* probiotic (0.55%) and nano-Se particles (0.3%) showed significantly reduced glucose, GOT, triglyceride, total cholesterol, and 3-MH levels. In contrast, total protein and HDL-cholesterol were increased.

In contrast to previous reports, Selim *et al.* [13] reported that the supplementation of nano-Se at 0.15 or 0.30 ppm in the broiler diets did not affect hematological parameters, humoral and cellular immunity. Besides, Ahmadi *et al.* [14] revealed that total protein and glucose concentrations in broiler blood plasma were not significantly altered by nano-Se supplementation (0.1-0.5mg/kg feed).

EFFECTS OF NANO-SELENIUM ON POULTRY ANTIOXIDANT STATUS

Selenium plays a main role in certain physiological pathways in the body. It is important for the glutathione peroxidase (GSH-Px) family which has a role in the immune system. Generally, Se-enriched diets increased GSH-Px activity in all tissues of human and animals. . Moreover, broiler diets enriched with nano-Se significantly increased GSH-Px concentration compared to the control diet [25, 27]. The use of 0.3mg nano-Se/kg diet as feed supplements boosted superoxide dismutase (SOD) and GSH-Px activity of layer chickens compared to the control or sodium selenite groups [9].

Likewise, Wang [28] reported that dietary sodium selenite and nano-Se to broiler diet augmented hepatic and serum GSH-Px activities. Cai *et al.* [22] reported that broilers that received 0.3 - 0.5 mg/kg nano-Se had a significant influence on free radical inhibition in serum, muscle and liver. On the other hand, the birds fed nano-Se (2.0 mg/kg) showed harmful effects on these parameters [22]. The addition of nano-Se (0.1875 mg/kg) in the broiler diet can improve the antioxidant enzyme activities and, thus, the oxidation resistance in the birds [10]. Dietary nano-Se (0.3) mg/kg diet supplementation might improve antioxidative status in broilers [8].

EFFECTS OF NANO-SELENIUM ON POULTRY GENE EXPRESSION

The mucins which are secreted and produced by goblet cells represent the main structure of the mucus layer in the intestinal epithelium. The mucus layer is part of the innate host response preventing gastrointestinal pathologies and participating in nutrient digestion and absorption. It has been reported that the nanoparticles of selenium supplemented to *in vitro* cultured crypt cells enhanced the mucin gene expression [29]. In turn, increased the epithelium cells' activity and enhanced the absorption of nutrients *via* epithelium membranes [30].The mRNA expression of glutathione peroxidase (GPX), fatty acid synthase (FAS) and delta-6 desaturase for broilers fed a mixture of selenium nano-particles (0.3%) and *Aspergillus awamori*(0.05%) were higher (P < 0.05) than those in control [19]. A dietary level of 0.1875 mg Se nanoparticles/kg increased the liver GSHPx1 mRNA gene expression in broiler chicken [11]. As well, mRNA expression levels of Selenoprotein P (SelP), glutathione peroxidase 4 (GPx4) and Selenoprotein W (SelW) genes were significantly increased after dietary supplementation of nano-Se compared to the sodium selenite and control groups [31].

EFFECTS OF NANO-SELENIUM ON IMMUNE RESPONSES

Several researches conducted in various animal tissues have well documented that Se is mostly accumulated in immune response organs such as liver, spleen, and lymph nodes [32]. In this regard, it has been reported that Se treatment can augment the production of antibodies and expand complement responses *via* various devices, which include various selenoproteins [32]. Yazdi *et al*. [33] suggested that biogenic SeNPs could be a stimulator for the immune system. SeNPs could enhance the respiratory burst activities and expanded neutrophils chemotactic compared with different organic selenium sources. The authors reflect the varied pharmacokinetics parameters of SeNPs compared to selenite for evaluation of immune stimulator functionality of SeNPs [32].

It has been reported that nano-Se (0.3mg/kg diet) supplements significantly increased CBH response after immunization and the antibody titers against sheep red blood cell (SRBC) of layer chickens compared to sodium selenite group or the control group [9]. The lymphoid organs' weights were not significantly different between various Se sources. Birds fed on diet supplemented with nano-Se (0.30 mg/kg) showed improved levels of IgM, IgG, malondialdehyde, glutathione peroxidase and glutathione in serum [22]. However, thymus, bursa and spleen indexes were unaffected by nano-Se supplementation. Also [23], reported that the addition of 0.30 mg/kg of nano-Se to broiler diet led to higher IgG and IgM levels in response to SRBC antibody.

In contrast, Peng *et al.* [34] stated that low dietary selenium decreased the thymus weight (%), augmented apoptosis of thymic cells, and reducted of T cells and impaired the cellular immune function in broilers. El-Deep *et al.* [8] noticed that supplementation of nano-Se at 0.3 ppm in the diets of broiler exposed to thermal stress had a beneficial influence on phagocytic activity (82% *vs.* 55%) and index (4.5 *vs.* 2.1). Lately, Moghaddam *et al.* [35] recorded enhancement in total anti-SRBC in birds supplemented with Nano-Se (0.3 mg/kg) compared to those supplemented with organic selenium. Wang [28] verified augmented antibodies titer against NDV by adding nano-Se at 0.15-1.2 mg/kg diet compared with the control group.

EFFECTS OF NANO-SELENIUM ON SEMEN CRITERIA

The inclusion of Nano-Se (0.3 ppm) in broiler diets that were exposed to thermal stress decreased the adverse influences of heat stress on semen criteria and improved the spermatozoa count and motility and reduced the percentage of dead spermatozoa when compared to control group [8]. Moreover, it was reported that the presence of 0.3 ppm Nano-Se in the roosters' diet enhanced the GSH-Px activity in plasma by more than two-fold as compared with control [8]. Sperm concentration, ejaculate volume and sperm forward motility were significantly augmented for local Sinai cocks fed a diet supplemented with Nano-Se (0.3 mg/kg diet) compared to those fed the control diet. Also, nano-Se significantly reduced abnormal and dead sperms compared with the control (without nano-Se) [36].

EFFECTS OF NANO-SELENIUM ON POULTRY MICROBIOTA

The main objective of the poultry industry was to enhance productivity by maintaining the health of flocks. Several approaches have been used to reduce the pathogens including antibiotics,vaccinations, biosecurity, natural compounds, plant extracts, and organic acids. Nanotechnology, as a new approach, not only destroys pathogenic bacteria but also gets rid of bioaccumulation and toxic effects. New metal nanoparticles can provide this pathogen decreasing impact when the most suitable and biocompatible nanomaterial was used . Gangadoo *et al.* [24] reported that nano-Se inclusion in broilers' dietbroilers' diets changed the microbial community of these birds, presenting a noteworthy increase of opportunistic pathogens Staphylococcus and turicibacter.

EFFECTS OF NANO-SELENIUM ON CARCASS TRAITS

Cai *et al.* [22] stated that adding nano-Se (0.3mg/kg feed) to broiler diet has a beneficial impact on chickens' meat quality by increasing the glutathione peroxidase activity in tissue, and as a result, reduced drip loss. This improvement of antioxidant response may support the maintaining of cell membrane integrity [37]and augmented the level of Se in muscle and liver.. Ahmadi *et al.* [14] found lower abdominal fat percentage in the nano-Se supplemented birds than the control. There were no significant differences between the nano-Se-fed groups and the control group in weights of edible organs (gizzard, liver and heart), non-edible organs (kidneys, lungs, testes, pancreas, crop, proventriculus, right and left cecum) and thymus as well as the width, length and the diameter of the right and left cecum [14].

GENERAL CONCLUSION

The studies confirmed that dietary nano-Se supplementation could improve immune function, meat quality, oxidation resistance, and the Se content in muscle and liver. Supplementation of Nano-Se at a level of 0.3 mg/kg demonstrated important effects with better responses. However, negative effects appeared at nano-Se levels above 1 mg/kg. These findings recommended the dietary supplementation of nano-Se to broilers at 0.3 to 0.5 mg/kg.

EFFECTS OF NANO-ZINC ON POULTRY PERFORMANCE

Nano zinc particles represent one such nanotechnological approach. . It has many beneficial effects, such as growth promoting, antibacterial, immunomodulation and and reproduction enhancing activities in poultry. Table **2** shows some different impacts of nano-Zn on poultry in available literature during the last five years.

It was reported that dietary supplementation of 40 mg/kg nano zinc oxide (nano-ZnO) to growing broilers' diet significantly enhanced BWG and feed efficiency compared to control [38]. This enhancement of growth performance might be related to the impact of Zn on leucine aminopeptidase activity in the small intestine resulting in improving the intestinal digestion and absorption of nutrients in broilers.

Table 2. Effects of nano-Zn on poultry (available literature during the last five years).

Dose	Size of Nanoparticles	Poultry Type and Age	Effects	Reference
60 and 30 ppm zinc oxide nanoparticles (ZnO-NPs)	30nm	Laying hen 55-56 weeks old	Increased egg production % Improved phagocytic activity and index Increased serum SOD and GSHPx activities	[39]

(Table 2) cont.....

Dose	Size of Nanoparticles	Poultry Type and Age	Effects	Reference
50, 75 and 100 mg nano-zinc-oxide per kg diet	35–45 nm	Laying hens 42-54 weeks old	Negative effects on the egg shell thickness and bone mechanical properties	[40]
40 ppm (nano ZnO)	27 nm	Broiler chicken 1-42 days old	Positive effect on the overall performance, serum Zn Improved economic efficiency	[41]
Nano- Zn (20, 40, 60 and 80 µg/egg)	< 100 nm	Broiler chicken *in ovo* (18th-day incubation)	No harmful effects on the developing embryo and hatchability	[7]
ZONPs (40 mg/kg diet)	39.2-41.3 nm	Broiler chicken 1-35 days old	Improved body weight gain, feed efficiency, villus height and crypt depth	[42]
nano-ZnO (50 mg/kg)	27 nm	Broiler chicken 1-42 days old	Increased iron and copper contents in the hepatic tissue and Zn content in the tibia Decreased malondialdehyde Increased SOD activity Positive effects on mRNA expression of insulin-like growth factor-1 and growth hormone genes	[43]
40 and 80 mg ZONPs	19.3 nm	Broiler chicken 1-35 days old	Increased villus height (VH), and villus surface area (VSA) of the small intestine Beneficial effects on intestinal and caecal tonsils micro architectural changes.	[44]
0.3, 0.06 and 0.03 ppm nano- Zn	N/A	Broiler chicken 1-42 days old	Improved health status	[45]
30, 60, 90 or 120 mg of ZONPs /kg diet	40nm	Broiler chicken Starter stage (1-21 days)	Improved oxidant state Positive effect on the several serum enzymes activity	[46]
100 and 200mg NPs-ZnO/kg	N/A	Broiler chickenStarter stage (1-21 days)	Improved carcasses yield, increase in relative weight of digestive and lymphoid organs	[47]
Nano zinc (15, 30 and 60 mg/kg)	N/A	Giriraja chicks, (a dual-purpose chicken) 1-56 days old	Improved growth performance	[48]
Nano-zinc (100, 50, 10 ppm)	N/A	Turkey 1-98 days old	Maintained homeostasis in turkey muscles as indicated by the activity of the aminopeptidases.	[49]

(Table 2) cont.....

Dose	Size of Nanoparticles	Poultry Type and Age	Effects	Reference
40, 60 and 80 ppm nano zinc	N/A	Broiler Chicken during Summer 1-42 days old	Better performance and immunity	[50]
0.04 and 0.08 mg nano-Zn oxide/egg	<100 nm	Broiler chicken *in ovo* (18th day incubation)	No effect on body weight gain, feed intake and FCR. No effect on cell-mediated immune response and humoral immune response. Reduction of hatchability	[51]

N/A = not available; GSHPx = gluthatione peroxidase; SOD = superoxidase dismutase.

Also, it is conceivable that zinc oxide supplementation in broilers reduced labile active molecules such as iron (redox-active molecule) by improving the antioxidant defense system in the intestine mucosal cell [52]. Additionally, it was proposed that dietary zinc oxide in broiler can increase sucrose concentration in the small intestine and result in enhanced nutrients absorption [52]. Enriched broiler diets with nano ZnO (20 or 40mg/kg feed), significantly declined ascites index and mortality [38]. It has been suggested that nano-ZnO exhibits certain protection to chicks' cardiac myocytes by reducing oxidative stress and MDA in liver and serum and consequently promoting antioxidant status [38, 53]. Dukare Sagar *et al.* [50] examined the different sources of Zinc nanoparticles (organic, inorganic, green synthesis of ZnO, and chemical synthesis of ZnO) in broiler diets and observed that the green synthesis of ZnO (60-80ppm) improved significantly BWG, feed intake as well as feed efficiency. In the same line, Olgun and Yildiz [40] examined the different levels (50, 75 or 100 mg/kg diet) and forms of Zinc (zinc oxide and zinc sulphate, as inorganic zinc and zinc glycine as an organic form; and nano zinc oxide) on laying hens' performance. Nano zinc oxide produced the highest values of egg weight in laying hens that received 100mg/kg. Likewise, Zhao *et al.* [54] noticed that supplementation of nano-ZnO at 20 and 60 mg/kg in the diets of broiler could promote BWG and achieve a better FCR compared with inorganic form (60 mg/kg ZnO). Fathi *et al.* [55] reported that broilers receiving nano-ZnO (10mg/kg) had a significantly greater average daily gain. On the other hand, the addition of nano-ZnO at 20 mg/kg had significantly lower feed efficiency than other groups.

In contrast, Bami *et al.* [56] evaluated different sources of Zinc (Zinc oxide 100mg; or Nanoparticles of Zinc, 25 or 50mg/kg diet) supplemented to broiler diets; they concluded that dietary zinc nanoparticles did not affect growth performance. In the same line, Olgun and Yildiz [40] revealed no significant effect on BWG and egg production . Also, hens received nano-ZnO reduced egg shell thickness compared to organic and inorganic forms. Higher levels of nanoZnO (100 mg/kg nano-ZnO) in broiler diets decreased BWG and decreased feed efficiency. With the continuation of the dietary treatment, these influences were exacerbated [16].

The previous data show that appropriate levels of nano-ZnO are better than conventional ZnO for improving growth performance and feed efficiency in poultry. Still, extra nano-ZnO may lead to a toxic effects and inhibit the growth of the bird.

EFFECTS OF NANO-ZINC ON INTESTINAL MORPHOLOGY

The health of the gastrointestinal tract is vital to the well-being and efficiency of poultry. Intestinal histomorphology status plays a pivotal role in the absorption of nutrients, so the large crypt signalized that tissue turnover is higher [57]. The addition of Zinc nanoparticles (25 or 50mg/kg diet) to broiler diets exhibited an increase (P<0.05) of crypt depth (CD), villi length (VL), and VL to CD ratio compared to untreated group [56]. Moreover, it was indicated that nano-ZnO were able to increase CD, VL, villi width and VL significantly to CD ratio in the jejunum of broiler [58], which may be due to the enhancement of absorption of Zn, and increasing in cell multiplying by the synthesis of protein in broiler intestine [56, 59].

EFFECTS OF NANO-ZINC ON BLOOD CONSTITUENTS

Feeding broiler with 20mg/kg nano-ZnO led to increasing HDL, cholesterol, SOD and alkaline phosphatase (ALP) activity in serum [55]. This increasing the levels of lipid profile in the serum may be attributed to zinc nanoparticles could promote fat absorption. It was well documented that the dietary zinc deficiency was accompanied by reduced plasma total cholesterol, HDL, LDL, and triglyceride levels [55, 60, 61]. El-Katcha *et al.* [39] illustrated that laying hens fed a diet containing 30 mg of nano zinc/kg had low liver enzymes (alanine transferase (ALT) and Aspartate transferase (AST) activities. No effects on triglycerides, total protein and albumin concentrations were detected after administration of nano-Zn. However, administration nano-Zn augmented serum zinc, phosphorus, high-density lipoprotein and total cholesterol concentrations. Dietary nano-ZnO (60 and 90 mg/kg) decreased serum ALP, AST, ALT and lactate dehydrogenase enzyme activity, and malondialdehyde significantly, but increased total antioxidant capacity and SOD compared with the control treatment [46]

Conversely, an experiment has been made by Fathi [38], who illustrated that adding nano-ZnO (20 or 40mg/kg) to broiler diets did not exert any significant effects on the blood parameters and liver enzymes (AST and ALT) and LDH activities. At the same time, both levels on naoZn reduced MDA concentration in plasma and liver. The accumulation of Zinc oxide nanoparticles in liver tissues was detected and caused toxicity.

EFFECTS OF NANO-ZINC ON IMMUNITY RESPONSES

Birds that received 60-80ppm of green synthesized ZnO increased immunity organ weights. The H/L ratio was also increased significantly by introducing 80 mg synthesized ZnOcompared with other sources of Zinc (organic, inorganic and chemical synthesis of ZnO) [50]. Feeding broiler with nano-ZnO (50mg/kg diet), increased ($P < 0.05$) the antibody titer against SRBC compared with zinc oxide (100mg), nano-ZnO (25mg) or control group [56]. Zn may serve as a modulator of the immune response and the alterations in Zn profiles of the body impaired the T T cell functions and the balance among the various T helper cell subsets [62]. Based on previous reports, Sunder *et al.* [63] and Bartlett and Smith [64] reported that the use of Zn in broiler diet showed positive influence on antibody titer against SRBC. The nano-ZnO has an effective role in the antioxidative status of broilers [54]. Previous reports in broilers proposed that 20 mg nano-ZnO/kg diet can stimulate antioxidative function, but 100 mg nano-ZnO/kg diet increased antioxidative function, and extra nano-ZnO addition can cause toxic effects and hepatocyte damage. This would elucidate the gradual decrease in total antioxidant capability detected in liver tissue in the experiment of Zhao *et al.* [54].

In contrast, the addition of 200 mg of ZnO-NPs to the diets of broiler significantly augmented the relative weight of the pancreas and proventriculus compared with other groups, while no significant changes in relative weight of lymphoid organs were detected in broiler [47]. It has been indicated that dietary supplementation of 20 mg nano-ZnO/kg diet had a similar result on the copper-zinc superoxide dismutase activity in liver tissue and serum as that of the control (60 mg ZnO/kg diet) [54]. Catalase is an antioxidant enzyme that can eliminate oxidative stress from the body and guard the mitochondrial membrane structure against damage [65 - 67]. The activity of catalase in the serum of broiler fed with 20 or 60mg nano-ZnO was increased significantly compared with 100mg nano-ZnO and control group [54]. Malondialdehyde (MDA) is an essential guide for oxidative damage and lipid peroxidation caused by ROS [68]. Zinc nanoparticles reduced MDA levels in liver tissue and serum significantly when birds fed with 20, 60, or 100mg of nano ZnO [54]. Feeding broiler with 20 mg/kg nano-ZnO significantly reduced MDA levels in serum [55].

EFFECTS OF NANO-COPPER ON POULTRY PERFORMANCE

Nano-copper (nano-Cu) shows a variety of effects on poultry performance. Recently, the use of nano-Cu has received much attention due to its high bioavailabilityand incorporation in poultry nutrition, because it can enhance the performance and health of poultry. Table **3** shows some impacts of nano-Cu on poultry in available literature during the last five years.

Dietary supplementation of copper-loaded chitosan nanoparticle (CNP-Cu) was investigated in the broiler, where broilers fed diets containing CNP-Cu (100 mg/kg) showed increased average daily gain by 7.79% compared with the untreated group [69]. Feed intake also was enhanced when broilers received CNP-Cu (100 and 150 mg/kg diet) [69]. It was observed that injection of nano-Cu induced higher (P < 0.05) live weight of broiler by 5.07% after 21 days of treatment compared with control [70]. The nano-Cu administration by injection in the broiler did not show alteration regarding the broiler liver's amino acid profile [70]. Dietary nano-Cu did not affect the growth performance of turkeys [71]. In the same line, feeding turkeys with different levels of nano-Cu (2-10 mg/kg diet) did not affect BWG after 14 weeks of treatment [72].

EFFECTS OF NANO-COPPER ON BLOOD CONSTITUENTS

Miroshnikov *et al.* [70] indicated that the injection of nano-Cu in broiler may promote protein level in blood serum. The authors reported that the platelets, erythrocyte, and hemoglobin levels were increased after introducing copper nanoparticles by 44.8%, 34.1% and 21.3%, respectively, compared with the control group. In *ovo* studies, egg treated with NanoCu (50ppm) by injection to the air cell increased the accumulation of Cu in the liver and breast after 42 days of rearing [73]. This elevation of copper levels in organs may be related to that nanoparticles administration led to enhanced Cu absorption *via* the epithelial cells in the gastrointestinal tract. Several *in vitro* studies demonstrated that nanoparticles had a high absorption rate in the stomach and intestines due to their size [74]. Besides, Wang *et al.* [69] demonstrated that the supplementation of 100 mg CNP-Cu/kg diet increased albumin and total protein significantly in broiler serum by 14.50% and 11.52%, respectively and also, reduced the urea level significantly in serum by 13.84%.

In contrast, El-Kassas *et al.* [75] observed no differences in the copper concentration between broilers fed diets supplemented either with copper oxide nanoparticles (CuONPs) or copper oxide (CuO) under normal temperature. However, higher Cu level was detected in serum after dietary supplementation of CuO-NPs under thermal stress (33 C±2) compared to moderate temperature. CuO-NPs stimulated a clear increase in Cu level in birds housed in moderate temperatures compared with those exposed to heat stress [75]. Dietary inclusion of CuO-NPs by 50% and 100% resulted in an insignificant modulation of H/L ratio compared to the supplementation of CuO under both normal or heat stress [75]. The Ross birds received CuO-NPs at both 100% and 50% of recommended

Cu during exposure to thermal stress, significantly upregulated lysozyme activity in the serum compared with the heat-stressed group that received 100% of copper requirements as CuO [75]. It was also observed that the supplementation of CuO-NPs at 50% of recommended copper level significantly augmented phagocytic activity in the chickens compared to 100% CuO.

Additionally, Wang *et al.* [69] found that no differences were presented in the values of Ca, P, glutamic-pyruvic transaminase, glutamic-oxaloacetic transaminase and alkaline phosphatase (ALP) as a result of dietary inclusion of CNP-Cu at different levels in broiler diets. Besides, it was found that dietary supplement of nano copper to the turkey diets had no effect on the levels of Cu, Zn, Ca, P and Mg in the blood [71]. Chickens that received the amount of 5, 10, and 15 mg/L drinking water of copper nanoparticles showed increased levels of copper in the intestinal walls and the blood plasma [78]. Based on the *in vitro* experiment, the accumulation of copper in intestinal walls could reduce the absorption of Ca and Zn, but does not affect the absorption of Fe [78].

Table 3. Effects of nano-Cu on poultry (available literature during the last five years).

Dose	Size of Nanoparticles	Poultry Type and Age	Effects	Reference
50 ppm	2–15 nm	Chicken embryo Injection (1st day of incubation)	Increased metabolic rate No harmful effect on embryo development	[76]
50 ppm	15–70 nm	Chicken embryo Injection (1st day of incubation)	Positive influence on chick performance and a higher percentage of breast and leg muscles	[77]
4, 8, 12 and 16 μg/egg	< 100 nm	Broiler chicken *in ovo* (18th-day of incubation)	No harmful effects on the developing embryo and hatchability	[7]
20, 10, 2 mg/kg		Turkey 1-98 days old	Maintained homeostasis in turkey muscles, as indicated by the activity of aminopeptidases.	[49]
5, 10, 15 mg/L drinking water	5 nm	Broiler Chicken 1-42 days old	Increased Cu content in the blood plasma Decreased absorption of Ca and Zn No effect on Fe absorption	[78]
200 μL/bird Intramuscular injection	103 and 937nm	Broiler chicken (14-35 days)	Stimulated growth and metabolic changes Increased red cell level, haemoglobin, Cu and protein in blood serum	[70]

(Table 3) cont.....

Dose	Size of Nanoparticles	Poultry Type and Age	Effects	Reference
50 ppm	N/A	Broiler chicken Injection (1st day of incubation)	The greatest accumulation of Cu observed in the liver and spleen organs and less in the breast muscle	[73]
100 mg/kg	N/A	Broiler chicken 1-32 days	No effect on the digestibility of nutrients and growth performance	[79]
5, 10, 15 mg/L drinking water	5 nm	Broiler chicken 1-42 days old	Increased Cu content in the blood plasma Reduced absorption of Ca and Zn No effect on iron absorption	[78]
50 mg/kg	37.3 nm	Chicken embryo Injection on 1st day of incubation	Nano-Cu had pro-angiogenic properties at a systemic level to a greater degree than $CuSO_4$. Affected mRNA concentration and gene expression	[80]

N/A = not available.

EFFECTS OF NANO-COPPER ON IMMUNE RESPONSES

The immune organ weights could be a good significant indicator of animals' immunity status. Wang *et al.* [69] postulated that adding 100 mg/kg of CNP-Cu to broiler diets enhanced some immunological characteristics such as bursa of Fabricus, spleen and thymus indices by 19.61, 22.64, and 31.27%, respectively, compared to the un-supplemented group. Results indicated that the addition of CNP-Cu to broiler diets augmented lysozyme levels, complements (C), and immunoglobulins in chicken's serum. Broilers received100 mg CNP-Cu/kg diet significantly augmented lysozyme levels, C3, C4, IgG, IgA, and IgM in blood serum compared with the control group [69]. This improvement of immune responses might be related to hydroxyl and reactive amino functional groups' attendance on chitosan, which could stimulate macrophages and prompt immunoglobulin and lysozyme [81]. Turkeys broiler fed with Cu-NP exhibited an increase of total glutathione concentrations [72], and decreased catalase activity and MDA levels in the blood plasma [71, 72].Conversely, Jankowski *et al.* [72] reported that the inclusion of Cu-NP (2 mg kg^{-1}) contributed to an increase in IL-6, blood MDA concentration and SOD activity compared with the unsupplemented group. More recently, the supplementation of Cu nanoparticles (6.5 or 3.25mg/kg diet) in the diet of mice as a model increased the ceruloplasmin activity, MDA and lipid peroxides and further decreased the total glutathione, catalase activity, 3-itrotyrosine, 8-hydroxydeoxyguanosine and protein carbonyl level [82].

EFFECTS OF NANO-COPPER ON POULTRY MICROBIOTA

Microbial communities in the intestinal tract have gained attention from scientists in the last years because of playing a pivotal role in host animals' immunological and nutritional functions [83, 84]. The Coliforms in animals' intestinal ecosystem are harmful to the hosts, whereas bifidobacteria and lactobacilli are valuable [85]. The populations of *Bifidobacterium and Lactobacillus* were significantly enhanced by 3.31 and 3.85%, respectively. In contrast, the Coliforms species' account was reduced by 5.71% in the cecal digesta of broiler that received100 mg/kg of CNP-Cu [69]. Moreover, Han *et al.* [86] reported that CNP-Cu could increase the bifidobacteria and lactobacilli counts in Sprague-Dawley rat's intestine and further prevent the growth of *E.coli* in *in vivo* experiment [87]. CNP-Cu was found to inhibit some of the microbiota that may establish a good environment for *Bifidobacterium and Lactobacillus* growth [86]. However, more research is needed to illustrate nanoparticles' potential impacts on the microbial ecosystem in animal intestines.

EFFECTS OF NANO-COPPER ON GENE EXPRESSION

Supplementing the diets with CuO-NPs to heat-stressed broiler did not affect the BAX mRNA transcript level. Supplementation of Cu at 50% and 100% of the recommended copper requirements as CuO-NPs to broiler exposed to high ambient temperature (33±2) resulted in 4.63 and 10.02 folds higher CASP8 expression level than those receiving the CuO form [75]. Nevertheless, CuO-NPs supplemented to Ross chickens failed to make significant alterations in CASP8 mRNA under normal temperature [75]. The high level of copper nanoparticles (6.5mg/kg diet) in mice diet exhibited a significant reduction in protein nitration and oxidation as well as DNA methylation and oxidation ; on the other hand, lowering the concentration of nano-Cu in the diet stimulated the oxidation of proteins and DNA methylation [86].The inclusion of CuO-NPs (100% or 50% Cu requirements) in broiler diets under normal environmental temperatures led to an increase in the expression of TGFβ by 75.88 and 4.21 folds and IFN-γ by 3.80 and 39.28 folds compared to 100% CuO and control group [75]. The reduction in copper dose resulted in a decline in the level of lipid peroxides (LOOH), CAT activity and GSH + GSSG activity; however, the level of protein carbonyl and methylated DNA were augmented.

CONCLUSION AND RECOMMENDATION

The use of nano-minerals in poultry nutrition showed good results in improving final products' quality and composition. Nanotechnology can be used in poultry nutrition to enhance performance, bioavailability of nutrients, and poultry's immune and antioxidant status. Nevertheless, more research is still needed to support the effectiveness of nanotechnology as well as its safety to avoid any negative impact on poultry, environment, and humans.

CONSENT FOR PUBLICATION

Not applicable.

CONFLICT OF INTEREST

The author declares no conflict of interest, financial or otherwise.

ACKNOWLEDGEMENTS

All the authors acknowledge and thank their respective Institutes and Universities.

REFERENCES

[1]   Singh A, Prasad SM. Nanotechnology and its role in agro-ecosystem: a strategic perspective. Int J Environ Sci Technol 2017; 14(10): 2277-300.
[http://dx.doi.org/10.1007/s13762-016-1062-8]

[2]   Uniyal S, Dutta N, Raza M, Jaiswal S, Sahoo J, Ashwin K. Application of nano minerals in the field of animal nutrition: A review. Bull Environ Pharmacol Life Sci 2017; 6: 4-8.

[3]   Reda FM, El-Saadony MT, Elnesr SS, Alagawany M, Tufarelli V. Effect of dietary supplementation of biological curcumin nanoparticles on growth and carcass traits, antioxidant status, immunity and caecal microbiota of japanese quails. Animals (Basel) 2020; 10(5): 754.
[http://dx.doi.org/10.3390/ani10050754] [PMID: 32357410]

[4]   Abd El-Hack ME, Alagawany M, Farag MR, *et al.* Nutritional and pharmaceutical applications of nanotechnology: trends and advances. Int J Pharmacol 2017; 13(4): 340-50.
[http://dx.doi.org/10.3923/ijp.2017.340.350]

[5]   Nguyen QK, Nguyen DD, Nguyen VK, *et al.* Impact of biogenic nanoscale metals Fe, Cu, Zn and Se on reproductive LV chickens. Adv Nat Sci: Nanosci Nanotechnol 2015; 6(3): 035017.
[http://dx.doi.org/10.1088/2043-6262/6/3/035017]

[6]   Sheiha AM, Abdelnour SA, Abd El-Hack ME, *et al.* Effects of dietary biological or chemical-synthesized nano-selenium supplementation on growing rabbits exposed to thermal stress. Animals (Basel) 2020; 10(3): 430.
[http://dx.doi.org/10.3390/ani10030430] [PMID: 32143370]

[7]   Joshua PP, Valli C, Balakrishnan V. Effect of *in ovo* supplementation of nano forms of zinc, copper, and selenium on post-hatch performance of broiler chicken. Vet World 2016; 9(3): 287-94.
[http://dx.doi.org/10.14202/vetworld.2016.287-294] [PMID: 27057113]

[8]   El-Deep M, Shabaan M, Assar M, Attia K, Sayed M. Comparative Effects of Different Dietary Selenium Sources on Productive Performance, Antioxidative Properties And Immunity in Local Laying Hens Exposed to High Ambient Temperature. J Anim Poult Prod 2017; 8(9): 335-43.
[http://dx.doi.org/10.21608/jappmu.2017.45998]

[9]   Mohapatra P, Swain R, Mishra S, *et al.* Effects of dietary nano-selenium on tissue selenium deposition, antioxidant status and immune functions in layer chicks. Int J Pharmacol 2014; 10(3): 160-7.
[http://dx.doi.org/10.3923/ijp.2014.160.167]

[10]   Aparna N, Karunakaran R. Effect of selenium nanoparticles supplementation on oxidation resistance of broiler chicken. Indian J Sci Technol 2016; 9(1): 1-5.
        [http://dx.doi.org/10.17485/ijst/2016/v9iS1/106334]

[11]   Aparna N, Karunakaran R, Parthiban M. Effect of Selenium Nano Particles on Glutathione Peroxidase mRNA Gene Expression in Broiler Chicken. Indian J Sci Technol 2017; 10(32): 1-5.
        [http://dx.doi.org/10.17485/ijst/2017/v10i32/106626]

[12]   Bagheri M, Golchin-Gelehdooni S, Mohamadi M, Tabidian A. Comparative effects of nano, mineral and organic selenium on growth performance, immunity responses and total antioxidant activity in broiler chickens. Int J Biol Pharm Allied Sci 2015; 4: 583-95. [IJBPAS].

[13]   Selim NA, Radwan NL, Youssef SF, Eldin TAS, Elwafa SA. Effect of inclusion inorganic, organic or nano selenium forms in broiler diets on: 2-physiological, immunological and toxicity statuses of broiler chicks. Int J Poult Sci 2015; 14(3): 144-55.
        [http://dx.doi.org/10.3923/ijps.2015.144.155]

[14]   Ahmadi M, Ahmadian A, Seidavi A. Effect of Different Levels of Nano-selenium on Performance, Blood Parameters, Immunity and Carcass Characteristics of BroilerChickens. Poult Sci J 2018; 6(1): 99-108.

[15]   Prasoon S. Jayanaik, Malathi V, Nagaraj CS, Narayanaswamy HD. 2018 Effects of dietary supplementation of inorganic, organic and nano selenium on meat Production and meat quality parameters of a dual purpose crossbred chicken. Int J Agric Sci 2018; 10(15): 6788-92.

[16]   Zhou X, Wang Y. Influence of dietary nano elemental selenium on growth performance, tissue selenium distribution, meat quality, and glutathione peroxidase activity in Guangxi Yellow chicken. Poult Sci 2011; 90(3): 680-6.
        [http://dx.doi.org/10.3382/ps.2010-00977] [PMID: 21325242]

[17]   Hu CH, Li YL, Xiong L, Zhang HM, Song J, Xia MS. Comparative effects of nano elemental selenium and sodium selenite on selenium retention in broiler chickens. Anim Feed Sci Technol 2012; 177(3-4): 204-10.
        [http://dx.doi.org/10.1016/j.anifeedsci.2012.08.010]

[18]   Hawkes WC, Keim NL. Dietary selenium intake modulates thyroid hormone and energy metabolism in men. J Nutr 2003; 133(11): 3443-8.
        [http://dx.doi.org/10.1093/jn/133.11.3443] [PMID: 14608056]

[19]   Saleh AA. Effect of dietary mixture of Aspergillus probiotic and selenium nano-particles on growth, nutrient digestibilities, selected blood parameters and muscle fatty acid profile in broiler chickens. Anim Sci Pap Rep 2014; 32(1): 65-79.

[20]   Payne RL, Southern LL. Comparison of inorganic and organic selenium sources for broilers. Poult Sci 2005; 84(6): 898-902.
        [http://dx.doi.org/10.1093/ps/84.6.898] [PMID: 15971527]

[21]   Ryu YC, Rhee MS, Lee KM, Kim BC. Effects of different levels of dietary supplemental selenium on performance, lipid oxidation, and color stability of broiler chicks. Poult Sci 2005; 84(5): 809-15.
        [http://dx.doi.org/10.1093/ps/84.5.809] [PMID: 15913195]

[22]   Cai SJ, Wu CX, Gong LM, Song T, Wu H, Zhang LY. Effects of nano-selenium on performance, meat quality, immune function, oxidation resistance, and tissue selenium content in broilers. Poult Sci 2012; 91(10): 2532-9.
        [http://dx.doi.org/10.3382/ps.2012-02160] [PMID: 22991539]

[23]   Boostani A, Sadeghi AA, Mousavi SN, Chamani M, Kashan N. Effects of organic, inorganic, and nano-Se on growth performance, antioxidant capacity, cellular and humoral immune responses in broiler chickens exposed to oxidative stress. Livest Sci 2015; 178: 330-6.
        [http://dx.doi.org/10.1016/j.livsci.2015.05.004]

[24]   Gangadoo S, Dinev I, Chapman J, *et al.* Selenium nanoparticles in poultry feed modify gut microbiota

and increase abundance of Faecalibacterium prausnitzii. Appl Microbiol Biotechnol 2018; 102(3): 66-1455.
[http://dx.doi.org/10.1007/s00253-017-8688-4]

[25]   Boostani A, Sadeghi AA, Mousavi SN, Chamani M, Kashan N. The effects of organic, inorganic, and nano-selenium on blood attributes in broiler chickens exposed to oxidative stress. Acta Sci Vet 2015; 43: 1264.

[26]   Nassir F, Moundras C, Bayle D, *et al.* Effect of selenium deficiency on hepatic lipid and lipoprotein metabolism in the rat. Br J Nutr 1997; 78(3): 493-500.
[http://dx.doi.org/10.1079/BJN19970166] [PMID: 9306889]

[27]   Bermingham EN, Hesketh JE, Sinclair BR, Koolaard JP, Roy NC. Selenium-enriched foods are more effective at increasing glutathione peroxidase (GPx) activity compared with selenomethionine: a meta-analysis. Nutrients 2014; 6(10): 4002-31.
[http://dx.doi.org/10.3390/nu6104002] [PMID: 25268836]

[28]   Wang Y. Differential effects of sodium selenite and nano-Se on growth performance, tissue se distribution, and glutathione peroxidase activity of avian broiler. Biol Trace Elem Res 2009; 128(2): 184-90.
[http://dx.doi.org/10.1007/s12011-008-8264-y] [PMID: 18972070]

[29]   Gowri AM, Abiroopa A, Vaishnavi AS, Nandhini S. Nano-selenium activates Mucin gene expression in intestinal crypt cells. Pharma Innovation Journal 2018; 7(11): 421-4.

[30]   Forstner J, Oliver M, Sylvester F. structure and biologic relevance of gastrointestinal mucins. New York: Infections of the gastrointestinal tract Raven Press 1995; pp. 71-88.

[31]   Jafarzadeh H, Allymehr M, Talebi A. ASRI REZAEI S, Soleimanzadeh A. Effects of nano-selenium and sodium selenite on SelP, GPx4 and SelW genes expression in testes of broiler breeder roosters. Bulg J Vet Med 2020; 23(2): 218-28.
[http://dx.doi.org/10.15547/bjvm.2208]

[32]   Amini SM, Mahabadi VP. Selenium nanoparticles role in organ systems functionality and disorder. Nanomed Res J 2018; 3(3): 117-24.

[33]   Yazdi MH, Mahdavi M, Setayesh N, Esfandyar M, Shahverdi AR. Selenium nanoparticle-enriched Lactobacillus brevis causes more efficient immune responses *in vivo* and reduces the liver metastasis in metastatic form of mouse breast cancer. Daru 2013; 21(1): 33.
[http://dx.doi.org/10.1186/2008-2231-21-33] [PMID: 23631392]

[34]   Peng X, Cui HM, Deng J, Zuo Z, Cui W. Low dietary selenium induce increased apoptotic thymic cells and alter peripheral blood T cell subsets in chicken. Biol Trace Elem Res 2011; 142(2): 167-73.
[http://dx.doi.org/10.1007/s12011-010-8756-4] [PMID: 20607441]

[35]   Zamani Moghaddam AK, Mehraei Hamzekolaei MH, Khajali F, Hassanpour H. Role of selenium from different sources in prevention of pulmonary arterial hypertension syndrome in broiler chickens. Biol Trace Elem Res 2017; 180(1): 164-70.
[http://dx.doi.org/10.1007/s12011-017-0993-3] [PMID: 28317078]

[36]   Rizk YS, Ibrahim AF, Mansour MK, Mohamed HS, El-Slamony AE, Soliman AAM. Effect of dietary source of selenium on productive and reproductive performance of Sinai laying hens under heat stress conditions. Egypt Poult Sci J 2018; 37(2): 461-89.

[37]   Cheah KS, Cheah AM, Krausgrill DI. Effect of dietary supplementation of vitamin E on pig meat quality. Meat Sci 1995; 39(2): 255-64.
[http://dx.doi.org/10.1016/0309-1740(94)P1826-H] [PMID: 22059831]

[38]   Fathi M. Effects of zinc oxide nanoparticles supplementation on mortality due to ascites and performance growth in broiler chickens. Iran J Appl Anim Sci 2016; 6(2): 389-94.

[39]   El-Katcha MI, Soltan MA, Arafa MM, Kawarei E-SR. Impact of dietary replacement of inorganic zinc by organic or nano sources on productive performance, immune response and some blood biochemical

constituents of laying hens. Alex J Vet Sci 2018; 59(1): 48-59.
[http://dx.doi.org/10.5455/ajvs.301885]

[40]   Olgun O, Yildiz AÖ. Effects of dietary supplementation of inorganic, organic or nano zinc forms on performance, eggshell quality, and bone characteristics in laying hens. Ann Anim Sci 2017; 17(2): 463-76.
[http://dx.doi.org/10.1515/aoas-2016-0055]

[41]   Badawi M, Ali M, Behairy A. Effects of zinc sources supplementation on performance of broiler chickens. J Am Sci 2017; 13(7): 35-40.

[42]   Hafez A, Hegazi S, Bakr A, Shishtawy H. Effect of zinc oxide nanoparticles on growth performance and absorptive capacity of the intestinal villi in broiler chickens. Life Sci J 2017; 14(11): 125-9.

[43]   Ibrahim D, Ali HA, El-Mandrawy SA. Effects of different zinc sources on performance, bio distribution of minerals and expression of genes related to metabolism of broiler chickens. Vet J 2017; 45(3): 292-304.
[http://dx.doi.org/10.21608/zvjz.2017.7954]

[44]   Ali S, Masood S, Zaneb H, *et al.* Supplementation of zinc oxide nanoparticles has beneficial effects on intestinal morphology in broiler chicken. Pak Vet J 2017; 37(3): 335-9.

[45]   Sahoo A, Swain R, Mishra SK. Effect of inorganic, organic and nano zinc supplemented diets on bioavailability and immunity status of broilers. Int J Adv Res (Indore) 2014; 2(11): 828-37.

[46]   Ahmadi F, Ebrahimnezjad Y, Ghalehkandi J, Sis N, Eds. The effect of dietary zinc oxide nanoparticles on the antioxidant state and serum enzymes activity in broiler chickens during starter stage.; International Conference on Biological, Civil and Environmental Engineering Dubai 2014.

[47]   Mohammadi F, Ahmadi F, Amiri A. Effect of zinc oxide nanoparticles on carcass parameters, relative weight of digestive and lymphoid organs of broiler fed wet diet during the starter period. Int J Biosci 2015; 6(2): 389-94.
[http://dx.doi.org/10.12692/ijb/6.2.389-394]

[48]   Pathak SS, Reddy KV, Prasoon S. Influence of different sources of zinc on growth performance of dual purpose chicken. J Bio Innov 2016; 5: 663-72.

[49]   Jóźwik A, Marchewka J, Strzałkowska N, *et al.* The effect of different levels of Cu, Zn and Mn nanoparticles in hen turkey diet on the activity of aminopeptidases. Molecules 2018; 23(5): 1150.
[http://dx.doi.org/10.3390/molecules23051150] [PMID: 29751626]

[50]   Dukare Sagar P, Mandal A, Akbar N, Dinani O. Effect of different levels and sources of zinc on growth performance and immunity of broiler chicken during summer. Int J Curr Microbiol Appl Sci 2018; 7(5): 459-71.
[http://dx.doi.org/10.20546/ijcmas.2018.705.058]

[51]   Jose N, Elangovan AV, Awachat VB, Shet D, Ghosh J, David CG. Response of *in ovo* administration of zinc on egg hatchability and immune response of commercial broiler chicken. J Anim Physiol Anim Nutr (Berl) 2018; 102(2): 591-5.
[http://dx.doi.org/10.1111/jpn.12777] [PMID: 28990230]

[52]   Ghalehkandi JG, Karamouz H, Nazhad HZA, Sis NM, Beheshti R. Effect of different levels of zinc oxide supplement on mucosal lucin aminopeptidase enzyme activity in small intestine of male broiler chicks. Int J Anim Vet Adv 2011; 3(5): 313-5.

[53]   Powell SR. The antioxidant properties of zinc. J Nutr 2000; 130(5S) (Suppl.): 1447S-54S.
[http://dx.doi.org/10.1093/jn/130.5.1447S] [PMID: 10801958]

[54]   Zhao C-Y, Tan S-X, Xiao X-Y, Qiu X-S, Pan J-Q, Tang Z-X. Effects of dietary zinc oxide nanoparticles on growth performance and antioxidative status in broilers. Biol Trace Elem Res 2014; 160(3): 361-7.
[http://dx.doi.org/10.1007/s12011-014-0052-2] [PMID: 24973873]

[55]   Fathi M, Haydari M, Tanha T. Effects of zinc oxide nanoparticles on antioxidant status, serum enzymes activities, biochemical parameters and performance in broiler chickens. J Livestock Sci Technol 2016; 4(2): 7-13.

[56]   Bami MK, Afsharmanesh M, Salarmoini M, Tavakoli H. Effect of zinc oxide nanoparticles and Bacillus coagulans as probiotic on growth, histomorphology of intestine, and immune parameters in broiler chickens. Comp Clin Pathol 2018; 27(2): 399-406.
[http://dx.doi.org/10.1007/s00580-017-2605-1]

[57]   Hu CH, Gu LY, Luan ZS, Song J, Zhu K. Effects of montmorillonite–zinc oxide hybrid on performance, diarrhea, intestinal permeability and morphology of weanling pigs. Anim Feed Sci Technol 2012; 177(1-2): 108-15.
[http://dx.doi.org/10.1016/j.anifeedsci.2012.07.028]

[58]   Ahmadi F, Ebrahimnezjad Y, Sis N, Ghalehkandi J, Eds. Effect of zinc oxide nanoparticles on the carcass traits and gut morphological of broiler chicks during starter phase. 3rd International Conference on Nanotek and Expo; Hampton 2013.

[59]   Tsai YH, Mao SY, Li MZ, Huang JT, Lien TF. Effects of nanosize zinc oxide on zinc retention, eggshell quality, immune response and serum parameters of aged laying hens. Anim Feed Sci Technol 2016; 213: 99-107.
[http://dx.doi.org/10.1016/j.anifeedsci.2016.01.009]

[60]   Al-Daraji HJ, Mahmood HMA. Effect of dietary zinc on certain blood traits of broiler breeder chickens. Int J Poult Sci 2011; 10(10): 807-13.
[http://dx.doi.org/10.3923/ijps.2011.807.813]

[61]   Wu Y, Sun Z, Che S, Chang H. Effects of zinc and selenium on the disorders of blood glucose and lipid metabolism and its molecular mechanism in diabetic rats. Wei Sheng Yan Jiu 2004; 33(1): 70-3.
[PMID: 15098483]

[62]   Bonaventura P, Benedetti G, Albarède F, Miossec P. Zinc and its role in immunity and inflammation. Autoimmun Rev 2015; 14(4): 277-85.
[http://dx.doi.org/10.1016/j.autrev.2014.11.008] [PMID: 25462582]

[63]   Sunder GS, Panda AK, Gopinath NCS, *et al.* Effects of higher levels of zinc supplementation on performance, mineral availability, and immune competence in broiler chickens. J Appl Poult Res 2008; 17(1): 79-86.
[http://dx.doi.org/10.3382/japr.2007-00029]

[64]   Bartlett JR, Smith MO. Effects of different levels of zinc on the performance and immunocompetence of broilers under heat stress. Poult Sci 2003; 82(10): 1580-8.
[http://dx.doi.org/10.1093/ps/82.10.1580] [PMID: 14601736]

[65]   Jiang Z, Lin Y, Zhou G, Luo L, Jiang S, Chen F. Effects of dietary selenomethionine supplementation on growth performance, meat quality and antioxidant property in yellow broilers. J Agric Food Chem 2009; 57(20): 9769-72.
[http://dx.doi.org/10.1021/jf902411c] [PMID: 19807096]

[66]   Sinzato YK, Lima PHO, Campos KE, Kiss AC, Rudge MV, Damasceno DC. Neonatally-induced diabetes: lipid profile outcomes and oxidative stress status in adult rats. Rev Assoc Med Bras (1992) 2009; 55(4): 384-8.
[http://dx.doi.org/10.1590/S0104-42302009000400010] [PMID: 19750302]

[67]   Duzguner V, Kaya S. Effect of zinc on the lipid peroxidation and the antioxidant defense systems of the alloxan-induced diabetic rabbits. Free Radic Biol Med 2007; 42(10): 1481-6.
[http://dx.doi.org/10.1016/j.freeradbiomed.2007.02.021] [PMID: 17448894]

[68]   Nielsen F, Mikkelsen BB, Nielsen JB, Andersen HR, Grandjean P. Plasma malondialdehyde as biomarker for oxidative stress: reference interval and effects of life-style factors. Clin Chem 1997; 43(7): 1209-14.

[http://dx.doi.org/10.1093/clinchem/43.7.1209] [PMID: 9216458]

[69]   Wang C, Wang MQ, Ye SS, Tao WJ, Du YJ. Effects of copper-loaded chitosan nanoparticles on growth and immunity in broilers. Poult Sci 2011; 90(10): 2223-8.
[http://dx.doi.org/10.3382/ps.2011-01511] [PMID: 21934004]

[70]   Miroshnikov S, Yausheva E, Sizova E, Miroshnikova E. Comparative assessment of effect of copper nano- and microparticles in chicken. Orient J Chem 2015; 31(4): 2327-36.
[http://dx.doi.org/10.13005/ojc/310461]

[71]   Kozłowski K, Jankowski J, Otowski K, Zduńczyk Z, Ognik K. Metabolic parameters in young turkeys fed diets with different inclusion levels of copper nanoparticles. Pol J Vet Sci 2018; 21(2): 245-53.
[PMID: 30450862]

[72]   Jankowski J, Kozłowski K, Ognik K, *et al.* Redox and immunological status of turkeys fed diets with different levels and sources of copper. Ann Anim Sci 2019; 19(1): 215-27.
[http://dx.doi.org/10.2478/aoas-2018-0054]

[73]   Mroczek-Sosnowska N, Lukasiewicz M, Wnuk A, Sawosz E, Niemiec J. Effect of copper nanoparticles and copper sulfate administered *in ovo* on copper content in breast muscle, liver and spleen of broiler chickens. Annals of Warsaw University of Life Sciences-SGGW Animal Science 2014; 53: 135-42.

[74]   Tomaszewska E, Muszyński S, Ognik K, *et al.* Comparison of the effect of dietary copper nanoparticles with copper (II) salt on bone geometric and structural parameters as well as material characteristics in a rat model. J Trace Elem Med Biol 2017; 42: 103-10.
[http://dx.doi.org/10.1016/j.jtemb.2017.05.002] [PMID: 28595781]

[75]   El-Kassas S, Abdo SE, El-Naggar K, Abdo W, Kirrella AAK, Nashar TO. Ameliorative effect of dietary supplementation of copper oxide nanoparticles on inflammatory and immune reponses in commercial broiler under normal and heat-stress housing conditions. J Therm Biol 2018; 78: 235-46.
[http://dx.doi.org/10.1016/j.jtherbio.2018.10.009] [PMID: 30509642]

[76]   Scott A, Vadalasetty KP, Sawosz E, *et al.* Effect of copper nanoparticles and copper sulphate on metabolic rate and development of broiler embryos. Anim Feed Sci Technol 2016; 220: 151-8.
[http://dx.doi.org/10.1016/j.anifeedsci.2016.08.009]

[77]   Mroczek-Sosnowska N, Sawosz E, Vadalasetty KP, *et al.* Nanoparticles of copper stimulate angiogenesis at systemic and molecular level. Int J Mol Sci 2015; 16(3): 4838-49.
[http://dx.doi.org/10.3390/ijms16034838] [PMID: 25741768]

[78]   Ognik K, Stępniowska A, Cholewińska E, Kozłowski K. The effect of administration of copper nanoparticles to chickens in drinking water on estimated intestinal absorption of iron, zinc, and calcium. Poult Sci 2016; 95(9): 2045-51.
[http://dx.doi.org/10.3382/ps/pew200] [PMID: 27307476]

[79]   Sarvestani S, Resvani M, Zamiri M, Shekarforoush S, Atashi H, Mosleh N. The effect of nanocopper and mannan oligosaccharide supplementation on nutrient digestibility and performance in broiler chickens. J Vet Res (Pulawy) 2016; 71(2): 153-61.

[80]   Mroczek-Sosnowska N, Łukasiewicz M, Wnuk A, *et al. In ovo* administration of copper nanoparticles and copper sulfate positively influences chicken performance. J Sci Food Agric 2016; 96(9): 3058-62.
[http://dx.doi.org/10.1002/jsfa.7477] [PMID: 26417698]

[81]   Dove CR, Ewan RC. Effect of vitamin E and copper on the vitamin E status and performance of growing pigs. J Anim Sci 1991; 69(6): 2516-23.
[http://dx.doi.org/10.2527/1991.6962516x] [PMID: 1885367]

[82]   Ognik K, Cholewińska E, Juśkiewicz J, Zduńczyk Z, Tutaj K, Szlązak R. The effect of copper nanoparticles and copper (II) salt on redox reactions and epigenetic changes in a rat model. J Anim Physiol Anim Nutr (Berl) 2019; 103(2): 675-86.
[http://dx.doi.org/10.1111/jpn.13025] [PMID: 30618103]

[83]   Rehman H, Hellweg P, Taras D, Zentek J. Effects of dietary inulin on the intestinal short chain fatty acids and microbial ecology in broiler chickens as revealed by denaturing gradient gel electrophoresis. Poult Sci 2008; 87(4): 783-9.
[http://dx.doi.org/10.3382/ps.2007-00271] [PMID: 18340001]

[84]   Ismail IE, Abdelnour SA, Shehata SA, *et al.* Effect of Dietary *Boswellia serrata* Resin on Growth Performance, Blood Biochemistry, and Cecal Microbiota of Growing Rabbits. Front Vet Sci 2019; 6: 471.
[http://dx.doi.org/10.3389/fvets.2019.00471] [PMID: 31921925]

[85]   Santos A, San Mauro M, Díaz DM. Prebiotics and their long-term influence on the microbial populations of the mouse bowel. Food Microbiol 2006; 23(5): 498-503.
[http://dx.doi.org/10.1016/j.fm.2005.07.004] [PMID: 16943043]

[86]   Han XY, Du WL, Fan CL, Xu ZR. Changes in composition a metabolism of caecal microbiota in rats fed diets supplemented with copper-loaded chitosan nanoparticles. J Anim Physiol Anim Nutr (Berl) 2010; 94(5): e138-44.
[http://dx.doi.org/10.1111/j.1439-0396.2010.00995.x] [PMID: 20546066]

[87]   Du W-L, Xu Y-L, Xu Z-R, Fan C-L. Preparation, characterization and antibacterial properties against E. coli K(88) of chitosan nanoparticle loaded copper ions. Nanotechnology 2008; 19(8): 085707.
[http://dx.doi.org/10.1088/0957-4484/19/8/085707] [PMID: 21730738]

SUBJECT INDEX

Resistance 6, 12, 14, 56, 112, 127, 204, 207, 242
  bacterial 12, 120, 204
  intestinal 112
  methicillin 127
  plasmid-mediated 6
Resistance genes 12
  transmission 12
Responses 11, 34, 214
  allergic 11
  delayed hypersensitivity 11
  immunological 34
  secondary 214
Resveratrol 202, 205, 206, 207, 208, 209
  dietary 208
RNA viruses 72
ROS and lipid peroxide concentration 209
Rosemary 36, 37, 41, 44, 177
  addition 41
  chemical composition 37
  oil 36
  plant 36, 44
  powder 177
  products 36
Rosmarinus officinalis 36, 38, 44

S

Saccharomyces 242, 244, 250
  boulardii 244, 250
  cerevisiae 242, 244
Salmonella 60, 98, 163, 251
  gallinarum 251
  indiana 98
  typhi 60, 163
Salmonellosis 14
Salvia officinalis 140
Saponins 68, 74, 77, 78, 80, 112, 113, 114, 158, 161, 162, 163, 164, 176, 181
  supplementary 114
  triterpene 68, 112
Secretion 75, 95, 160, 164, 204, 207, 228
  bicarbonate 164
  pancreatic 228
  pepsin 95

Seeds 56, 57, 59, 61, 107, 112, 139, 141, 156, 157, 158, 177, 178, 180
  anise 177
  compressed 57
  white 141
Serum 42, 44, 160, 180, 208, 209, 270
  antioxidant enzymes 208
  creatinine 42
  enzymes activity 270
  glutamic oxaloacetic transaminase 42
  IgG concentration 209
  lipid profile 44, 160
  protein 180
Sheep red blood cells (SRBCs) 41, 214, 264, 267, 273
Shigella 62
  dysenteriae 62
  flrxneri 62
  sonne 62
Shikimate dehydrogenase 126
Short-chain fatty acids (SCFA) 9
Skin 11, 38, 155, 156, 157, 165
  allergies 38
  diseases 155, 156, 157
  reactions 11
Staphylococcus lutea 62
Steroids 158, 163
Stevens-Johnson syndrome 11
Streptococcus agalactiae 126
Stress 36, 67, 97, 181, 208, 209, 268, 274
  anti-heat 67
  heat 97, 209, 268, 274
  mediated mobilization 181
Stressors, oxidative 206
Stronger neo-minophagen C (SNMC) 71
Surface Plasmon Resonance (SPR) 17
Synthesis 5, 6, 7, 8, 67, 73, 74, 75, 76, 91, 123, 126, 165, 166, 167, 206
  andenhanced intestinal mucus 91
  biotechnological 206
  chemical 206
  decreasing DNA 73
  estradiol 74
  prostaglandin 165
Synthetic 36, 180

www.ingramcontent.com/pod-product-compliance
Lightning Source LLC
Chambersburg PA
CBHW050810220326

41598CB00006B/172